Springer Series on
REHABILITATION

Carolyn L. Vash, Ph. D. has extensive experience as a counseling and clinical psychologist, administrator, researcher, and educator, and is former Chief Deputy Director of the California State Department of Rehabilitation. She previously developed a comprehensive vocational rehabilitation program at Rancho Los Amigos Hospital in Downey, California. The author of numerous books and articles, she also serves on the advisory boards of several rehabilitation projects and government commissions. Dr. Vash received the Ph. D. in psychology from the University of California at Los Angeles in 1964. Severely disabled herself, she currently divides her time between serving as vice president of the Institute for Information Studies in Falls Church, Virginia, and conducting a private consulting practice in Altadena, California.

The Psychology of Disability

Carolyn L. Vash, Ph.D.

Foreword by
George W. Hohmann, Ph.D.

Springer Publishing Company
New York

To my husband, Dick Vash,
and to the memory of my mother, Sibyl Conine

Springer Publishing Company, Inc.
536 Broadway
New York, New York 10012

   87 88 89 90 5 4

Library of Congress Cataloging in Publication Data

Vash, Carolyn L.
  The psychology of disability.

(Springer series on rehabilitation; v. 1)
  Bibliography: p.
  Includes index.
  1. Physically handicapped—Psychology. 2. Physically
handicapped—Rehabilitation. I. Title. II. Series.
HV3011.V37   362.4   81-13576
ISBN 0-8261-3340-1   AACR2
ISBN 0-8261-3341-X (pbk.)

Printed in the United States of America

CONTENTS

FOREWORD

It has been a quarter of a century since Carolyn Vash came to my office to discuss the feasibility of becoming a psychologist. She was a senior at Long Beach State College and I was a newly arrived staff psychologist at the adjoining campus of the Long Beach VA Hospital. I encouraged her ambitions, but warned that the graduate program which she sought had a record of rejecting some otherwise qualified seriously disabled students and that employment possibilities were very limited. Time proved me wrong on both counts. So much for my predictions.

In her Preface to this new work, Dr. Vash sets the goal of sharing her experience relative to the psychology of disability: "fifty years of learning on the part of the author: thirty years as a severely disabled individual, overlapping twenty years as a rehabilitation psychologist . . ." Thus setting the tone for an experiential report, the author is freed to use her great ability as a creative writer to produce a book that is eminently readable and avoids the ponderous style that characterizes much of the psychological literature. The neophyte reader can easily grasp the principles of what we "really know" about the psychology of disability by case examples from Dr. Vash's vast experience. The experienced reader will find ambiguous issues and principles made explicit and may even have a few preconceptions dislodged, freeing him/her to attempt new and creative solutions. *The Psychology of Disability* is also very instructive reading for many disabled people. It makes generous use of individual experiences, delineates individual organismic variables versus environmental influences and the interaction between them, and presents psychological principles that will help all thoughtful readers to make sense of the "disability experience."

It seems to me there are four issues that make this work significant and enduring. First, it is solidly based on the established psychological principle that behavior is a function of the individual interacting with the environment ($B = I \times E$) and disability is just one of the many variables that affect this equation. Until the last decade, the psychology of disability concerned itself primarily with such individual variables as phases of adjustment, reaction to loss, and ways of adapting the individual to function in the environment. With the advent of the civil and human rights movements of the 1960s and early 1970s, emphasis shifted to examination of environmental effects on the disabled person—everything from the "medical model," institutionalization, attitudinal barriers, and physical barriers, to legal and constitutional rights. Now our attention is directed to both the individual *and* to those environmental factors that influence the behavior of disabled individuals (and groups—another area about which we know very little), and especially to the interaction of these factors.

The second important issue to which Dr. Vash directs attention is the many subjectively important experiences of severely disabled individuals. For nearly two decades rehabilitation specialists have shared the concentration of other groups of psychologists in studying objective, observable behavior. It is almost with embarrassment, if at all, that we direct attention to such subjective phenomena as beliefs, values, fantasies, and spirituality ("cognitive structures" sounds better these days) as they affect the behavior of disabled persons. An example may clarify. I share the author's experience that most thoughtful disabled people, and particularly those with sudden, catastrophic onset of disability, have the feeling of somehow having cheated death. Most also report that this feeling helps them handle the problems of living. The thought runs something like this: "When trouble strikes, I remind myself that by all odds I should be dead. This problem isn't so bad, when I think of all the good things I have experienced since my disability." We know pitifully little about how such belief systems develop or influence behavior and adjustment. Are these subjective phenomena factors that strengthen the ego? What role does blame placing play in adapting to disability? How do disabled people deal with the existential (or spiritual) question, "What's it all about?"

Another important issue confronted here is that of psychological development in long-term living with severe disability. Virtually all of the rehabilitation psychology literature (and, for that matter, rehabilitation literature in general) concerns itself with the newly disabled or, in the case of the congenitally disabled, those who enter a rehabilitation program for the first time. Precious little is known about the interaction between a long-standing, severe disability and, for example, a mid-life crisis. It is as though we have assumed that once a person is "rehabilitated," "adjusted," or "retrained," his/her life will proceed along the same course as that of a nondisabled person, the disability playing no further role. Perhaps we have oversold such clichés as "just like everyone else."

Finally, to me the most valuable contribution Dr. Vash makes here is the notion of "embracing the disability" and transcending it. Several years ago, Carolyn Vash, Nancy Kerr, and I (all seriously disabled, all rehabilitation psychologists) were having a drink together in a bar in Kansas City, when Carolyn introduced this notion into our conversation. It was not the first time I had heard it. Thirty years before, a friend of mine who is paraplegic, a former stevedore, and poorly educated said to me, "I wouldn't have missed being a God-damned paraplegic for anything." I thought him completely mad at the time. It took me many years to understand what this simple and wise man had discovered in two years—that a disability can be a unique aspect of oneself that offers additional opportunities for experience, growth, maturation, and self-actualization. I had been thoroughly trained by the rehabilitation process in the notion that my disability was the enemy—to be defeated, controlled, minimized, compensated for, and, yes, denied. It was never, never OK to like being what I was (among other things): disabled.

Very practical rehabilitation practices and procedures flow from this notion. The philosophy and goal of rehabilitation that the best rehabilitation is that which encourages the return of the disabled to the closest possible approximation to "normal" emphasizes procedures like brace walking, natural appearing (if ineffective) prostheses, and disguised orthotics, all of which are designed to make the disabled a pale image of the normal. For example, some time ago I found myself being irrationally irate at the widespread practice of insertion of penile prostheses in newly spinal-cord-injured men—sometimes without either the awareness or concurrence of the spouse. Such action was once more saying to the recipient, "it's *not* OK to be disabled (unique, different) and the only way to be a real whole man (acceptable to yourself and others) is by having this pale, artificial, awkward approximation of erectile function." Another put-down in a most sensitive area!

A different approach follows from the viewpoint that Dr. Vash proposes. If the therapist understands or even expects that many disabled people can, with time, "embrace" the disability, then the energies of the rehabilitation process can be directed toward training the person in the most effective way of taking care of the chores of living with a disability. Energy may be freed from compensating for the disability, or trying to be "normal," or hating the disability, or denying it, and be directed toward more joyous aspects of life such as experiencing, learning, producing, loving, and knowing, thereby transcending the effects of the disability. For this hopeful view of the psychology of disability Dr. Vash deserves our gratitude.

George W. Hohmann, Ph.D.

PREFACE

The Psychology of Disability is an effort to share fifty years of learning on the part of the author: thirty years as a severely disabled individual, overlapping twenty years as a rehabilitation psychologist, researcher, educator, and administrator. Hopefully, the overlay of these several perspectives will give helpful, added dimension to issues that are sometimes difficult to appreciate from a single vantage point.

This is the time to acknowledge the dozens of individuals (whose names have been changed) whom readers will "meet" in this volume: people whose stories I have followed personally and have related here as a way of illustrating the principles and issues discussed. I also want to acknowledge a number of individuals who have been especially helpful critics and contributors of ideas: Jacqueline Sanchez, Herbert Rigoni, Barbara Waxman, Diana De Bro, Robert and Patricia Hadley, Gregory Kimberlin, Sanford Bernstein, John Millen, Jerry Kuns, Maria French, Edward Roberts, Elizabeth Pan, Thomas Backer, Barbara Morrione, Harry Grace, Bryan Kemp, Edward Workman, Tony Hickey, Pam Kauss, and Danleigh Spievak.

A special acknowledgment is made to my typist, Carolyn Scotton. Actually, Carolyn Scotton passed from existence in 1958, but her initials live on, on everything I type for myself. I am now divulging a long-held secret. The inscription "CLV:cs," found at the end of anything I type that is letter perfect, is a private joke. The two individuals are one. The initials "cs" stand for Carolyn Scotton, my name when I was rejected for service, at the age of nineteen, by the state–federal VR program, because I refused to abandon my "unrealistic" goal of becoming a psychologist for the "practical" one of becoming a secretary. It serves as a reminder of how wrong people on both sides of the desk can be. At the time, less than three years postonset of polio, I thought the counselor must be crazy to think that I, with my upper-extremity weakness, could ever learn how to type. He thought I was equally foolish to aspire to a high-level goal that had eluded him. We were both entrammeled in preconceptions that clouded our abilities to see.

The major intent of this volume is to dislodge preconceptions, thus opening up new ways of looking at the disability experience. It is my firm conviction that, once this is accomplished, new ways of dealing with it will follow.

INTRODUCTION*

Some dangers inhere in even acknowledging the validity of the concept "the psychology of disability," since, in the past, it has led to unhelpful exaggerations of the perceived differences between people with disabilities and those without. The fact is, human beings are more alike than different, regardless of variances in their physical bodies, sensory capacities, or intellectual abilities. To illustrate, a disabled person is said to experience a sense of loss over the functional abilities that an illness or injury has destroyed. Similarly, a nondisabled person may experience a sense of loss over something s/he once had and now has lost. The stimulus is different, but the sense of loss, the fear that life will be painful or meaningless without the lost element, are virtually the same. Viewed in this light, the psychology of disability is little different from the psychology of being human. That is, when the nature of the basic Stimulus–Organism–Response relationships—the building blocks of scientific psychology—are understood, there should be no residual to study separately in order to understand why people with disabilities behave as they do.

The definition of the psychology of disability underlying the material in this book follows such a line of reasoning. It is considered here to be largely, though not entirely, the study of how human organisms respond to a set of stimulus conditions associated with disability. Stated somewhat differently, one could say that, in general, it is the study of *normative responses* from (psychologically) *normal organisms* to *abnormal stimuli*.

Some of these abnormal stimuli are biological, such as being paralyzed. Some are environmental, such as inaccessible entrances. Others are social, such as having a salesperson ask your companion, not you, what size you wear. Not being able to get a job is an economic example. Some stimuli are obvious,

*Portions of this introduction have been adapted from an earlier monograph (Vash, 1975).

such as a restroom door you can't get through, while others are subtle, like people not using the word "cripple" when you are around. Some are pleasant, such as being allowed to board an airplane first. Some are unpleasant, such as not being allowed to board at all. Pages could be filled with such examples, which in itself illustrates the unusual stimulus situation the disabled person is in: a continual flow of perceptions and experiences that cannot be validated by the majority of people around one. Thus, isolation and lack of consensus for one's ideas and feelings are added to the list of unusual stimulus conditions. And so it goes.

Following from this, the psychology of disability becomes bifurcated as an applied science. One branch is a rather typical applied behavioral science, embodied in a group of professionals who use the findings of research and clinical experience to help people with disabilities cope with, adapt to, and adjust to other unusual stimuli. The other branch is embodied in an activist movement by a group of people determined to alter the stimulus conditions because the world needs "treatment" as badly as the people with disabilities.

This latter branch is a relatively new development. It emerged slowly after World War II, when medical science found ways to save wounded soldiers who then returned, significantly disabled, to a society that felt it owed them something. Acknowledging a debt and paying it are two different things, however, and little progress was made. The civil rights movement pointed the way, and, oddly enough, the 1965 Watts riots added impetus. A segment of the black population in south central Los Angeles engaged in violent, self-destructive behavior for six days; somehow, one of the results of it was that blacks all over the country, other racial minorities, women, people with disabilities, and multitudes of other groups who had accepted powerlessness and half-filled cups all of their lives began to scream. They saw more clearly that society, even an indebted one, is not going to fix itself for you. The folks with the problem must come up with the solution. They also rediscovered the Constitution. Everyone had known all along that blacks were deprived regularly of their constitutional rights, but whoever thought people with disabilities were? The "expectation explosion" became a chain reaction, and "consciousness raising" tried to ensure that everyone's expectations were as high as they should be.

A very few years ago, the preponderant emphasis in rehabilitation was on modifying the "patient" to fit into the world as it was. Patients were modified by medicine, surgery, physical therapy, occupational therapy, psychotherapy, vocational counseling, social casework, prosthetic and orthotic devices, education, training, and much, much more. Family homes were remodeled, occasionally at public expense; but to expect all housing to be built accessible to people with disabilities would have been viewed as an idealistic delusion, about as likely as having a black mayor in Los Angeles. The motto was, "If a round peg doesn't fit in a square hole, you square the peg, you don't ream out the hole."

Some changes are being made. The "other half" of the psychology of disability has become the *politics* of disability, which may be just as it should be. It's not very good for people, psychologically speaking, to be deprived of their constitutional rights. If the applied psychology of disability is to be a helpful discipline, then it must tend to the business of altering destructive stimulus conditions, as well as modifying disabled individuals and their responses.

Scope and Purpose

The Psychology of Disability is intended to serve as a textbook or collateral reading source for students engaged in the study of the psychological aspects of disability, as well as a general resource for rehabilitation professionals in the full spectrum of allied health and vocational service disciplines. The material is presented in two parts, which might be labeled "What it's like to be disabled" and "What people who are inclined to help can do."

Part I, "The Disability Experience," is an effort to admit the reader into sundry corners of the experiential worlds of people with disabilities. It is a phenomenological accounting of the ways in which disabled people confront and are confronted by the world and of how they go about the business of living under the sometimes peculiar circumstances disability can generate. It attempts to present the psychological experience from the perspectives of people who have disabilities; the inner states and processes, the interpersonal situations and operations, and the behavioral mechanisms and patterns that emerge. The eight chapters of Part I chronicle both the objective and subjective experiences associated with being a disabled person in a handicapping world and how these affect the basic life functions of surviving, loving, working, playing, and—for some at least—transcending both the disability and the more troubling aspects of the world.

Part II, "Interventions," is a response to the problems and sources of psychological pain that are exposed by the discussions in Part I. It describes some major ways in which changes can be wrought; some are designed to improve the world, and others are intended to help disabled individuals react constructively to the conditions life has proffered. Interventions aimed at changing the world are not thought of generally as psychological services, but they may have a profound effect on the psychological well-being of an individual. Therefore, some of the major efforts being made are discussed in the first chapter of Part II. The remaining five chapters are devoted to intervention strategies used by psychologically trained professionals (for example, psychologists, rehabilitation counselors, social workers, psychiatrists, speech pathologists), other rehabilitation professionals (for example, nurses, occupational therapists, physical therapists, physicians), peer providers (for example, peer counselors), and social/behavioral scientists. Four of these chapters deal with ways to help disabled people improve the quality of their lives by working on themselves (as opposed to changing the world). The last deals with the future—ways of preventing disablement caused by behavioral or psychological processes, and research frontiers.

Unavoidably, the choice of subject matter and manner of presentation reflect the author's belief system regarding what the psychology of disability is all about, thus determining the issues considered important enough to include, the programs viewed as successful, and the policy decisions suggested. Moreover, the author's personal and professional experience has been preponderantly weighted in the area of motor disabilities; therefore, the selected issues and case examples may reflect this experiential loading despite conscious efforts to the contrary.

The Issues

The commonality of experience among people with different types of disabilities is great because the processes of being devaluated as a result of having a disability and learning to accept all that disablement entails are shared by all. It may be too sweeping a statement, but devaluation and acceptance seem to constitute the underlying cause and inherent solution to most of the specific psychological problems associated with disability. The form of a disability, however, does shape the manifest problems, so it is necessary to examine the specific ways in which various impairments impact people's lives. For example, deafness or even blindness may impede a person's participation in a conversation, whereas severe physical disability might prevent one from attending the gathering at all.

Probing further, although sensory, motor, and internal disabilities have significantly different impacts, they all reflect bodily dysfunctions, as opposed to impaired mental processes. With disabilities such as these, one can adopt rather comfortably the definition stated earlier: the psychology of disability is the study of normative responses from psychologically normal organisms to abnormal stimuli. Naturally, there are exceptions; people who could not be considered "psychologically normal" become disabled, too, and occasionally disablement proves to be the stress that pushes a vulnerable individual into neurosis or psychosis. More to the point, many people have disabilities that are explicitly psychological in nature, such as mental retardation or mental illness. While it would not be reasonable to assert that they are "psychologi-

cally normal organisms," it is still true that many of the psychological problems experienced are not due to the mental disabilities per se, but to such
abnormal stimuli as being devaluated in the eyes of others. In this light, it is
important to focus on abnormalities in stimulus situations before ascribing
abnormality to the psyches of disabled individuals, even when the disability is
mental in nature. Although the "letter" of the definition must be altered
somewhat to accommodate this portion of the disabled population, the "spirit"
of the definition is equally applicable.

Devaluation and acceptance: these are considered the pivotal variables
in adjusting to life when it is complicated by disability. Let us look at each in
more detail.

Devaluation

Following close behind outright oppression in terms of psychologically
damaging consequences is devaluation, that is, being regarded as a lesser
being, inferior, not very capable, not very useful, possibly burdensome,
unaesthetic, and, generally, one down. People with disabilities consistently
experience devaluation in the eyes of others, and their own. This is true
regardless of the nature of the disability, whether it impairs physical, sensory,
or mental functioning. The phenomenon was illustrated powerfully at a
rehabilitation conference held in California in 1974. Dr. William Rader—
psychiatrist, psychodramatist, and public performer par excellence—began
an arousing display of the tragic, even deadly, effects of communication
misfires between helpers and helpees with a simple routine. He addressed
the audience, alternately standing up and then sitting in a wheelchair, all the
while challenging them to deny that their perceptions of his competence
fluctuated as he stood and sat, stood and sat. There was much discussion
afterward, and virtually all in attendance, from able-bodied to very severely
disabled, acknowledged that their views of his competence *had* changed, had
alternated dizzyingly as he stood and sat; that he had appeared more credible,
more worthy of attention when he stood. It was an emotionally draining
experience for many. It was a confrontation of prejudice they had ignored or
denied for a long time. Why such an impact from recognizing that one does,
indeed, devaluate people with disabilities? Can it be changed? Probably not,
unless it is first acknowledged and examined in every aspect.

The first line of inquiry addresses whether such prejudice is biologically
based. Does the human species instinctively shun damaged organisms because their perpetuation could threaten the survival of the species? The
anthropological observation that numerous primitive tribes leave aged or
injured members to die because efforts to save them would endanger larger
numbers is familiar to many. Is it possible that biological mechanisms which

once operated for species protection have not caught up with an affluent and technologically advanced civilization that has rendered them anachronistic? No one knows.

The second line of inquiry is psychosocial, but the content is similar. People tend to shun, be prejudiced against, or devaluate individuals who are different. This is more so if the difference occurs at the low end of the distribution, that is, if the individual has less of something than most people have. But people who are too beautiful or too brilliant or too rich or even too kind come in for their share of suspicion and punishment as well. This phenomenon may have biological substrates also, since it appears to have been "learned" by almost every culture on earth. Can people learn to tolerate a wider range of differences? How?

The third line of inquiry is politicoeconomic. In an affluent, technologically advanced society, saving lives and improving the quality of life for those saved but left damaged is not going to threaten the survival of the species. It can, however, reduce the sum total of goods available for the rest. People with disabilities, especially severe ones, are viewed as a group of "takers" who don't put much back into the system, into the family, the community, or the larger society.

Considering materialistic values only, this may be a valid notion. If severely disabled individuals lack the inner resources or miss the strokes of fortune leading to jobs paying enough to support high-cost needs, then the issue is not whether the public pays, but how. Should there be a tax-supported welfare system or should the person be subsidized through an employer who, in turn, passes the cost on to the public in increased prices for goods and services? In terms of the long-run impact on the purses of the people, there may be little difference. In terms of the psychological well-being of the disabled people affected, the difference may be great.

If one looks beyond the material to spiritual values, the issue becomes meaningless. If one has faith, or at least adopts the belief, that the purpose of life is spiritual development rather than materialistic acquisition, then sharing of goods with those unable to produce their own is not inconsistent with enlightened self-interest. The reason for this is an associated faith that we are all parts of the same universal spirit, wherein selfishness and unselfishness become, paradoxically, the same. Just as one must "selfishly" pursue one's own development—and sometimes deny others—if one is to become a truly beneficial influence for others, so must one also pursue the removal of hindrances to others' development, because to do otherwise is ultimately to impair one's own. There is no reason to believe that people with disabilities put less into this system than anyone else.

In recent years, numerous surveys have been conducted to assess the service needs of severely disabled people. The reports make few references to needs for psychological services. That of one national study (Urban Institute,

1975) highlighted the fact that psychological services were *not* among those most sought after by respondents. The top priorities went to vocational assistance, transportation, and physical therapy; however, the report did make the point that people's views of themselves are often diminished by the presence of a handicap. In other words, they devaluate themselves.

This is a psychologically sophisticated age. A large segment of the population is aware of the potential destructiveness, to self and others, of impaired or undeveloped self-esteem. It is well known that many psychiatric disorders are outgrowths of this. Newspaper accounts of people who commit "senseless crimes" relate histories of impaired self-respect, as well as early efforts, which interviewed relatives recall, on the part of the criminals to prove that they "were somebody." Books like *I'm OK, You're OK* (Harris, 1967) proliferate and sell millions of copies. We are this wise, and yet the respondents didn't ask for help in dealing with their feelings of devaluation. As will be seen later, providers frequently offer only the most cursory efforts to help in this way. Why?

First, the sophistication is solely intellectual. When the need becomes an emotional reality, people are still both inwardly and outwardly directed to handle that part of the adjustment process themselves. A great deal of physical help and dependency are accepted because there is no other choice consonant with survival. To need still further help, implying emotional as well as physical dependency, is unacceptable, so the need is denied. Beyond this, the social sanctions against getting psychological or psychiatric help interfere with asking even when the need is recognized.

Second, it is not easy to relate help provided in this area to savings of public dollars. Physical restoration can demonstrably reduce the lifelong medical costs for which the public pays. Vocational rehabilitation can reduce welfare costs and get some tax money coming into the system as well. If physical restoration and vocational rehabilitation can do that, who is going to worry about *feelings?*

Apart from humanistic concerns about quality of life, it is possible that sufficient attention to such soft data of rehabilitation—from the earliest moments postonset through the entire life process—could further reduce medical, welfare, and related costs to a degree barely conceived of today. People who feel badly about themselves generate needs that must be served. Unfortunately, it too often happens after the person is in such deep psychological trouble that the effects are being felt by others as well.

Acceptance of Disability

In the earlier days of the rehabilitation movement, there was a great deal of talk about the importance of "accepting one's disability." This sometimes meant the absence of the defense mechanism "denial." At other times, it simply meant acknowledging one's loss without feeling rotten about it. Acceptance was good. People were never supposed to *like* their disabilities, however; that was considered worse than denial. Profits reaped were labeled "secondary gain" and secondary gain was a no-no. This required the disabled person to know exactly where the line between acceptance and enjoyment lay, and to be eternally vigilant not to cross over. Acceptance was biting the bullet and smiling at the same time, and about equally easy.

By the late 1950s, it was becoming unfashionable to talk about accepting disability. The literature explained to anyone gauche enough to use such language that it did not make sense to expect a person to accept disablement and that the professionals of a prior era had "laid a bum trip" on disabled people. No one should be enjoined to accept something that meant settling for second-rate hopes and goals. "Adapting to" and "coping with" became the preferred terminology.

Actually, it was this thinking that led, in part, to the advocacy revolution. Some realistic souls saw that counseling would not solve the problem if, at the end of it, disabled people still could not get from one point to another because there were stairs or no accessible buses in between. Life still would not be very much fun because the world was not a very reasonable place to live. Thus began the shift of emphasis from modification of the person to modification of the world; the new recommendations were for removing the stairs and the discriminatory hiring practices instead of counseling disabled people to stop liking upstairs restaurants and start liking the few jobs they would be allowed to do.

Now, as the 1980s dawn, a long-elusive but critically important distinction is finally becoming clear. If the disability cannot be changed, then it must be accepted, as must any other reality, pleasant or unpleasant, if the person is to survive and grow. What need *not* be accepted is the unnecessary handicapping imposed on disabled people by a poorly designed or unaccommodating world or by their own failures to accept what is and go on from there. These are the causes of second-rate dreams, and they should be summarily rejected.

This volume is not a compendium of indisputable facts. It is an overview of one author's observations on the experiences of people with disabilities and of individuals who try to help them with the harder parts. It is hoped that it will provide a useful base of information to students and practitioners in the wide range of rehabilitation disciplines wherein understanding of the psychological aspects of disability is integral to the work.

I
The Disability Experience

1 The Person

Reactions to Disablement

Some people are born with disabilities. They grow gradually into the recognition that they are different from most other people and in ways that are negatively evaluated. Something everyone else can do, they cannot. The realization of having been shortchanged comes slowly; it is their parents who may experience sudden shock. Other people become disabled after a lifetime—whether brief or long—of being more or less like everyone else. It may happen in a catastrophic moment, or it may take days, weeks, months, or years of illness to develop.

The reactions to the facts of disablement depend in part on when and how it happens and in part on a host of other factors to be explored in this initial chapter. The long-range response patterns, variously referred to as "adjusting to," "coping with," or "accepting" disability, will be dealt with in later chapters devoted to specific areas of human functioning. Here, the focus will be on the more immediate emotional and behavioral reactions of people who find themselves disabled, and on the array of personal characteristics and situations that determine the types and intensities of their reactions to the lack or loss of capabilities ordinarily taken for granted.

Just as "when and how it happens" contribute to determining a person's reactions to disablement, so also do such widely ranging factors as the type of disability, its severity, its stability, the person's sex, inner resources, temperament, self-image, self-esteem, the presence of family support, income, the available technology, and government funding trends. This sampling of causal factors associated with reactions to disablement illustrates four general classes of reaction determiners: (1) those emanating from the disability itself, (2) those linked to the person who becomes disabled, (3) those present in the person's immediate environment, and (4) those that are part of the larger cultural context.

Although Chapter 2 deals explicitly with the external forces impinging on people with disabilities, it is impossible to totally separate "the person" from "the world." To illustrate, George Hohmann, a rehabilitation psychologist who learned about spinal-cord injury first hand, points out that spinal-cord injury simply isn't as depressing today as it was three decades ago when he was injured (personal communication). The reasons he cites are the medical and technological advances, increased federal funding for needed programs, and the passage of protective civil rights legislation that have come about in the intervening years.

Thus, many different variables influence the types and intensities of reactions to disablement, and all of these variables interact with one another to create still greater complexity. To begin to understand what happens, let us look at what several people have had to say about their own reactions to disability.

Mike is mildly mentally retarded. He works in a rehabilitation facility as a custodian, and has reading skills comparable to the average second grader. His social skills are remarkable; he is poised and at ease and has a special gift for mediating other people's arguments. He speaks unhesitatingly about being a "slow learner" and how it felt when he first recognized that fact.

> The kids around home made fun of me because I couldn't catch on to things like they did. At first I cried, then I just stayed by myself. My folks put me in a special school where all the kids were like me. I was one of the smartest ones. I helped the kids who were slower than me. I really hated those kids that laughed at me. I still don't think people should laugh at slow learners. We're people like everyone else.

Mike's "folks" were actually his grandparents. His parents had sought to have him institutionalized when he was three, so the grandparents offered to take him. They were among the concerned citizens who established the facility in which he now works.

Nan was born with cerebral palsy. She was the first child of a ten-year marriage and highly prized by her parents. She believes her family's upper-class status in a Central American country, coupled with strong (Catholic) religious ties, served to facilitate their acceptance of and dedication to a disabled child. They moved to the United States when she was eight to avail themselves of better services for her.

For the first thirteen years of her life, she was taught to believe that she was "as good as anyone else and could do anything she wanted to do." This gave her the self-confidence to disregard the taunting of other children, to whom she attributed ignorance. She learned to walk, albeit awkwardly and at a fast pace to keep her balance, and learned to speak understandably to most listeners. She suffered such traumas as being placed in a school program for retarded youngsters until her intellectual gifts were recognized. In the main, however, she was a happy and energetic youngster who felt good about herself.

She says she can speak knowledgeably about both birth disorder and later-life disablement because at the age of thirteen, she fell and broke her hip. Thenceforward, she was unable to walk independently and, in her words,

> All of the teachings of my first thirteen years were undone. My parents couldn't understand why I couldn't walk anymore (and it was only a few years ago that a doctor explained it to me) and they accused me of being lazy and ungrateful. I realized that I wasn't really a human being to them, I was a project that had been set back. Then, when a teacher encouraged me to go to college and I told them, I found that they had never believed all those things they had told me about being able to do anything I wanted to. They didn't believe I could do anything, really . . . not drive, and certainly not go to college.

Today, Nan is a happy and effective schoolteacher, the only severely disabled teacher to be hired *after* onset by a large, city school system. She says those early years of confidence helped her combat the doubts and rejections she experienced later on, even though they were in one sense "undone." She believes having cerebral palsy forced her to mature quickly and to be less vulnerable to many of the emotional terrors that plague teenagers and young adults. She acknowledges that

> People with my disability don't find it easy to get dates, and you can't be as bold as other women or you'll scare men off. Maybe I'll find someone and maybe I won't. Either way, I know and like who I am, and, for the first time in my life, I now have good friends who accept me. Later on, I may adopt an older child with a disability, whether I'm married or not.

She believes there is a status hierarchy of disabilities in which polio and spinal-cord injury are at the top and mental retardation and cerebral palsy are at the bottom. She considers this less a function of time of onset than the nature of the impairments; however, she laughingly recalls claiming that her disability resulted from "falling down and breaking my hip" for several years after that happened.

Dana, who got polio at the age of sixteen, was present when Nan described her experiences. She agreed that her disability was freer from stigma than Nan's, but quipped that any advantage was overshadowed by Nan's greater maturity. She especially marveled at how "together" Nan appears to be with respect to her impaired status on the marriage market. Essentially triplegic, with considerable weakness in her "good" arm, Dana indicated this was her most painful area of reaction to disability.

She, too, experienced singular acceptance within her (very scholarly) family and also within a wide circle of friends. Having planned since junior high school to get an advanced degree, she had little more than the usual doubts about her ability to "make it" in her chosen career. However, she recalled a long and tortuous process of dealing with angry disappointment and consciousness-consuming fears about being "damaged merchandise on the marriage market." Of this she says,

> Mother always assumed I would get a Ph.D. in something because it was "the thing to do." But she also conveyed that the most important thing in life was to be a good wife and mother. A Ph.D. could be a cushion to fall back on in case you were widowed or divorced, but it wasn't a matter of trade training. When the doctor told us I would be permanently paralyzed, one of her first attempts to reassure me was, "Well, honey, think of it this way; you'll never have to wash dishes and your hands will always be lovely and smooth." I read the message, "Hopefully, you'll still be attractive enough to get a good husband."
>
> As soon as I could be up in a wheelchair, she started pushing me downtown to buy new clothes to fit my thinner frame. She would excitedly repeat appreciative comments she overheard from passing males. I now think they may have been apocryphal, but I believed them then and her strategy worked. I felt confident that, wheelchair or no, I was a pretty young girl who could expect to go on having lots of dates, and somehow believing it made it so. I determined never to do anything I couldn't look graceful doing, and I was off on a new career of proving to myself and the world that despite being in a wheelchair, I was still desirable.
>
> That neurotic adventure consumed a large part of the next sixteen years of my life. In my spare time, I got the expected Ph.D. and developed a successful career, but most of my consciousness was going into countless lovers and a couple of husbands. When my second marriage imploded, I went to a shrink and started getting the whole silly script rewritten.
>
> I've now been happily married to my third husband for over ten years, the Ph.D. is in "cushion" status, and my husband forced me to learn to cook *and* wash the dishes. I make Nan look as graceful as a ballerina when I start working in the kitchen. Sometimes, when I'm struggling to lift a heavy pot or something, I think back on the days when I wouldn't do anything that might look awkward. The irony is, it took so much craziness to come full circle. My present lifestyle is just about what mother had in mind. It makes you wonder about destiny.

Morris, who had been diagnosed as having multiple sclerosis a few years earlier, read what Nan and Dana had shared about themselves and remarked,

> I envy them both; at least they know that what they see today is what they've got tomorrow. With this crazy thing [MS], you never know whether you'll be better or worse a year from now or even the next day. I get a lot of the same rejection Nan does; I walk and talk like a drunk, and I've been going through a lot of the same shit Dana has—because I used to be quite the ladies' man. Now I'm afraid to even ask for a date. I may be kidding myself, but I think that when women see me in class,

they think, "Hey, he's pretty good looking." But when I start to talk or get up to walk, they back off fast. I did ask one girl to a movie, but she thought I was weird when I wouldn't take her out to eat afterward. I just haven't gotten to the point where I can ask a girl to cut up my food for me . . . and when I do it myself, I'm not exactly Mr. Cool. Nan and Dana should just be glad they're not men. It's OK for women to be helpless, but it doesn't look too good on a guy. I used to get really turned off in movies where some guy gets shot up and then goes on and on about being "half a man." But I tell you, that's not just schmaltz; that's really the way it feels sometimes.

Harris, who has been deaf since an explosion occurred near him in Korea, speaks of different kinds of reactions from those described by Nan, Dana, and Morris, all of whom have motor disabilities. He described the loneliness of being "left out" even when physically present in a group and his anger at being ignored when a conversation partner seeks the easier path of talking with the interpreter instead of him. He described his disbelief, years earlier, when he worked for the first time as a deaf person in the produce section of a supermarket. A customer, calling to him repeatedly from behind, grew increasingly frustrated and angry at getting no response. Harris first became aware that his attention was being sought when he was hit in the back of the head by a pound of hamburger, which the customer had lobbed at him. Boredom also is a problem when he travels and doesn't have his work or other pursuits available to absorb his consciousness. He says hearing people don't appreciate how much they amuse themselves by simply listening to the ambient sounds.

Reaction to loss can take many forms, and so can loss itself. Earl's story illustrates this.

Earl spent his twenties becoming blind. Although he always had done strenuous physical work, he was exceedingly bright and says he was able to adjust to college and a professional career with relative ease. He had been totally blind for seven years when his vision was significantly restored by surgery. He was delighted, of course, but totally unprepared for the adjustment agonies in store. He put it this way:

I had become a superblindman. Everyone marveled at how well I could manage every aspect of my life. My traveling skills were so good that a lot of people joked that I was faking it. They couldn't imagine how a blind man could get around so well, even without a cane. Then, all of a sudden, I was just an average guy again; no big deal, nothing super about me. I'd lost my special status and there was no support coming from anywhere for what I was going through. When I tried to tell people how I felt, they would shut me up, saying, "I don't want to hear this. You're spoiling my fantasies about the wonderful thing that has happened to you." Obviously, I don't want to be blind again, but I'd like a little understanding that

what's happened to me isn't totally the magical happy ending without any adjustment problems of its own. It's not pleasant having people regard you as some kind
of nut.

Mary knew that problem well. She had a "nervous breakdown" when she
was twenty-three years old and and for the next four years she was hospitalized intermittently about half of the time. She no longer considers herself
mentally ill, but believes she carries with her a residual lifelong disability. She
says,

> I am not sick now, but I will always be very vulnerable to stress, and I have to pay
> attention to that so I don't end up getting sick again. I've learned to do that pretty
> well. The harder part is dealing with the way other people treat you when they
> know that you've had a mental problem in the past. Some of them act scared, and
> some just discredit you—like your opinions and judgment can't be trusted any
> more. I am in a group living situation, not a halfway house run by institutional
> types who run your life for you, just a group of four people who got acquainted
> when we were all patients at the same hospital. We know we need each other's
> support to stay out of the hospital, and, with it, we *can*. We're all working, but
> none of our employers knows we've been in a mental hospital. If you lie about
> it and get caught, you can get fired. But if you don't lie about it, you'll never
> get hired in the first place. The anxiety of being found out is what's really
> disabling.

Frank had his second stroke when he was sixty-three. He was an old
sixty-three, having had a first stroke and a heart attack three and five years
earlier. His hearing was very poor in one ear, and he had to use a magnifying
glass to read the newspaper. Both strokes affected the left side of his body and
spared his speech, which he used mainly to say, "Poor Papa." Self-pity had
been a way of life since he was forty. Having been a successful, young,
small-town banker, he never recovered, psychologically or economically,
after his bank failed. Now, living in an extended-family household with his
wife, a divorced daughter, a divorced son, and a granddaughter, he settled,
uncomplainingly, for the occasional attention they paid him and showed no
inclination to broaden his activities beyond watching ball games on television
and muttering, "Poor Papa." He died two years later, following a second heart
attack, leaving a guilt-laden, grief-stricken family. His gentle nature was
deeply loved, but he had been easy to ignore.

As these vignettes illustrate, disablement has the power to elicit the full
range of human emotions, from fear, anger, and sorrow to relief and even joy.
Almost universally experienced are anxiety about survival and episodes of
rage. Some people rage against themselves, their own incompetence to do
what everyone else takes for granted; others rage against the universe for

being unjust. Some turn their rage against other people for failing to help. While the spectrum of human emotions may be limited, the ways of manifesting or expressing emotions are virtually infinite. Also reflecting enormous variation are the specific triggers to emotionality from one person to another. What hurts or angers one may seem inconsequential to another. As with human variation generally, the question of determination arises: *what* causes *whom* to react, and *how*?

The ensuing pages will refer to the foregoing vignettes, and to other "case examples" as well, in the course of delineating factors that determine (1) how, and how intensely, different individuals feel about their disabled status and (2) how their feelings affect a wide range of their behavior.

Determiners: The Nature of the Disability

This chapter began with the observation that both time and type of disability onset influence how the person reacts. In addition, other influences relating to the nature of the disability are the types of functions that are impaired, the severity and visibility of the disability, its stability over time, and the presence (or absence) of pain.

Time of Onset

As Nan suggests, self-concept may be influenced by whether a disability was present from birth or happened later to a previously "normal" individual. To her, having been born disabled seemed somehow less respectable than to have acquired a disability adventitiously later on. Although such feelings appear to be fairly common among people with disabilities, the matter is seldom discussed unless it makes a functional difference—as in deafness and, to a lesser degree, blindness. Never to have seen objects in space puts a congenitally blind person at a learning disadvantage compared with those who have visual memories, and the far greater difficulty in learning to speak intelligibly for people who were deaf before language acquisition is well known.

One's stage of life when adventitious disablement occurs influences the kinds of reactions that will be experienced. This is so partly because it affects the way one is perceived and reacted to by others and partly because different developmental tasks are interrupted during different life stages. The person who becomes disabled in infancy or childhood may, like the person born with a disability, be subjected to isolation, unusual child-rearing practices (such as overprotection or rejection), and separation from the mainstream in family life, play, and education. The person who becomes disabled later on may not have to face these same issues, but will have different ones to confront.

Dana's story illustrates one way of reacting to having been "nipped in the bud" just as the wonders and pleasures of womanhood were becoming realities. Earl, who became disabled after completing the developmental task of establishing himself vocationally, found he had to do it all over again. Frank was well into the "decline" stage of his life when he experienced disability; he no longer had the motivational resources necessary to react in any but a passive way.

Type of Onset

The experience of a close brush with death may be a powerful influence on a person's life, and many disabled people feel they cheated the grim reaper by surviving their disabling accidents or illnesses. It seems strange that so little attention has been paid to this issue within rehabilitation circles, especially in view of the importance assigned to the topics of death and dying in both the popular and professional presses in recent years. The claims of some disabled people that they were "given up for dead" tend to be discounted as melodramatic bids for attention, and no further probing is done to learn how an actual or perceived near-death experience might influence their emotions, values, beliefs, and behavior.

The reaction to nearly dying, or believing that one has nearly died, is complexly interwoven with such other variables as religiosity and self-concept. Dana, for example, reported that for years she felt guilty for having survived to be a burden.

> I felt I had been slated to die but somehow tricked the great scythe wielder and lived . . . to be a damn drag on a number of people. A lot of my achievement trip was feeling I had to earn and re-earn my right to a place on the planet. What looked like ambition was actually paying penance for not having been gracious enough to just die.

A very different reaction was shared by Lillian, who is paraplegic as a result of spinal meningitis. A devout Mormon, Lillian related that the sense of having been spared led to an intensification of her faith and purpose, which was especially helpful to her when she was abandoned by her husband following disablement.

A year after experiencing a cardiac arrest, Emma was still reliving the terror and frustration of hearing herself pronounced dead and being unable to signal otherwise. She says that nearly every time she is confronted by her memory losses or impaired coordination and strength she recalls the operating table comments and consensus that, "It's just as well, she'd be a vegetable if she lived anyway." She says she sometimes thinks she fooled them and at other times thinks they were right.

The type of onset also is associated with greater and lesser degrees of placing blame for the disabling outcome. Accidents, in which an official designation of responsibility is made, are simply the most obvious case. To believe that a permanent disability resulted from a momentary, foolish act of one's own may strongly affect reaction to the disability itself—at least until the feelings of self-blame are resolved. Blaming someone else may have an even stronger impact. Keith, who lost a leg when the motorcycle he was riding collided with a truck, became consumed with hatred toward the truck driver, especially after the courts found him not at fault. Fred, shot in the spine accidentally by his younger brother, believes both of their lives would have been better if their parents had permitted him to express the anger he felt. Kathy remembers wondering childishly why her parents wouldn't do whatever they were supposed to do to make her get better when she had polio as a child. They had always done so when she was sick before.

There are no formulae to describe how a sudden versus prolonged onset or a self- versus other-induced injury generally will affect reactions to disability. In all cases, it will depend on other variables present and how they interact with the type-of-onset variables. Keith, to cite an extreme example, had been previously diagnosed a "paranoid personality." Another person would not necessarily react as he did.

Functions Impaired

The body–mind system affected is the most central issue and almost too obvious to mention. In spite of the commonalities across all types of disablement, it is nonetheless clear that losing your eyesight, your hearing, or your ability to move is going to generate different reactions because each creates different problems. Impaired mental functioning or energy reserves create different problems still. This can be illustrated, in part, by what happened at a party at the author's home when a fuse blew and all of the lights went out. Among the 200 guests were a number of people who use wheelchairs, are deaf, or are blind. The wheelchair users tried to dodge effectively when walking party goers stumbled over their chairs and fell into their laps. The deaf guests definitely were not amused when their only means of communication was cut off. Those who were blind simply chuckled and asked, "So what's the problem?"

Typically, when nondisabled people are asked what disability they most dread, the majority responds, "Blindness." This reaction may be one reason why legislation for blind people in nearly all countries seems to be ahead of that for people with other disabilities. Even as adults, it seems, we are most afraid of the dark. People with motor-system impairments tend to respond as nondisabled people do; no matter how severely immobilized they might be, the concordance is that blindness would be worse. Blind and deaf people offer different opinions, however. Blind people, who have "been there," are much less apt to think that blindness is the worst disability that can happen. From a different perspective, deaf people often declare that blindness would be preferable to their disability and note ruefully that nondeaf people have little appreciation for the implications of being unable to hear.

Beyond these general observations, most of the impact of the impaired function is tied to characteristics of the disabled individual. For example, an "auditory" person—one who learns better from lectures than from a text and loves music better than the visual arts—is likely to be far more devastated by the loss of hearing than a "visual" person with the opposite pattern.

An additional aspect worthy of mention here is the extent to which a disability interferes with physical attractiveness. It is well known to psychologists and the laity alike that physical beauty is a very functional attribute to possess. Sensitivity to its lack or loss sometimes can exceed the pain felt about the more obviously functional impediments disability entails. Aesthetic displeasure with oneself also may be compounded by the reactions of others when disfigurement or deformity is extreme.

Severity of Disability

It has become a truism among rehabilitation professionals that there is not a one-to-one relationship between severity of disability and the intensity of reaction (or quality of adjustment) to it. One person can assimilate total paralysis with fair equanimity, while another is devastated by the loss of a finger. They have their reasons, and some of them will be explored in a later section (see Determiners: The Person); however, varying degrees of severity do create different kinds of situations for disabled people to respond to, somewhat independently of personal dynamics. A young woman with one partially paralyzed leg will not experience the fear associated with the realization of total dependency on others for survival; and the totally paralyzed person will not experience the embarrassment of being swung impetuously onto a dance floor by a handsome stranger. Similarly, a mildly retarded person will not know what it is like to be so severely damaged that life is an incomprehensible blur, and the profoundly retarded person will (presumably) escape the pain that comes from awareness of unwelcome limitations to learning ability.

Visibility of Disability

Closely related to the issue of severity is the visibility to others of the functional impairment. The young woman with the mild disability of a partially paralyzed leg was put in an embarrassing situation because her disability was not visible to her would-be dance partner. Morris, too, illustrated the issue of visibility when he noted that women seem interested in him until he speaks or gets up to walk. Invisible disabilities can be very difficult, interpersonally, simply because you appear to be what you are not. Ken, a husky-looking, barrel-chested man, related that he is often asked to help when something heavy is being moved. However, his barrel chest is a result of emphysema and he must reply, "I'm sorry, I can't." He says he is tired of explaining because "They always act like they think I'm just lazy and making excuses anyway . . . they can't figure anyone who looks so strong could really be too weak to lift one end of a couch."

Stability of the Disability

Ken's condition exemplifies another aspect of the disability itself, one that influences reactions: the extent to which it changes over time. Emphysema is known to have a downward course leading to a hastened death. It also fluctuates, now better, now worse, as it moves along that path. The same is true for numerous other conditions affecting virtually every body system. This creates a very different situation from that experienced by the person with, say, a spinal-cord injury, wherein the disablement occurs rapidly, improvements take place and reach a plateau, and then stability is reached.

Not all progressive disorders reduce longevity. For example, retinal detachment is a degenerative condition that has run its course when the individual becomes totally blind; no threat to life or other body systems is entailed. During the degenerative phase, the person merely has to wonder how long the residual vision will hold out. Multiple sclerosis, on the other hand, has more pervasive implications, including a less predictable and therefore potentially more unnerving end to anticipate. Reactions to such disabilities are shaped by these realities and by what the affected people tell themselves about their projected futures.

An important point in either case is that people with progressive disabilities are dealing with more than residual disablement; they confront an active disease process *plus* whatever residual disablement follows in its wake. Also a potent stimulus to reaction, cessations of symptoms and remissions sometimes occur, encouraging hope for containment or cure. When neither is forthcoming, a new round of disappointment, fear, anger, or other reactions may take place.

Pain

Arthritis is a progressive condition prototypic of the last nature-of-disability factor being considered here. A cardinal symptom is pain. Joint stiffness and deformity are surely undesirable, but pain tends to usurp consciousness, depending on its degree, whenever it is present. Progressive disorders are not the only ones to have associated pain; people with such stabilized conditions as spinal-cord injuries and amputations have their share of pain as well. Whatever the stimulus, when pain occurs, it is certain to influence a person's feelings and behavior. It is hard to be jolly, creative, or maybe even civil, when you hurt—but some can learn to do so. The extent to which pain is prepotent over other stimuli in capturing consciousness depends largely on the extent to which such learning has occurred. This reflects individual differences among people, which leads to the next topic for discussion.

Determiners: The Person

Emotional and behavioral reactions to disablement also depend importantly on characteristics of the people who become disabled. What remaining resources do they have for developing effective and gratifying lifestyles? For those whose disabilities occur adventitiously, what activities and behavior patterns are interrupted by disablement, and how central are these to their happiness? What kinds of temperaments do they have? What is the spiritual or philosophical base in their lives? What personality traits do they have that will influence the type and intensity of their reactions to disablement? Specific aspects of such determiners as these will be explored next.

Sex

Perhaps the most obvious person variable affecting reaction to disablement is the individual's sex. It is important to stress at the outset that being male or female does not necessarily imply better or worse reactions, only different ones. Morris pointed out a sex-related difference that he considered crucial: the greater social acceptance of a passive, dependent lifestyle for women than for men. He believes, therefore, that when disablement forces such a lifestyle upon someone, it is less disruptive of self-concept for women than men. This he holds is true even if the woman had not been a passive or dependent person before, simply because she will be punished less by society for assuming those traits after disablement.

Karen, a disabled feminist whose work centers about sexual counseling for disabled women, acknowledged (ruefully) that such a viewpoint has validity, but countered that the advantage is virtually destroyed by the far greater demand placed on women to be beautiful, physically perfect specimens in face and figure. She points out that by definition, disabled women cannot hope to meet this social ideal.

In ways such as these the two sexes have somewhat different burdens to bear and their reactions will vary accordingly.

Activities Affected

The story about the executive secretary who lost both legs and went right back to doing her job, compared with the violinist who lost his little finger and was destroyed forever as a concert performer, may be the oldest cliché in the rehabilitation business. Clichés come about, however, because there is repeatable truth in them, and this hackneyed tale conveys an important fact. The impact of disablement is largely contingent on the extent to which it interferes with what you are doing.

Earl was operating a ranch when he began losing his eyesight; when she contracted polio, Dana was rehearsing for a modern-dance exhibition. Both valued and engaged in vigorous activities that no longer would be possible for them, and they reacted with grief. Dana mourned for many years the loss of her prime outlet for physical energy and creative expression. Olivia, on the other hand, was a stenographer whose hobbies were chess and gem cutting before she lost both legs in an accident, and none of these activities was significantly affected. Although she assuredly reacted to her loss with considerable emotion, her ability to resume previously rewarding activities helped to mitigate a prolonged reaction of grief.

A rare but not unique occurrence is illustrated by Stephen. This seventeen year old had been a "behavior problem" throughout his school years, and much of his trouble was attributed to his father's disdain for his lack of athletic prowess. Following a spinal-cord injury, Stephen seemed less troubled than before, as if he now had an acceptable reason for being unable to meet his father's expectations.

It is not only the actual, ongoing activities interrupted by disablement that influence a person's reactions. Activities never engaged in but held out as goals for the future may be equally powerful determinants.

Interests, Values, and Goals

An irony often pointed out is that people who sustain spinal-cord injuries through adventurous, potentially dangerous activities are apt to be singularly intolerant of a sedentary life. If quiet pastimes turned them on, they wouldn't have chosen downhill skiing, surfing, auto racing, gang fighting, or armed robbery in the first place. It also is observed that people from cultures placing high valuation on physical or sexual prowess are more devastated by this disability than those whose traditions stress, say, scholarly pursuits. Whether one's goal is to climb the Matterhorn or break records set by Fanny Hill or Don Juan, if it is quashed by disablement, the "loss" may be as painful as the forfeiture of extant activities. This applies not only to people with spinal-cord injuries; similarly, interests, values, and goals can influence responses to the whole range of disabilities.

People with unifocal interests probably are going to react quite strongly to a disability that obliterates their expression, while people may adjust more easily if their interests range across several modalities: physical, intellectual, vigorous, rigorous, passive, active, and so forth. The chances are that the latter will have some interest areas that are spared. As the phenomenon of interest testing shows, however, people are not always aware of their interests, values, and potentially rewarding goals. Manifest interests at the time disablement occurs may reflect only a small part of the pattern of appreciations that could offer gratifying activity. The more varied this potential, the more protected is the individual from frustration and dejection over being disabled.

Dana, for example, had a variety of previously recognized intellectual interests to compensate her loss of dancing, at least in part. Others require a process of interest discovery to help them identify new directions and goals. Dana's value system, which already ranked scholasticism high, was ready to accommodate demanded changes; however, when an individual's values are invested almost totally in functions that are lost, the reactions to disablement and subsequent difficulties in learning to adjust are magnified accordingly.

Remaining Resources

The extent to which a person is devastated by the loss of function also is determined by what other resources for coping and enjoying are left. This can be illustrated by a conversation that took place between a rehabilitation hospital patient and a similarly disabled staff member who had been held out by other staff as an example of what could be aspired to. After a very brief time together, the patient blurted, "Hell, if I had your brains and looks I wouldn't be depressed either!" In this instance, the staff member had had many more years to adjust to her disability; however, all else being equal, a quadriplegic with an IQ of 140 probably does have better prospects for the future than a quadriplegic with an IQ of 100. When capacities for physical activity are severely reduced, it helps to have the option of developing a "cerebral" kind of life. The staff member cited also had other resources that helped temper the intensity of her reactions; a naturally high level of energy, strong career motivations, a life history of emotional stability, numerous artistic talents, social poise, and considerable potential for leadership. All of these inner strengths can be used to build a secure and satisfying life. Recognizing that such resources, and the alternatives they create, exist can do much to alleviate fears and other erosive emotions.

Some of the strengths just listed are employment resources, that is, capacities that can be developed to a level worthy of drawing a wage. Resources such as these will be considered in detail in Chapter 5. Others might be subsumed under a more general rubric of character resources, those qualities of personality or temperament that can influence reaction to disablement and subsequent adjustment in any realm of life.

Other Personality Variables

Interests, values, and most of the inner resources discussed previously are personality variables, and there are many additional ones that influence reaction to disablement. Depending on who defines the term and for what purpose, "personality" is imbued with a variety of meanings. Researchers define it operationally, writers define it literarily, and both groups do so idiosyncratically, to suit the purposes at hand. This book offers no exception. "Personality" is used here as an umbrella term, designating a constellation of interrelated constructs such as "personality traits (factors)," "behavioral patterns," "response tendencies," and "temperament." The use of the word "temperament" requires a little explaining, too, since it is not in high fashion today in either scientific or professional circles. This author has a response tendency to use "temperament" whenever a connotation of biological determination exists. Emotionality and energy or activation level serve as examples.

Considerable research has been done to discover what personality traits harbinger good or poor adjustment to disability in the long run, but virtually none has examined their effect on more immediate emotional/behavioral reactivity. One problem is the need for preonset personality data in the study of such relationships, and it is seldom available. Nonetheless, these reactions are important because they set the climate in which adjustive efforts take place.

To give an illustrative sampling, such variables as flexibility, adaptability, maturity, and the polar opposites of these appear to influence reaction to change generally, and this includes changes imposed by disability. The relative strengths of an individual's needs also will influence reaction style. To cite a fairly obvious example, a person with high needs for succorance and little need to nurture others should experience less discomfiture over enforced dependency than a person with the opposite pattern. This does not imply an easier or more successful adjustment to disability; quite the opposite could be true if other factors failed to prevent the person from lapsing into passive acceptance of helplessness.

Countless other personality variables bearing *prima facie* relevance to style of reacting could be mentioned. A number of those measured by standard personality tests and research instruments will be discussed in Chapter 10 with respect to their impact on long-range adjustment. Here, we will consider just one last set of personality variables that seem to be particularly powerful determiners of disability-related reactions.

Spiritual and Philosophical Base

One's spiritual belief system and philosophy of life shape the meaning of disablement for each affected person; this, in turn, influences the ways in which one reacts. The person who views disablement as a punishment from God for past sins assuredly will feel differently about it than will a person who views it as a test or an opportunity for spiritual development. The person who sees it as a purely chance occurrence in a probabilistic universe will respond differently still. The "will to meaning" has been regarded as an important shaping force since Viktor Frankl wrote of his suffering in a Nazi concentration camp and the avenues through which he found salvation (Frankl, 1970).

A psychologist who contracted Guillain-Barré syndrome drew from Frankl's Logotherapeutic concepts to describe her own experience, which she considered analogous to his world-famous ordeal. She writes,

> Seven months ago I was hospitalized with . . . Guillain-Barré syndrome. It was actually a great relief that was felt, rather than dismay at this diagnosis, just as the concentration camp victims felt relieved of their anticipatory anxiety when the hiding was over. . . . I was told by a well-recognized neurologist . . . that mine was most certainly a case of hysteria . . . and that I needed many years of intense, in-depth psychoanalysis. . . . I felt myself much too sophisticated to conjure up such an affliction. . . . I knew my own system and knew that something was physically wrong. . . .
>
> The paralysis [became] extensive. . . . I was dependent on hospital staff for every need. A virtual prisoner in a metal-railed bed, lonely and isolated. Friends came initially as a matter of concern and, perhaps, curiosity. There were many at first, but the human condition prevailed. Like its counterpart in the animal world, the weakened member was left to its own demise while the fit continued with their own kind. [Hayman, 1975]

She points out that the categorical disease societies, such as the Multiple Sclerosis Foundation, adopt a posture not unlike that of Frankl's "medical ministry," facilitating acceptance of a permanently altered state by familiarizing people with their own attitudes and their freedom of choice. She quotes Frankl's statement, "Man is, and always remains, capable of resisting and braving even the worst conditions. To detach oneself from even the worst conditions is a uniquely human capability." She relates how she accomplished this in her own situation.

> I was detaching myself from the painfully lonely situation through humor, though at the time I called it hilarity! And, I must have succeeded in detaching myself from myself as well, since there was intense pain accompanying the destruction of the diseased nerves. . . .
>
> Even though I was convinced that I would eventually walk, the uncertainty of

how long it would take was a most depressing factor. Dr. Frankl refers to this phenomenon in terms of a "provisional existence of unknown limit," and charges it with being the most depressing influence of all. . . .

One day the tears of exasperation broke through in the presence of a very perceptive Sister. . . . This wise lady sensed my need to look beyond myself at a critical moment of spiritual distress, or existential frustration, as the will to meaning in my life was most certainly being frustrated at this time. [Hayman, 1975]

Hayman takes care to separate spirituality from religiosity in her treatise, and this seems an important distinction. Acknowledging a spiritual aspect of life and having a life philosophy into which disablement can be meaningfully integrated appear rather consistently to ameliorate destructive reactions to disability. Specific religious beliefs may or may not prove helpful. For example, no cases are known to this author wherein equating disability with divine punishment has aided an individual; the help has come when such a belief has been cast off. A belief that a disability is somehow part of God's purpose can be helpful, but belief in God is not requisite if the experience can be imbued with meaning or purpose in other terms. Diane, severely paralyzed and agnostic, illustrates this when she says,

My disability has a purpose, but I don't consider it God's purpose; it is *mine*. My disability forced me to go to college and it's toughened up aspects of my personality that were a whole lot weaker than my legs and arms are now. No way do I like being paralyzed, but I do like a lot of the things that have come from it. Sometimes, when I start to get really mad at myself for being unable to do simple things, I think of that and simmer down.

Determiners: The Environment

Reactions to disablement are determined not only by characteristics of the disabilities and the people who have them, but also by what is going on in the environment. Both the immediate environment and the broader cultural context exert powerful influences on emotional and behavioral reactions to disability. Such immediate environment variables as family acceptance and support, income, available community resources, and the presence or absence of loyal friends have a great deal to do with how a person feels about being disabled. Whether or not one is institutionalized and, if so, what the characteristics of the institution are are particularly potent determiners. For example, an almost totally paralyzed government administrator relates (Roberts, 1977) that "The affront, indignity, and impersonalness of mealtime situations in the hospital" had once triggered "a terrible rage that I could neither deal with myself, nor express for fear of reprisals. Mealtimes would leave me tired and defeated. . . I was deeply depressed and resolved repeatedly to die."

Whether or not your culture is characterized by a high degree of technology that could resolve (some of) your functional problems, sufficient funding of the programs you need and enforceable laws to protect your rights also will influence how you feel. It was the changing cultural context of which Hohmann spoke when he said that disability isn't as depressing now as it was thirty years ago (personal communication).

Since both types of environmental determinant will be explored in depth in the following chapter, they will only be mentioned here. This chapter will close with a poem chosen to highlight the fact that reaction to disability goes on as long as the person and the disability do. It doesn't stop at some point in time when the person has "adjusted," it simply changes with each step in the learning (adjustment) process. It was written by Dana after seventeen years of disability experience, on a lonely night after her second marriage had ended. She says that reading it the next morning was what prompted her to seek psychotherapy.

Requiem for Spring

One day, when she was thirty-three and had tasted some of the
     joys of life and several sorrows,
She pondered briefly, a matter of three days, and made a
     decision.
She would not destroy herself because she preferred to keep
     her weakness everyone else's assumption
And only her certain knowledge.

This decision firm, and, God knows, it had been twenty years
     in the making,
She looked up from the desk she had tidied while she thought
     and into the overgrowth of plantings that loomed above the
     windows, criss-crossing and falling.
Now, she said silently, what now?

It is not as if I had a choice, she reassured herself
     and quickly added that perhaps this was not true.
I still have a modicum of beauty and
     sufficient wit to appear intelligent.
No, Quasimodo loved only beautiful women and there is no choice
     and there is no hope.

Day before yesterday a great man died . . .
    today the flags are lowered . . .
    tomorrow workers get a day to mourn, rejoicing . . .
While I, relentlessly wishing, pitiable small thing,
    mourn the loss of passion.

One day when she was sixteen and had tasted all of the joys
    of life and none of the sorrows,
She hesitated in her step and fell.
Sprawled across the dancing floors and propped against a
    fencepost in the corral,
Sitting woodenly watching elsewhere and elsewhere,
She smiled and nodded and convinced a number of people that
    pain was not pain.

At the age of eleven, it first occurred to her that
    death must be sweet.
Dark juvenile poems mark the way.
Miss Budd discouraged that sort of thing and so, two years later,
    did Miss Watson, who considered despair an inappropriate emotion.
Particularly during pubescence.

Liberated oceans drench me. Soon again they will rise from
    the sea and fall on me.
A tree sips from earth its anodyne while I, obsessed,
    protest my own apostasy.
Once a lover, now dispassionate, the dark affords no solace.
I have disavowed you darkness! is my cry.
No more the phantom comfort of the lonelier than I.

Ophelia, Ophelia, where have you been so long?
Off in the meadow, drinking wine,
Wandering, dreaming of an ancient song . . .
Sinking slowly into oblivion, having dreamed too long.

    Dana's poem also points out an important caution, not everything labeled
"reaction to disability" is precisely that. Dana reveals a dark side to her nature
that predated her disability by at least five years. She says now that rehabilitation workers should not let their patients or clients "get by with making
everything a disability issue," that she only began to unravel what was making
her unhappy when she stopped blaming her disability for every unpleasant
moment.

2　The World

Disabled People in a Handicapping World

To be disabled is one thing. To be handicapped is quite another. Now that disabled people are coming out of the closet and proclaiming, "I am, therefore, I think," one of the things they think about is the effect of language on how they are perceived by others and how they perceive themselves. One camp abjures the term "disabled." They say it reminds them of a defunct automobile resting uselessly by the side of the road. They insist on being called "handicapped." Another camp abjures the word "handicapped." They say it reminds them of pitiful poster children looking up gratefully at benefactors dropping dimes into the can. They insist on being called "disabled." Still another group signals thumbs down on both terms. "Inconvenienced" is their word. A fourth favors "impaired."

Sound familiar? Just when we're getting straight between "Black" and "Negro," along comes someone who insists on "African." It's the same battle all over again; the reasons are the same and they are good ones. Words have the power to shape images of the referenced objects and their choice is important in building or breaking down stereotypes. A group is oppressed, hidden, stripped of power, and made to feel ashamed of the nature of its being. Then social conditions shift in a way that permits the lid of oppression to be lifted a bit. A few of the stronger members climb out and hold the lid aside so that more can follow. Before you know it, you have a "movement," and one of the first orders of business is negotiating acceptable language by which to identify the members when it becomes necessary.

The author belongs to a fifth camp that uses the terms "disability" and "handicap" to convey two different meanings. This can be made clearest by first defining a third term, "illness." Illness refers to an active disease process. Disability refers to any residual impairment of physiological, anatomical, or psychological functioning that results from an illness, injury, or birth defect. It is defined in terms of individual functioning and, assuming there is no

22

longer an active disease process, is relatively unchanging for a given individual. Thus, it makes sense to speak of "a disabled person." Handicap refers to the interference a disability creates in an individual's efforts to perform in a given life area. It is defined in terms of social consequences and may vary greatly, depending on what the person is trying to do. Thus, it does *not* make sense to speak of a "handicapped person" in a global way.

To illustrate, Carol is a severely disabled person. About seventy percent of her muscles are paralyzed, and that is unchanging. But she is not always handicapped. Paralyzed muscles have little to do with thinking, talking, reading, writing, and listening, which are most of what she does in her work. On a dance floor, she is definitely handicapped. In the kitchen, her handicap varies from mild, when she makes a "whatever you've got, throw into the pot" stew, to severe, when she tries something that requires split-second timing, like a soufflé. Thus, while disabilities remain constant, handicaps appear in varying degrees and disappear, depending on what the person is trying to do.

Handicaps don't always come from disabilities. A big, burly college professor, whose worst disability is the farsightedness that often comes with middle age, commented one day that he is handicapped with respect to becoming a jockey. He mused, "That may seem a pretty trivial point, but what if I'd been born into a society where everyone else is jockey-sized and anyone who couldn't become one got put down?" People belonging to ethnic minorities are handicapped, not by disabilities, but by highly visible physical characteristics that are socially devaluated. Observations such as these led to the title for the present chapter: Disabled People in a Handicapping World.

Much of the handicapping that disabled people experience is imposed by (1) the humanmade parts of the physical environment and (2) social customs, values, attitudes, and expectations. Not all of it is; Carol never will be able to climb a mountain and there is nothing anyone can do about that; however, it is unnecessary for her to be stymied by flights of stairs when ramps and elevators can serve the same purpose. Stairs are a part of the physical world, but their continuing existence in architectural design—now that the problems they pose for a sizeable segment of the population have been recognized—is a function of social values and attitudes. It is these unnecessary handicapping effects of the humanmade world that the activist branch of the applied psychology of disability is attempting to correct.

The world that disabled people must reckon with is comprised, then, of two major aspects: physical objects and other people. The physical world is by far the less complicated. Conceptually, the topic of "other people" ranges from simple interactions between two human beings to the complex machinations of transnational organizations. Emotionally, it spans the cynicism of Jean Paul Sartre's "Hell is other people" and the beauty of John Donne's "No man is an island."

The remainder of this chapter will review environmental phenomena and events that interact directly or indirectly with disabled people to determine their reactions to disability and how little or how much they are handicapped in the various areas of life performance. To begin, a series of experiences had by Sally, disabled by rheumatoid arthritis, will illustrate several lines of force that impinge on disabled people from without.

Getting Up and Off to Work.   It takes Sally nearly two hours to get up, bathed, toileted, dressed, groomed, and breakfasted each morning. It used to take her ten to fifteen minutes to button her blouse until she discovered a device that reduced it to three. There may be other assistive devices she could profit from learning about.

Transportation.   It was hard enough for her to find a job, but it turned out to be harder still to find a way to get there each morning. She can't drive, she couldn't get her wheelchair onto the bus, and it didn't fit into the trunks of otherwise willing carpoolers who could have given her a ride.

The Work Plant.   She finally got a ride from a person who had to drop her off half an hour before her plant's opening time. She got cold waiting outside for the first husky male arrival to haul her up three stairs into the building. She was allowed to use the spacious restroom adjoining the executive's office, since the women's restroom was not accessible, but she says she always felt so foolish going in there.

The Job Site.   This was a miracle, which is why she put up with all the rest. Her counselor got a rehabilitation engineer to design a special desk for her so she could reach what she needed to operate independently. In the evening while waiting for her ride, she set everything up for the next day. Usually, someone stayed to help her.

More Transportation.   A big day arrived. Sally was invited to attend an out-of-state meeting that could have impact on her chances for promotion. She arranged for a ride to the airport and to be met at the other end. When she arrived at the gate, she was told that she would not be permitted to fly without an attendant.

Shopping.   She has a friend who drives her and helps her with her shopping every Saturday. Imagine her surprise when she found a new barrier, designed to prevent the theft of shopping carts at the supermarket, which also kept her from entering. The barriers were removed after a few months because nondisabled shoppers objected to leaving their groceries unattended while they went for their cars. She says the "Handicapped Only" parking spaces are always filled, but she has only once seen another discernibly disabled shopper in the store.

Recreation.   Sally used to ice skate before her arthritis got too severe, and she loves the follies. She never used to go because of the accessibility problems. As soon as the auditorium announced "new special arrangements for the handicapped," she got a group of friends interested in going with her. They sat together in the regular seating area. She sat alone in the area marked, and enforced, "Handicapped Only."

Housing.   She finally got an opportunity for advancement with another firm, which required her to move. She went in debt the first three months paying an attendant to help her until she could locate an accessible apartment in which she could live independently. While she stayed in a hotel, a deaf friend visited her and noticed the fire alarm bell. He pointed out that a bell wouldn't help him much, and asked her to mention to management that a flashing light also should be installed.

These experiences could be depressing to even read about unless note is taken that such frustrating "Catch 22s" are signs of progress. A few years earlier, she might not have bothered to leave the house at all because she'd have known there would be little to expect. Enough progress has been made to make it realistic to try, and the "Catch 22s" are transitional phenomena that we hope will disappear in time.

Sally was confronted by a series of barriers to living independently, working, and enjoying leisure time. Some of the barriers were physical, such as the stairs and inaccessible restrooms. Others were attitudinal, such as the airline policy that assumed disabled travelers don't know their own needs. Happily, her experiences included helps as well as hindrances: employers who were willing to hire her, friends who cared and would offer assistance, even the auditorium that accommodated her physical, if not her social, needs.

How people react and adjust to disability is partly determined by the mix of helps and hindrances they encounter in their lives. As pointed out in the previous chapter, environmental determiners of reaction to disability can be divided into two major types: those that are palpably present in the person's immediate environment and those that are interwoven more subtly into the larger cultural context. The former may vary sharply from one individual to another; the latter tend to be uniform for all individuals in a given time, culture, or subculture. In this chapter, environmental influences have been divided in still another way: those relating to the physical world and those relating to other people.

These distinctions are useful for comprehending the totality of interacting external influences that shape behavior; but, true to life, they do not remain in neat categories when in operation. The physical stairs cannot be separated from the architect who designed them, and the architect cannot be separated from years upon years of tradition in design.

With this disclaimer regarding the precision of categorization in mind, the ensuing pages will discuss first the environmental influences seen mainly as cultural context determiners and therefore as exerting similar influence on all disabled people in a given time and place. Second, we will explore influences that are tied to individuals' personal situations and therefore reflect marked variation from one person to another.

The Cultural Context

It may go without saying that the cultural context referred to in this volume is the United States of America in the last quarter of the twentieth century. A few cross-cultural comparisons will be drawn, but, unless otherwise specified, the previous assumption can be made. The fact is, some of the most powerful influences on reactions and adjustment to disability may be *pan*cultural, suggesting that they are, *au fond*, rooted in human nature. A large portion of the introductory chapter was devoted to what is considered the most potent negative influence of all: devaluation. There it was admitted that the genesis of devaluation, whether biological or culturally learned, is unknown. Being unable to discern which determiners are immutable aspects of human nature and which are potentially alterable products of human culture, all are arbitrarily assigned here to "the cultural context."

A few isolated instances in which disabilities (or disabled individuals) have been revered rather than devaluated can be cited. The best known example is epilepsy, regarded in earlier times as "the sacred disease." This elevated status was probably a result of the fact that epilepsy was very common among the ruling classes, and these rulers had little tolerance for being the brunt of devaluative statements. In addition, a few individuals scattered throughout history have been regarded as almost holy for reasons directly related to their disabilities. A current example is a mentally retarded artist in Japan whose exquisite works are revered not only because of their superb quality but also because of the childlike innocent who produces them.

Exceptions aside, the rule is devaluation, and its form and degree are heavily influenced by the surrounding culture. Devaluation can be blatant or it can be subtle. The Nazis, to give a clear example of blatancy, killed disabled people. Other societies, for the greatest part, have been so subtle that their devaluative practices went unrecognized as such for generations, until the new breed of activists started pointing them out. The creation of separate, segregated educational and work systems provide prime examples in both the Eastern and Western hemispheres.

Devaluation also may be tough, or it may be tender. Treating disabled people as pariahs and forcing them to sit outside the city gates to beg was a very tough stance to take. This attitude followed from a belief that "the afflicted" were sinners in the eyes of God and deserved to be punished. A more tender approach is to consider people with disabilities as unfortunates, not outcasts, and worthy of pity rather than contempt. Blatant or subtle, tough or tender, devaluation is devaluation and this is well understood by the objects of either attitude. Such awareness is illustrated by the comments of a severely disabled woman who had just been introduced as a keynote speaker. Invited to speak because she has clearly made a success of her life, she acknowledged her introduction by saying, "I guess I will never stop being surprised to hear myself referred to as 'someone less fortunate than the rest of us.'"

Not only the form but the degree of devaluation is shaped by the prevailing philosophy of the culture. A dominant element of the Nazi philosophy is the principle of Aryan superiority, which leaves no room for damaged specimens, especially among Aryans. On the other hand, the principle of reincarnation, which is embraced by many cultures, allows for no misfortunes. An important element of the latter is that one chooses one's body, one's parents, one's total life situation for the purpose of "working out karma." Thus, one *chooses* to live in a disabled condition for reasons related to spiritual development; one is not the victim of a regrettable accident. A rehabilitation administrator who has come to embrace the principle of reincarnation commented one day that, as one result, when she meets a person who is mentally retarded she no longer feels the pangs of pity she once did. She doesn't think of herself as more fortunate than (and therefore superior to) an unfortunate (and therefore inferior) person. She relates as a peer, a colleague spirit, and finds herself asking, albeit quietly to herself, "Ho there . . . what are you working out this time? I wonder if you are at a higher level of development than I for having come to such a test."

Attitudinal Barriers

This widely used term says, in essence, that disabled people tend to be rejected by other people. The most forceful rejectors used to be other disabled people who didn't want to "identify," but the movement is changing that. Perhaps the commonest attitudinal barrier is the tendency to overgeneralize about what "they" are like, whether "they" can be helped, whether "they" can communicate directly with salesclerks or need nondisabled intermediaries, whether damaged bodies can coexist with undamaged minds and the reverse. Only rarely are attitudinal barriers manifested openly and directly, such as in expressions of distaste or avoidance of eye contact, conversation, touching, or even proximity. They are more apt to be manifested indirectly, in the form of exclusionary practices deemed "necessary" for the safety or convenience of people in general. The term "attitudinal barriers" combines, in a sense, the effects of devaluative attitudes and discriminatory behavior.

In order to understand why attitudinal barriers exist, it is necessary to consider what qualities are venerated by a culture and are found lacking in certain groups. Some of the issues selected for review appear to be specific to our culture; others are so pervasive across geography and history as to suggest that they emanate from human nature itself.

Overvaluation of Rational Intellect. Since the seventeenth-century beginnings of the age of reason, Western society has placed an increasingly high premium on the particular type of intellect referred to as logicodeductive, sequential, rational, or linear-thinking. Another type, which earlier in history was greatly prized, concomitantly came to be ignored or even derogated. "Woman's intuition" was for long nearly the only reference made to the inductive, simultaneous, intuitive, or nonlinear thinking mode that was once considered *the* path to Truth. It did not serve well in the growing physical sciences (and their mathematization) and, over the course of three centuries, was declared illegitimate and practically forgotten.

Partly as a function of societal dismay over where science and technology have led, and partly as a function of their very progress in the field of brain research, intuition is in the process of being relegitimized. Some researcher–theorists believe the two types of intellect can be assigned to the left (linear-reasoning) and right (nonlinear-thinking) hemispheres of the brain. As a direct result, intuition is gaining scientific respectability. As an indirect result, we are beginning to recognize that certain people, those intuitive souls who are lacking in logicodeductive reasoning ability, have been unnecessarily handicapped with respect to mental functioning simply because their kind of gift was disdained.

People labeled "mentally retarded" are sometimes gifted in terms of nonlinear, instantaneous data processing ability, and Mike appears to be one such person. His ability to penetrate immediately the obfuscations that generate and escalate misunderstandings between people is the talent that allows him to mediate others' arguments effectively. He does not reason through the haze in stepwise fashion; he appears to intuit at once what has gone wrong. His gift has become recognized in the light of recent attention to this other type of intellect, but it is important to note that it is rewarded only as an interesting oddity. This society as yet offers only the rarest opportunities for acknowledgment equivalent to that given sequential reasoning; specifically, there are few jobs that explicitly draw on such talents and pay living wages to individuals so gifted.

Overvaluation of Physique. Physical beauty and prowess are not only very highly prized in society, most cultures also set stereotyped, narrow bands of standards as to what "makes the grade." Here, today, men should be tall, tanned, and muscular, with copious character in their rugged faces. Women should have gigantic breasts but no fat anywhere else and a minimum of character lines to mar delicate, regular, facial features. Ideally, both should appear youthful regardless of their chronological age, but for women it is a must. Athletic prowess is a must for men and highly desirable for women, if not taken to extremes. Women have more latitude here; if she can't play a decent game of tennis, a woman is okay if she can dance or wiggle nicely when she walks. Such values are so deeply inculcated that merely to associate a product with youthful movement and beauty is to elevate its sales. We all want "the image" for ourselves. Most of us feel, in varying degrees, that we must at least approach it in order to be happy. But some of us don't. As Kathy pointed out, people with disabilities are almost automatically disqualified.

The counterculture of the sixties was a helpful ally in combatting this barrier in that it rejected the traditional standards and attempted to widen the range of acceptable physical attributes by (social) force. But according to well-publicized recent research, there is still a strong correlation between physical attractiveness and such hard-to-define but universally desired conditions as success, happiness, and life satisfaction. It doesn't help to label it shallow, irrelevant, inhumane, and undemocratic. It is a force to be reckoned with, and some ways for doing that will be discussed in Chapter 11.

Undervaluation of Spirituality.   Just as modern society appears to have overstressed the importance of rational intellect and physique, at the same time it has reduced emphasis on matters of spirituality. These are natural outgrowths of the age of reason, with its advancing science, technology, and preeminent materialism. Descartes gave us the concept of mind–body duality in the seventeenth century, and we have been using and misusing it ever since. Somewhere along the line, the spiritual aspect of our being was mislaid. Like intuition, it is in the process of being rediscovered, and for essentially the same reasons. Again, a segment of the counterculture contributed substantially to initiating the shift.

Disabled people are handicapped differently by a materialistic society than by a spiritually oriented one. A society which combined the technological advantages of the West with the spiritual values of the East might not handicap its disabled members so much. When you conceive of yourself as nothing more than mind and body, and one or both of those has been damaged irreparably, it doesn't leave you very much that is stable and intact. The balance changes, however, when credence is given to the spirit, which seems to be impervious to the onslaughts of disablement.

The degree to which a culture is materialistically oriented influences societal reactions to disabled individuals in a number of practical ways. Along with technological advancement, the levels of industrialization and affluence rise, yielding many benefits. Concomitantly, the ethic encapsulated by the phrase, "I am my brother's keeper" diminishes, to be replaced by a welfare system. When responsibilities formerly carried by the family and the church are shifted to the state, a businesslike atmosphere, rather than a loving climate, is created for recipients of care. These and other cultural influences relating to style and level of social and technological development will be examined next.

Blaming the Victim. It is very difficult for humans to acknowledge how utterly capricious fate can be. Such an admission carries with it a disturbing awareness that we are not always in control of our own destinies. "If the fickle finger could point at *them*, it could someday point at *me*." To protect ourselves from the sense of impending vulnerability, we work things around in our minds to make misfortune the bearer's own fault. "He must have brought it on himself. I'm not bringing anything like that on myself; therefore, I needn't worry, it won't happen to me."

A very popular form of blaming the victim is the attribution of masochism to people who are victimized by serial misfortune. We don't like to believe that fate could really be so unfair. We search for other explanations and find one that is sanctified by modern psychology: the urge toward self-destruction. However unexplainable that might be, it is preferable to giving up what Jules Masserman (1955) has called an essential, human delusion of invulnerability.

Like devaluation, the method of blaming the victim is sometimes blatant, sometimes subtle, sometimes tough, and sometimes tender. "I'm not surprised, she's always been accident prone!" "Arthritis occurs with people who are filled up with pent-up hostility." "He deserves it for trying to rob that store in the first place!" "Poor thing, if she'd just been able to think a little faster, the accident could have been avoided."

Unfortunately, after thus reassuring ourselves, we start looking askance at the "unfortunates." Nowhere is this seen so clearly as with disabled people who develop one complication after another or additional, unrelated disorders. Family, friends, and rehabilitation workers alike find themselves saying, "It can't just be happening; she (or he) *must* be doing something to cause all of this." Whether s/he is or whether s/he isn't, fate is thereby dealing one more blow for her/him to react to.

Insistence on Mourning. We humans also have a tendency to assume that anyone who has lost something that we hold dear must be mourning its loss, be it physical prowess, money, power, or anything else. Allowing for the possibility of easy relinquishment seems to suggest that what we possess may be unimportant. *Au fond,* it may be less what we possess than what we strive for that stimulates this insistence on mourning. When we dedicate our energies and consciousness to amassing wealth or building the body beautiful or gaining influence and power, we may not want to hear that someone else has discovered—in one way or another—that goals of these sorts are not, after all, essential to happiness. What is the meaning of our struggles, then? To preserve the meaning we have ascribed to our own lives and efforts, we thus make the assumption of "sensible mourning." It is viewed as only sensible that a person would mourn, perhaps unremittingly, the loss of an essential ingredient of a satisfactory life.

This simply isn't always a valid assumption. Earl, for example, found that he mourned the loss of his disability—a process no one else could understand—more than he had mourned the loss of his vision. Stephen's disability also brought a compensatory trade-off in relieving him of the pain of failing in his father's eyes. That mitigated his mourning substantially. Even Dana, who mourned more expectably for a number of years, eventually surpassed mere reconciliation in an avowed embracement of all of her life experiences, including disability. Diehards may insist that this is "sweet lemon rationalization," but it does not seem sensible to believe that someone who has not experienced disability knows more about how it feels than somene who has.

Technological Level

In recent years, the United States Government has made a concerted effort to take mainland rehabilitation know-how to the islands in the Pacific. As a result, a number of rehabilitation experts have experienced directly the dramatic impact of cultural development on the lives of people with disabilities. Taking a spinal-cord injury as an example, in Micronesia the concerns must include getting the person into a canoe to reach a ship that can take her/him to a hospital in Hawaii, preventing pressure sores when s/he sleeps on a grass mat on a dirt floor, and finding a wheelchair that can withstand more than six months of the high humidity and rough terrain. One expert also observed that mainland values do not mesh well with life in Micronesia. She commented,

> The only real work there is gathering copra, which physically disabled people obviously can't do. But in order to be eligible for vocational rehabilitation funds to get the needed medical care, they are "punished" by being forced to go to work doing *something* . . . something that has no meaning in their frames of reference.

To those of us imbued with modern technological and materialistic standards, it would seem clearly preferable to be disabled in a culture with the technological means to circumvent many of the functional problems disability generates. Having grown used to the convenience and independence offered by motorized wheelchairs, powered lifts, electronic magnifiers, talking calculators, and portable teletypewriters, it would be hard to go back to a lifestyle bereft of spin-offs from the aerospace industry. A story about motorized wheelchairs provides a striking example of how the application of technology can influence not only the ways individuals feel about having disabilities, but their efforts to adjust and build satisfying lives as well.

Until the late 1950s, a number of rehabilitation hospitals had policies of discouraging the use of motorized wheelchairs. It was reasoned that people with weak upper extremities would profit from the exercise of wheeling manual chairs. Lost in this trend were those with so much upper-extremity weakness that they could not propel manual chairs at all. Rather suddenly, a change in philosophy came about, and the "personality changes" observed in many affected individuals were remarkable. Several years later, Bob related how his new wheelchair affected him.

> I got polio when I was too young to remember. As long as I have known me, I've been almost totally paralyzed. I'd spent all my life at [hospital] until a couple of years ago. They didn't know what else to do with me. I went all the way through high school there, and everyone used to tell me, "You're so bright, you should go on to college," but I just couldn't imagine it. After I finished school, I just sat in the hallway all day and talked with whoever came by.
>
> When they first asked me if I'd like to have an electric wheelchair, I said, "No." It seemed freaky, somehow, and I was afraid I might lose control of it. But they kept after me and boy! what a change in my life! All of a sudden, for the first time, I could go wherever I wanted to whenever I wanted to . . . I didn't have to wait for a "gray lady" or escort service to push me. I went all over the hospital, down the street to where some shops were, and I finally enrolled in college. Somehow, being able to move around on my own, I could imagine doing it. I've done really well in school and just moved out into my own apartment.

It also turned out that the no-motorized-wheelchairs policy had been a disservice to people who could wheel their chairs, but with enormous energy expenditure. The hospital staff member cited earlier went through the same philosophical transition and relates that, after adopting the use of a motorized chair, she greatly increased her artistic and domestic activities because she at last had the energy to pursue them. A policy designed to maximize independence had proved to have had the opposite effect.

Even more centrally influential on the quality of life for disabled people is the degree of industrialization and affluence that technological development permits. For example, new kinds of jobs are created, as technology advances, that do not require workers to move or manipulate physical objects—"thing jobs," in the terminology of the *Dictionary of Occupational Titles* (1965). "People (service) jobs" and "data jobs" come into being, jobs that workers unable to use their bodies as primary work resources are able to do. Moreover, an affluent culture can better afford to absorb the costs engendered by people with disabilities, restoring their functioning or supporting their additional needs when restoration is not possible.

On the problematical side, as the tempo of technological development increases, the rate at which jobs obsolesce is stepped up accordingly. This creates retraining needs among both nondisabled and disabled workers, but narrowed options make such transitions more difficult for the latter.

Socioeconomic and Political Style

Relatively independent of level of technological development, societies may diverge, or change over time, in political philosophy and socioeconomic style. The extent to which a society chooses to direct some of its resources toward the betterment of life for disabled individuals by creating/enriching a welfare system, passing protective legislation, and channeling monies into service programs has powerful impact on what it means to experience disability.

As an example, only a little over two decades ago, United States' citizens so severely disabled as to require the help of an attendant had only two potential options: to be cared for by family or friends or to live in a maintenance-care institution. The alternative of being provided with funds to live as an independent adult did not exist yet. Today, independent living is becoming the norm as a result of legislation creating an enriched welfare system that takes cognizance of both human and monetary needs. (Some of the ways in which this same system breaks down, from functional and psychological viewpoints, will be examined in Chapter 3.)

All of these cultural influences on reactions and adjustment to disablement are relatively uniform for people who experience disability within the same society during a particular period of time. The following section will take these as givens and explore other environmental determiners that are more variable from one individual's situation to another's.

The Immediate Environment

A counselor specializing in the problems of people with very severe physical disabilities summed up his years of experience by expressing the opinion that

> The main problem with being disabled is being *poor*. If you were rich enough, you could buy all the fancy gadgets available to do what they can, and whatever was left, you could pay other people to do. I don't think being disabled would be so bad if I had a valet, a chauffeur, a personal secretary, a big, accessible home, a van with *everything*, and no worries about grubbing for a job.

This counselor has not experienced disability, and some of those who have may feel he is missing some important points, but he also is making one: how rich or how poor you are has considerable impact on how miserable disability can make you. Moreover, one of the problems with disability is that it tends to make or keep you poor. Available income may not be *the* problem associated with disability, but it is surely an important determiner of reactions and adjustment to it.

Family Influences

Income is but one aspect of the familial milieu surrounding a person with a disability. Other relevant variables relating to family structure and dynamics include the family's social standing and power base in the community, parental acceptance, spousal loyalty, and the proferring of practical and/or moral support. Having a family member who is skillful and assertive in mastering crisis, a name that is recognized by local agency personnel, or a relative who plays golf with the major employers in the community can alter materially the negative ramifications of most any disability. The effects of these and many other aspects of family capability and interaction will be examined in detail in Chapter 4.

The Influence of the Community

Just as one's position within the community makes a difference in the consequences of a disability, numerous aspects of the community itself influence disability-related experience. Perhaps most basic are the community's size and location. A small town may offer a quality of human support that is lost in the big city, yet lack the sophisticated paraphernalia and services the latter provides. The differing demands made upon rehabilitation systems by rural and urban communities are felt most keenly by those in rural areas, since most service models are designed in and for the denser population centers with their relative wealth of medical, educational, psychosocial/vocational, and other resources.

The extent to which a given community has responded to protective legislation by eliminating mobility barriers, mainstreaming disabled youngsters in the public schools, and other such actions, also will have significant impact. So will the existence of voluntary service organizations and the service orientation of local churches. Does the local television station provide captions for nonhearing viewers? Does the transit authority have buses with lifts or at least a demand-response option for those unable to board standard buses? Does the responsible department of local government try to enforce existing protective legislation? Is there someone with a significant disability among the ranks of elected officials? Does an active disabled consumer organization exist? The answers to all of these questions portend much concerning the quality of life for disabled individuals in a given community. These are the problem areas being attacked by the activists determined to alter the stimulus conditions "out there," all of which they view as stemming fundamentally from the attitudes and actions of "other people."

Institutionalization

Most people with disabilities have occasion to experience that unique kind of community known as "an institution." This may be limited to hospital stay during the acute treatment; or it may include additional time in a hospital for rehabilitation. For some, an institution becomes home for a major period of their lives.

However Utopian an institutional setting might be, the inhabitants are not there by choice. Ordinarily, institutionalization is grudgingly accepted as an unavoidable necessity for accomplishing some other goal, such as rehabilitation. In point of fact, few, if any, institutions *are* Utopian; by their very nature they tend to restrict the degree of freedom and violate the privacy of the people who dwell in them. Depending on specific institutional policies, procedures, and personnel, these effects may be minimized or magnified.

Erving Goffman (1961), in his well-known work *Asylums,* described what he called the "mortification process" wherein institutional residents are deprived not only of their privacy but of their power over themselves, usually for the convenience and efficiency of those running the institution. Rules that would be considered intolerable if imposed on noninstitutionalized citizens are enforced and accepted. That they are behaviorally accepted does not indicate an absence of psychologically damaging consequences. Yielding self-mastery, even for a time, may have long-lasting, negative effects. Staff in rehabilitation hospitals have become alerted to the irony that the patients most willing to cooperate with medical usurpation of crucial decision making about their lives during institutionalization may be the least well prepared to resume effective, assertive self-mastery when they return to the ordinary world.

Psychologically speaking, it may be that the irony to end all ironies is the fact that, in hospitals, the staff member most important to the patient is the one considered least important, if prestige, remuneration, and care in selection are indices, to the rest of the staff. A long-term follow-up study (Kemp & Vash, 1971) reported that the vast majority of a sample of fifty spinal-cord-injured individuals interviewed five to ten years after hospitalization, when asked to recall their "brightest memories associated with being in [hospital]," responded with recollections concerning particularly caring members of the nursing *attendant* staff. Obversely, their "grimmest recollections," in the main, concerned attendants who were cruel or demeaning. The more prestigious and highly paid staff were not once mentioned. It is the attendants who carry out the most intimate ministrations; it is they who are there at the end of the day when memories and doubts flood consciousness, and on the weekends when no visitors have appeared. Yet in many settings, these employees are still selected and paid in the same ways as the housekeeping staff who take care of the physical plant.

Roberts' observations on the indignities to which he was subjected during mealtimes in an institution (see Chapter 1) suggest that some of the care-givers he experienced might have been better suited to building-maintenance tasks. Using feeding as a potent example of the emotionally loaded interactions between attendants and patients, it is important to note that not all of the error is made in the direction of uncaring or hostility-laden practices. Baby talk accompanying the feeding of an adult patient can have equally destructive effects. (Whether infantilization of this sort is also a form of hostility belongs to another book.)

Agencies

Contact with institutions doesn't end when one is no longer a resident of one. After return to the community, people with disabilities often continue to interact with other types of institutions, called "bureaucracies" or "agencies." These provide vitally important services and are appreciated for that reason, but the mortification process goes on. In order to receive the benefits allowing survival outside of a residential institution, disabled people still must tell all, hand over the reins, and oftentimes swallow much, possibly for a very long time. The widely publicized suicide of Lynn Thompson in 1978 galvanized the disabled community into a coalition determined to alter the laws and agency procedures that triggered her conclusion that death would be preferable to the life she foresaw upon being forced to return to a residential institution.

Chapter 3 will treat these and related subjects in more detail, and Part II will take the further step of exploring ways in which problems cited can be minimized.

Regional Differences

Just as legislative thrusts and government funding trends affect disabled people in relatively uniform ways, so may similar phenomena influence *subgroups* of people, as defined by their localities or in various other ways. Marked regional differences have been noted in the nature and effectiveness of national programs from one state or locality to another, but disabled people seldom have the choice to live where the services are best. One effort may be reflected in the tendency for motorically disabled people to migrate to California. This is not solely a result of more extensive health-related services, however; the Mediterranean climate and relatively accessible architectural style offer sufficient lure. The happenstances of geography, climate, and building style can have significant impact on how one reacts to a disability. For example, having to cope with snow when you're blind or use crutches can take its toll on your safety, your independence, and your sense of humor.

As always, it is not just the physical facts that create or eliminate problems, but also how people respond to them. In the western states, for example, if your home doesn't "work" for you after you begin using a wheelchair, the chances are you simply will move into another that does. This is not so in New England and other parts of the Eastern Seaboard. The tradition of the family home is far more sacrosanct there than in the West, and a home that has served a family for several generations will not be relinquished lightly, however difficult it may be to get a wheelchair in and out, or up and down the stairs.

Exotica

An influence that affected positively a particular subgroup of disabled people for a number of years is worthy of mention because of its implications for future reform vis-à-vis environmental influences in adjusting to disability. This was the operating style of the National Foundation for Infantile Paralysis. The families of children (or adults) who contracted poliomyelitis were given the financial help they needed to deal with catastrophic illness, but they were not subjected to the mortification process that accompanies recipiency of such government-administered aid as Supplemental Security Income. The program was "abused" in a way that consternated almost no one: because only polio patients were eligible, some physicians are thought to have intentionally misdiagnosed cases of Guillain-Barré or infectious neuronitis, which have very similar symptoms. It saddened rehabilitation workers to see patients with still other disabilities having nowhere to go for comparable help. Today, the generations of "polio kids" who are now adults can appreciate the Foundation that helped without imposing elaborate screening/monitoring systems that shatter the peace of mind financial aid should bring, by destroying dignity and privacy during a time of extreme emotional vulnerability.

3 Surviving

Living Independently

The previous two chapters have described and placed the disabled person in the context of a world comprised of the physical environment and other people. This chapter will begin the process of examining what happens when that person tries to partake of the American ideal in a world wherein survival (life) and independence (liberty) are prerequisite to the pursuit of happiness. As shown in Chapter 2, that pursuit is seriously impeded for some, and life and liberty may be in continual jeopardy. What does this do to an individual, psychologically speaking? Before exploring answers to this question, let us examine several ways in which "survival" and "independence" are interpreted.

The dictionary defines "survive" as meaning "to remain alive or in existence, as after an event or the death of another." This definition clearly implies biological survival; however, in conversational practice, the word is used to mean much more. Survival of the ego is implied sometimes, or survival of a preferred lifestyle, economic base, normalcy, or feelings of well-being. Such is the essence of the commonly made distinction between "merely existing" as opposed to "really living." The word "survival" will be imbued with this broader meaning here. The fact is, biological survival issues are the rarest kind encountered as one moves past the acute stage of an illness or injury—usually a brief period—and on to the years and decades of living with a disability in the community.

"Independence" is a controversial term. "There's no such thing; we are all *inter*dependent" is a familiar voicing of the discomfort felt with the concept. Again turning to the dictionary, we find "independence" to mean "freedom from the influence, control, or determination of another or others." This is not a difficult definition to accept; what is often rejected is an added connotation of "ability to survive alone, without the aid of others or respect to their actions." Disabled activists in the burgeoning consumer movement are endorsing the limits of the dictionary definition when they explain that independence, to them, does not imply being able to survive without the help of other people or assistive devices; it simply means freedom of decision making and the power of self-determination. It would be impossible to write about this topic without using the term in both of these ways, since the embellished connotation is prevalent within rehabilitation circles. ("Independent" is used often as a synonym for "unassisted," such as in independent dressing or transfer activities.) It is expected, however, that the context will make clear the sense in which "independence" is meant.

The processes of surviving and living independently after the event of disablement can be viewed from infinite perspectives. The following is but one alternative way of conceptualizing what happens, without and within. Maximizing one's health and capabilities, mastering the physical world, interacting with other people, striving for normalization, and taking charge of one's life—all the while altering conditions affecting disabled people generally—will be discussed in turn.

Maximizing Health and Capabilities

At the most primitive level of existence, the ability to locomote to find food and shelter is the basic requirement for independent survival. However, as civilization creates interdependencies, communication with other individuals also becomes essential. Disabilities impair one or both of these capacities; rehabilitation attempts to replace or restore them. When a disability is present at birth or develops gradually over time, rehabilitation efforts begin whenever the individual, a parent, a physician, or some other observer notices the need or believes the time is ripe. When the onset is sudden, rehabilitation ordinarily begins immediately after the acute medical care has ended, regardless of the individual's readiness for such procedures. Newly disabled people may be transferred directly from an acute-care hospital to a longer-term rehabilitation center with no intervening period of returning to familiar surroundings. As a result, they seldom understand accurately what they need to learn during rehabilitation in order to return to their previous lifestyles or move on to improved ones. Most rehabilitation programs assume that the professionals know what must be learned—an assumption that may be flawed.

Too often, all of the newly disabled people in a given rehabilitation facility are offered a standard ("shotgun") battery of rehabilitative services which proves later to have missed the mark because it was not individualized to each person's particular lifestyle and needs. In addition, many are still too emotionally distraught to make valid decisions about what offerings to accept or to make good use of whatever was offered. As a sign of progress, some thought is being given now to providing a briefer, general rehabilitation

program immediately after the acute-care phase, followed by a more extensive, individually tailored program once the person has had opportunities to
assess his/her specific needs, in terms of emotions as well as practical task
performance. However, less attention still is paid to the person's state of
consciousness, at whatever stage of treatment, than should be the case.

This is particularly regressive in light of current attention to holistic
health care. Today's intelligentsia is becoming exceedingly sophisticated
about individual responsibility in maintaining health as a state of positive
wellness, not simply the absence of disease. The importance of exercise,
nutrition, behavior (health-affecting habits), and state of consciousness in this
area are highly touted. Nonetheless, little is heard of such matters within most
rehabilitation settings. State of consciousness and health-affecting behavior
are largely ignored; exercises are focused more on strengthening weak muscles than on tuning general physiological functioning; diet is seldom stressed
unless it is clearly responsible for disease symptoms, as in diabetes. It is a rare
rehabilitation program that gives more than cursory mention to the fact that
eating habits must be dramatically altered when a person changes from a
robust lifestyle to a sedentary one. Thousands of overweight wheelchair users
attest to the need for consultation and intervention, while hospital canteens
continue vending junk food to patients needing to make every calorie count,
nutritionally. As a result, many people with disabilities are handicapped
further by impaired general health or having their limited energy drained
through poor nutrition, excess weight, poor habits of rest and exercise, and
inattention to their own states of consciousness. These issues will be discussed
further in Part II of this volume.

The reasons for maximizing general health and functional capabilities
relate to reckoning with the world. The less external help needed to accomplish day-to-day tasks, the more spontaneously and economically life can be
lived. The next two sections will explore a sampling of issues that arise when
people cannot achieve total independence from the aid of other individuals,
"the government," or assistive devices, even after health and functionality
have been maximized.

Mastering the Physical World

The physical environment offers enormous obstacles to people who have
motor or visual disabilities. Those with hearing or mental disabilities are
somewhat less affected because their locomotion abilities are not so directly
impaired. For them, mastery of the physical environment devolves upon
communication capacities, to be addressed in a subsequent section.

The prime environmental mastery issue for motorically disabled people
is accessibility, whereas safety is the major problem for people who are

visually impaired. On the surface it might seem, then, that motorically disabled individuals would be most vulnerable to the angry emotions, whereas blind people would experience fear more frequently. To an extent this is true, but the matter is more complex. Inaccessibility has implications for survival. To illustrate, if you can't get into a building, you can't take a job there, and the prospect of endless unemployment can be frightening as well as aggravating. At the same time, having to forego important or pleasurable activities because needed safety factors are lacking can engender ample irritation.

Accessibility and Safety

The commonest ways in which disabled people cope with the problems of inaccessible or unsafe facilities are by (1) minimizing their own handicaps by developing every feasible adaptive skill and (2) keeping up the good fight to get remaining environmental barriers removed. Some physically disabled people are interested in the development of wheelchairs that climb stairs, but most prefer to see stairs disappear from architecture altogether. External ramping for multistory buildings still is rare, but the idea no longer is treated as ludicrous. Good evacuation systems for disabled inhabitants of skyscrapers are rarer still, but feasible plans exist, and implementation may not be too far away. Here and there a bus system agrees to install visual street-name displays for deaf passengers, and more promise to do so in the future. Blind people are making themselves heard when they explain that procedures for aiding motorically disabled passengers to board aircraft should not apply to them because they are not needed.

The current era is one of fulminating improvements and opportunities for people with disabilities; however, this is bringing with it new varieties of exquisite frustrations. The crux of these is being lulled into expecting accessibility and safety and then suddenly, periodically, being confronted with their troublesome or dangerous absence. The deaths of blind and otherwise severely disabled people under such circumstances are reported regularly. Unpublicized are the untold numbers of "near misses" that leave individuals emotionally shattered for long periods of time.

A less dramatic but more typical example of what happens follows. Let's say you've grown accustomed to going, spontaneously, to restaurants without making prior calls to confirm accessibility. When you and your date discover five steps down after entering the restaurant, you are embarrassed and angry. The restaurant was built after statutes requiring accessibility were in effect, and the target of your anger is out of compliance with the law. Some dates might enjoy watching you confront management; others would be "turned off." You feel considerable pressure in judging what to do. In a comparable example, Harris relates with mock amazement the fact that a government commission on disability, of which he is a member, has been unable to persuade the officials who created the commission to install in their administrative building a TTY telephone for use by deaf people.

Periodic fear, embarrassment, or righteous indignation are improvements over chronic depression, but they, too, exact their tolls from a person's happiness. Many of today's disabled people could be termed an angry generation, expecting change to come faster than it ever does and seething inside when it doesn't. Then they must deal with the perplexing realization that even justified anger isn't very good for them, yet they need its impetus to sustain their demands for change.

Delays in achieving accessibility goals are perhaps tolerable, but the elimination of safety hazards is urgent, now that mainstreaming is exposing hundreds of thousands of formerly sheltered people to increasing risks. Hanging on to life is not a background variable for people with disabilities, especially when severe. People who have learned the hard way that "it *can* happen here" are frequently confronted by additional jeopardy. Moreover, it seems that as social or scientific advances eliminate one source of anxiety, another emerges to take its place. For example, less and less often now does a wheelchair user have to risk further injury by being hauled up a flight of stairs or sailing down an overly steep ramp. At the same time, the emerging energy shortage problem is producing the threat of brown-outs, which would immobilize electrically-powered assistive devices and life-support or environmental-control systems—a threat that disrupts the inner peace of people who rely on them.

Assistive Devices

Occasional anxiety about the actual or potential breakdown of assistive devices is a small price to pay for the practical and psychological benefits being enjoyed by their users. Just as widespread usage of motorized wheelchairs by people with impaired upper extremities produced a quantum leap in their quality of life (and may have been a causal factor in the closely following advent of the consumer movement), so is the accelerating production and use of other assistive devices upgrading the quality of life for more and more severely disabled people.

Mac, who is totally blind, is a gifted mathematician. He chose a career in counseling, however, because he could not work competitively as a mathematician in the early sixties when his work life began. A decade later, the "talking calculator" changed that and he returned to college to prepare for a second career in the field of his choice. Carol, quadriparetic from polio, reports that an electrical lift that allows her to do unassisted toilet transfers has saved her a significant monthly output for attendant help. It also has changed the nature of her dreams. Before acquiring the lift, she says about ten percent of her dreams had some anxiety-laden representation of her dependency on others for attending to toilet needs. Within two weeks after obtaining it, all such dream symbolism had disappeared. Perhaps unimportant in itself, the changed dreaming pattern reflects a highly important and deeply experienced reduction of disability-related anxiety.

Although Mac, Carol, and many others eagerly embrace new assistive devices, numerous disabled people resist them for a variety of reasons. Some say they feel dehumanized by mechanical aids or that they are leary of hardware. Others express fears that they will "turn off" other people by appearing "freaky" or comical. Ned drew an analogy between a device suggested for him and Charlie Chaplin's feeding machine in the silent film classic *Modern Times*. Loved ones who "need to be needed" may resist, too. The process of accepting assistive devices runs parallel to the acceptance of disability, involving a gradual admittance to consciousness of the way things are that is coupled with sufficiently strong desires to do what you want to do.

As noted earlier, people with impaired hearing have their share of anxieties about the physical world, too. Warning signals are frequently auditory and thus pose safety problems, and many events are "inaccessible" because no visual readout or interpreter services are provided. However, most of the problems "out there" for deaf people might better be subsumed under the rubric "other people," since communication is the capability impaired.

Interacting with Other People

The term "communication" is used here in the most general way, encompassing all aspects of information exchange: the transmission and reception of speech, writing, and miscellaneous other auditory (for example, screeching tires) and visual (for example, "body English") data. Blind people have problems with reception of writing and other visual data; deaf people have a primary problem with reception of speech and other auditory data and sometimes a secondary problem with transmission of speech. Speech dysfunction also occurs with a number of neuromuscular disorders, and people with mental disabilities may have trouble with all aspects of communication due to failure to interpret data in consensus with others.

The communication problems of deaf people are yielding more slowly to technological intervention than those of people who are blind, much to the angry dismay of some members of the deaf community. Braille, audiotape, and optical or electronic devices have reduced greatly the need for personal services (readers, primarily) for visually-impaired people, but hearing-impaired individuals continue to need interpreters to convey any auditorily presented information. Signing is a tiring activity and ideally is done by pairs who alternate turns. Marta, a deaf administrator, says,

> It was hard for me to accept the notion that I'm worth having two whole human beings to accompany me to meetings. My feelings are still confused, frankly. One minute I'm overwhelmed with gratitude that my little corner of the universe is willing to make this investment, and the next minute I'm angry because it doesn't make more. More pressure should be put on schools to make sign language as much a part of the core curriculum as English, and more funding should be directed toward developing portable devices that will decode speech and turn it into a visual readout. These are the only kinds of solutions that will work in the long run. Two-for-one is okay as a stopgap, but it can't go on forever.

A critical problem area for hearing-impaired individuals involves the legal–judicial system. Innumerable instances have been reported of police mistreatment of deaf people for failing to comply with commands they didn't hear, and the rights of hearing-impaired people to have adequate interpreter services during court proceedings are only beginning to be recognized. Individuals thus affected express fear and rage over the threats of harm and injustice entailed in these situations. Less critical but more pervasive in effect is the inaccessibility of televised information when no closed captioning or signed inserts are provided. Whether programming is considered good or poor, television serves as today's primary channel of current information, and to be deprived of it is socially handicapping.

If the deaf community is to have captioned television as a rule rather than a rare exception, then "they gotta ask." And they are asking, occasionally through the medium of lawsuits. The disabled community has grown quite capable of asking, as a group, for changes needed by disabled citizens at large. At the same time, however, disabled individuals often find it difficult to solicit help for themselves.

Asking for Help

Peter Leech, a psychiatric social worker who participated in the establishment of the Center for Independent Living in Berkeley, California, captures the inward recognition of many disabled people when he describes an insight-provoking experience he had soon after returning to school following disablement. He was sitting outdoors on campus when it began to rain. Unable to propel his wheelchair at that time, he waited for a passerby whom he could ask for a push to shelter. Several people came and went, but he was unable to ask. He explains,

> I was getting drenched in the rain, but I still couldn't ask anyone to give me a push. Suddenly, it hit me that I was waiting for someone to make eye contact with me and *then* I could ask. Somehow, I couldn't reach out through the "dark" and force my presence on someone who hadn't acknowledged me . . . especially when I was looking for a favor. Then I said to myself, "This is ridiculous!" and the next person by got collared. I thought about it later and came to the conclusion that the reason people don't make eye contact with disabled people is that they got punished for doing it when they were little kids. "Don't stare at cripples, Johnny!" says some flustered mother as she yanks him away by the arm. So he obeys, and never looks at a cripple again. I encourage kids to look and ask questions . . . and try to reassure their moms when they lunge in to drag the kids away. Maybe when they grow up they'll be looking at someone like me when he needs help.

Another of Leech's observations bears upon the wider issue of other people's reactions to those with disabilities. It also validates, somewhat, the fears expressed by disabled people who are reluctant to use assistive devices. He notes that people tend to see and respond to the *clutter* of a wheelchair, crutches and braces, or other appliances in evidence *before* they see and respond to the individual using them. This places heavy demands on each disabled person to have so prepotent a personality or such astounding good looks as to neutralize this perceptual tendency. Such demands are seriously handicapping since very few people, disabled or nondisabled, can develop and maintain without enormous effort maximal attractiveness plus consummate poise, charm, and assertiveness. The last of these attributes, assertiveness, is so critical to survival as to require further examination.

Asserting Oneself

Certain of the problems just discussed are moving toward solution fairly rapidly, now that the people who "own" the disabilities are asserting themselves and demanding their rights rather than leaving this job to professional rehabilitators and other concerned advocates who are not themselves disabled. The need for assertiveness, leavened with irreproachable diplomacy, is nowhere more evident than in dealing with people whose positions of authority allow them to determine the directions and quality of others' lives. For example, knowing how to "interview" taciturn physicians to obtain medical information on which to base one's own decisions is a valuable survival skill; so is the ability to secure helpful cooperation from teachers when one is physically unable to fulfill course requirements in the ordinary ways. Perhaps the most challenging test of interpersonal survival skill is the ability to extract from agencies help to which one is entitled, without stimulating resistance on the parts of agency workers.

Disabled people, especially those whose disabilities are severe, often rely on funds and services from public agencies to continue living normative lifestyles in the community. Failure to obtain either can mean institutionalization or being trapped in poverty. Some people get everything to which they are entitled and a little bit more; others fail to secure even the minimum for which they are eligible. The former may have propitious contacts, but success and failure are both determined significantly by personality variables. A severely disabled woman who skillfully avails herself of every existing benefit grinned and revealed,

> My mother always told me, "You can catch more flies with honey than with vinegar," and I'm here to tell you she was right. The most important thing to remember is that those workers are so drained by the teeming hordes of downtrodden souls they have to deal with daily that they have no tolerance for anger. If you can lighten it up with a little humor, you can get by with showing your exasperation, but it's better to keep your cool. You *have* to be well informed. The workers usually don't know as much about the rules and regulations as you do if you've been around for awhile, because their turnover is so high. Also, of course, they don't *care* as much . . . it's not their lives that hang in the balance. You have to know what you're talking about, be very firm, and, at the same time, make with the sunny disposition. If you can do all that, you at least have a chance of getting what you need and deserve. 'Course if you *can* do all that, chances are you have a great job somewhere and don't need any help!

This illustrates the wide range of knowledge, skills, and personal qualifications needed, and it does not bode well for the novice or the person with merely average poise, verbal fluency, cheerfulness, or ability to feign it. Few rehabilitation programs prepare their patients or clients for "agency management," but consumer-run independent living programs have begun filling this gap for people who've discovered that their skills in this area are deficient. On the light side: the clients of a consumer-run independent living program in one of the western states were given a course in "Assertiveness Training." Within a few weeks, the counselors in the local rehabilitation agency were asking their psychological consultant for assertiveness training to help them cope appropriately with these newly assertive clients.

The quality of assertiveness also is helpful in dealing with the general public. Salesclerks might tend to ignore a disabled shopper if permitted to do so, or strangers inclined to help may actually hinder. The ability to put people at ease when they fear their own words in conversation with a disabled person, or to firmly decline assistance while simultaneously showing genuine appreciation of the helping motive, are more than survival skills. They can radically elevate the quality of a disabled person's life.

Issues related to the most central interpersonal relationships in people's lives will be discussed extensively in subsequent chapters dealing with families, friends, lovers, and employers. Here we will consider just one group of individuals who are particularly important to survival for people with severe disabilities.

Personal Service Providers

Many people with severe disabilities find themselves in a situation ordinarily reserved for the relatively well-to-do. They must hire and supervise one or more personal employees. Instead of personal secretaries or domestic staff, their employees are attendants, readers, drivers, and interpreters. Problems arise for several reasons.

First, the selection and supervision of employees, especially when they provide intimate or crucial services such as attendants do, require employers to have various high-level skills and personal qualifications. Well-to-do individuals are more likely to have developed the skills, acumen, and assertiveness underlying success in these activities, by the time they are necessary, than are average people, often fairly young and inexperienced, who suddenly must employ personal assistants because of disabling conditions. Moreover, the employer–employee relationship is more delicately balanced because servants for the well-to-do constitute luxuries, whereas the personal employees of disabled people are essential to continuing survival. To illustrate, when an applicant with excessive power needs, or an alcohol problem, is not assessed accurately and is hired as an attendant, the employer is less free to terminate the worker peremptorily when unsatisfactory performance becomes evident. The "cost" will not be reckoned in terms of having to clean house or prepare meals until a replacement is found; it might be having no way to eat, get out of danger, get into bed, or go to the bathroom.

Second, well-to-do employers have a psychological advantage in gaining respect and compliance from personal employees, simply because the latter know the former are able to pay their salaries. Many disabled people are not; the employees know their salaries come from public or charitable sources and the balance of perceived power betwen the two is affected accordingly, to the disadvantage of the disabled employer. This makes the job of supervision even more taxing, especially for people who question their own self-worth in the first place. Mistreatment, unreliability, exploitation, defection without notice, subtle cruelties of withholding help, and countless other abuses are reported regularly about attendants for severely disabled individuals. They occur when disabled employers don't know how to screen out the "bad apples" at the outset or how to create a rewarding job for those they do hire. It is absolutely essential that the jobs be made intrinsically rewarding because the public funds provided do not constitute a living wage. A society that transmits the message, "You're worth taking care of, but only by someone who will work for less than an adequate wage," is not clear in its values, and the consequences must be managed.

Finally, many disabled employers are so anxious about finding help quickly, before other aspects of their support systems fall apart, that they often say "yes" to the first person who applies. Then they don't know how, or are afraid, to fire unsatisfactory workers, so the abuse goes on. Awareness that one's survival is contingent on the good will of others sometimes leads to fearfulness about rejecting *anyone*—at least explicitly. Unfortunately, what often happens is that the fearful individual's resentments emerge in indirect ways, leading to the very alienation that is feared.

Such problems are more prevalent with respect to attendants than the other classes of personal employees for disabled people. Interpreters for the deaf, for example, possess well-paid skills and make significant commitments to the type of work they do by developing those skills. Such is seldom true for attendants. Many feel trapped in their employment situations and would prefer other work if they could obtain it. This, in itself, strains the perhaps already impaired self-esteem of each party. Nonetheless, interpreters also can pose problems for their deaf employers; for example, some "take over" conversations and others distort meanings to serve their own ends. The critical difference can be summed up in this way: readers and drivers for the blind and interpreters for deaf individuals are extremely important aids to independent living, but attendants for severely disabled people may be essential to their biological survival. The potential of such a dependency to affect both persons' lives is not always fully appreciated.

Thus, to survive, psychologically as well as physically, disabled people using personal service providers must develop skill in their selection and supervision. However, interferences with good supervisory practice and harmonious coexistence, especially when live-in providers are required, arise as much from mood and self-concept problems as from skill deficits. Therefore, the material in Chapter 8 on transcending the erosive emotions associated with disability will be highly pertinent to this issue. Also relating significantly to the matters of self-esteem and feelings of well-being is the concept of normalization.

Striving for Normalization

The goal of the inner and outer struggles recounted so far is to live a more or less normal life in a more or less normal community and to break out of poverty and restrictive environments offering nothing to do and no one to do it with. It is to stay out of institutions and back bedrooms and break into the mainstream of *everything*—school, work, politics, and love affairs.

Disabled people now know that they have the right to participate, to give and receive, take risks like anyone else, and dramatically demonstrate when their requests or demands are not met.

Conflicting "Rights"

For the most part, "other people" are cooperative and helpful, expressing dismay over having been unaware in the past, and vowing to correct what they can in the future. At least this is true when the economic impact of implementing needed changes is either negligible or affects someone else.

When significant costs are entailed, however, resistances rise rapidly, often accompanied by the rhetoric of politicoeconomic conservatism. An illustrative example came from a field deputy of a very conservative state senator. In a telephone interview following an address he gave before an assembly of rehabilitation workers, he was informed that his remarks had outraged attendees, and he was asked to clarify. It was assumed that he had been seriously misinterpreted. He had not. In paraphrase, the following encapsulates his explanation.

> The State Architect has promulgated regulations requiring that 80 percent of a restaurant must be accessible to wheelchairs. This would impose costly changes on the owners of existing restaurants (if they were included) and it restricts the freedom of choice for those building new ones. If a businessman likes stairs in his restaurant, he should be free to have them. After all, if it weren't for the people with risk capital to build such businesses, none of us would have them to enjoy. If disabled people don't like restaurants with stairs, they are free not to go to them. There always will be plenty of restaurants that they *can* get into. The Senator believes that it is not right to use the law to promote one group's interest at the expense of another's, and this is what all these laws about architectural barriers in privately-owned buildings are attempting to do: promote the interests of disabled people at the expense of businessmen's. Frankly, the world could get along better without disabled people than it could without businessmen.

For those who may wonder: no, he did not see that a parallel exists between the disabled population and ethnic minorities who successfully challenged businesses' freedom of choice not so many years ago. The reason: "No one has ever *hated* disabled people." Also, of course, it doesn't impinge on aesthetic preferences in architectural style to accommodate ethnic minorities, nor are alteration costs on existing facilities entailed.

Interestingly, members of the disabled community in this deputy's state are well aware that the senator he serves has long held the appreciation of the food-service industry, and yet they expressed hurt as much as anger at these pronouncements. Sheltering assumes many forms and one form that is resistant to extinction is protection from the fact that certain sectors of society "couldn't care less." Many disabled people have been beguiled by predominant contact with "other people" who are in sympathy with the underdog; they are caught off guard by the disdain of those with different value systems and motives. The blunt pronouncements of individuals sharing this senator's views come as shocks, creating alarm and fear among people who can only wonder what will become of their improving conditions if such views become widespread. In a more personal way, it simply hurts to be told, just as you're beginning to believe that perhaps you *are* as worthwhile as anyone else, that to some, you're worth far less than a businessman's fancy for split-level restaurants.

This issue forms the basis of a controversy within the disabled community over the advisability of encouraging the development of fully accessible, service-rich housing arrangements explicitly for people with (usually severe) disabilities.

Independent Living Arrangements

Some people fear that the creation of independent living arrangement (ILA) projects will detract from the perceived responsibility of the total community to eliminate mobility (and other) barriers from the world at large. They foresee ghettoization of disabled people with accessible subcommunities and progressive lessening of movement between them and the mainstream of housing, shopping, work, and recreation. Equality is considered unfathomable in microcosm; and separate, even if equal, is abjured. Others would prefer to forego the remote, future possibility of general access in favor of creating a more immediate, accessible universe allowing unhindered living *now*. This camp cites the opportunities such communities offer for economical sharing of attendants and expensive equipment, as well as the preference of some to associate predominantly with others who share the disability experience.

This last turn of phrase reflects an important aspect of the newly emerging consciousness within the disabled community. In the past, many disabled people who wanted to make their marks on the world believed they should dissociate themselves from others with disabilities and thus avoid being sterotyped as "another of the unfortunate ones" by the nondisabled majority. More than this, they also felt that disabled people were inferior beings, and to be forced into their sole company was to be deprived of the privilege of consorting with interesting, worthwhile people. However, just as black became beautiful and led to the positive choices of some to live in segregated communities, a similar process is taking place among people with disabilities. In contrast with the past, valued camaraderie issuing from common experience is cited more often as the reason for preferring association with other disabled people than is discomfort or feeling inferior to those who are not.

Independent living arrangements can be as large and formal as a complex of several hundred accessible, fully equipped apartments that offer extensive personal services and are planned in conjunction with adjacent accessible shopping and employment facilities. They can be as small and informal as one disabled person living in an ordinary apartment and having an agreement with a neighbor to provide needed morning and evening attendant care. There is fledgling agreement in the disabled community that the full range of possibilities should be made available to allow for individual choice.

Individual choice: that is the crux of independence—having options to exert. The ILA concept specifically includes the provision of needed assistance from other individuals which, when given, allows even very severely disabled people to live free from the control or determination of others. As more alternative ILA styles are discovered and publicized, increasing numbers of disabled people are finding it feasible, psychologically as well as physically, to take charge of their own lives and contribute to an improved destiny for disabled people generally.

Taking Charge of One's Life

Legislative advocacy, by and for people who are blind, was fully operational by the 1930s. A comparable thrust for other disability groups could not be said to have existed before the 1960s. The last two decades have seen accelerating efforts among all disability groups to secure promised constitutional protection of their rights through the legal–judicial system and through public education in their communities.

The Organized Disabled

Most of the early advocacy efforts were made by disabled individuals fortunate enough to have broken into the establishment through familial, professional, or business channels. Gradually, other disabled people also became involved. Although they might not be working, they had the foresight, time, and motivation to press for needed changes. As some of the changes came about, still more disabled people were enabled to join the fight. The few, scattered social clubs for disabled members came to be complemented, occasionally absorbed, and, finally, vastly outnumbered by political action organizations wherein socialization and recreation constituted no more than secondary goals.

They recruited, expanded, hired paid staff, coalesced, and created chapters; in short, the disabled *organized*. They started finding each other and discovered that they were not alone. They started talking to each other and learned that other disabled people are *okay*, that they themselves weren't the only exceptions to a negative stereotype they'd accepted, and that all had valuable experience and information to share. Then they started taking action together and discovered that, indeed, in unity there is strength. Together, they have made significant progress toward reducing the full range of barriers to a quality existence—in the law, welfare, education, architecture, transportation, employment, housing, shopping, recreation, and much, much more. The strength issuing forth from an organized constituency has made possible still another phenomenon, which is radically altering the very core of what it means to have a disability.

Independent Living as a Movement

The advent of the "independent living movement," as the consumer movement of disabled citizens is called, may be the most dramatic happening in the history of rehabilitation. After centuries of being isolated, downtrodden, ignored, managed, manipulated, and "taken care of," the people who own the problem finally are saying that they'd "rather do it themselves." "You gave us your dimes; now give us our rights" is a trenchant expression of the new deal being sought.

Disabled activists have made their needs known to governing bodies at all levels of societal organization, and, little by little, efforts are being made to see that somehow these needs are met at least somewhat better. The validity of the claim that those sharing the needs are uniquely qualified to plan ways of meeting them is being recognized. As a result, consumer-dominated advisory boards to professionally-run agencies have become integral parts of standard operating procedure, and the consumers are advising whether invited to do so or not. More important, all across the country the reins of service provision are being turned over to the consumers themselves, through the medium of growing support for a new breed of service organization: independent living programs operated *by* and *for* the disabled.

Growing pains among these programs are severe and the reasons are familiar. Similar to what occurred in "poverty programs" for ethnic minority groups a few years earlier is the fact that staff frequently are catapulted into more responsible jobs than their absent or impoverished work histories have prepared them for. A severely disabled, recent college graduate who had never held a job before suddenly found himself employed as the executive director of an independent living center. He was totally unprepared to handle the administrative complexities of managing nearly twenty employees engaged in widely diverse forms of service and advocacy, and so he shortly alienated both his board of directors and his poorly selected employees. After recovering from the shock of being fired, he described himself, with rueful humor, as a case of "instant Peter Principle."

Also reminiscent of a phenomenon from the 1960s, nondisabled staff report feeling rejected and unappreciated simply because they are not members of the "in" group—the disabled majority. Disabled people have needed for a long time skills for putting nondisabled people at ease in their presence. Now, however, they must learn to make nondisabled colleagues feel accepted, worthwhile valued contributors. An extremist contingent declines to do so, explicitly denouncing the involvement of nondisabled individuals in any phase of service provision beyond the allocating of necessary funds.

In spite of the problems, consumer-run programs are maturing to offer a wealth of previously unobtainable services to people with virtually every type of disability. Experienced, well-informed advocates intercede for clients trying to wind their ways through bureaucratic red tape and regulatory obstacles. Just knowing that someone is there to help or at least explain, understandably, the basis of a dispute with an agency, brings considerable relief to people overwhelmed with frustration, helplessly believing they are getting the "run around." Attendant counselors are available to help severely disabled individuals locate, select, and supervise suitable attendants; and housing counselors help with locating the best a community offers in low-cost, accessible housing. Local transportation may be offered, as may captioned movies and interpreter services for deaf participants. Rap groups and other peer counseling services commonly are provided and will be discussed in detail in Chapter 12.

Thus it goes that disabled people struggle to survive and live independently in the community. To succeed in doing so is to have an opportunity to engage in the life functions explored in the next four chapters: loving, working, and playing. Because it appears to be most central to the core of a person's being, the matter of loving will be taken up next.

4 Loving

The Family

The great Western psychologist, Abraham Maslow, and the Eastern mystical writings from which he drew placed the needs for belonging and loving in about the middle of the hierarchy of human needs (Maslow & Mittelman, 1951). More basic are those for survival, safety, and security. More transcendental are those for self-actualization and spiritual awakening. The needs to love and be loved, to generate and enjoy a sense of connectedness with other human beings, occupy the central range of Maslow's now-famous "need ladder."

Most of us had our first experiences with belonging, loving, and being loved in the contexts of our parental families. Later, similar urges would lead us to break away from those groups to form new families of our own—issues to be covered in Chapter 5. Love relationships with friends are also of great importance and will be discussed in Chapter 7. The present chapter is devoted to the ways in which disablement affects and interacts with family relationships and functioning. It will examine the reactions, resources, coping strategies, pitfalls, and special issues that arise.

Disability: A Family Affair

Just as illness or injury disrupts the physiological homeostasis of the affected individual, so do they and their sequelae disrupt the homeostatic balance of the family unit. When disability occurs, the total family begins an adaptive struggle to regain its equilibrium. In other words, although only one member of the family "owns" the disability, all family members are affected and, to some extent, handicapped by it. The birth of a disabled child, the discovery of a degenerative disease in a youth, the catastrophic injury of a parent, or any other disablement befalling any member of a family can have as far-reaching and intense an impact on the others as on the one who becomes disabled. All experience shock and fear over the event or recognition of disablement, and the pain and anxiety of wondering what the future implications will be. The disability of one may alter the lifestyles of family members as much or more than that of the disabled individual: schedules, duties, plans, and roles all change. All experience loss—of a fully functioning cog in the family wheel— which generates disappointment, frustration, and anger, as freedom and time for fun disappear. At base, the family members must learn to deal with the same dimensions as the disabled person: their own reactions, the physical world, and other people. Although guilt is an issue with which disabled people must ofttimes reckon, especially when responsibility for an accident or unmet obligations are at stake, it is an almost universal problem for the loved ones of a person who becomes disabled.

Guilt

To begin with the obvious and proceed to the more subtle, parents who produce children with birth defects experience guilt, shame, and embarrassment, as well as disappointment, sorrow, and anger that their offspring are imperfect. Genetic and behavioral antecedents that may have contributed to the defect are sought, and unless a clear hereditary cause is found in the father's lineage, it is usually the mother who suffers most in this way. The guilt may be adopted as one's own, or it may be foisted onto the shoulders of another by blaming the doctor, the hospital, or the grandparents for passing on a genetic defect manifested in a later generation. The struggle to absorb versus repulse guilt and blame may go on for a very long time. When it is known that poor nutrition, drugs ingested during pregnancy, or other improper prenatal care have caused or contributed to a birth defect, the parents—and especially the mother—may face a particularly tortuous battle to overcome the guilt engendered.

Self-blame for the disablement of a child is in no way limited to those whose children are born with disabilities. When older children become ill or injured, self-blame occurs, too. Recriminations over failure to observe signs that might have led to earlier diagnosis and better prognosis, or over inadequacies of supervision that could have prevented an accident are not the exception but the rule.

Applicable when any family member becomes disabled is an aspect of guilt that arises from the ambivalent nature of love relationships, especially when lives are interdependent, as in a family. That is, past angry thoughts about the person who has become disabled are apt to be recalled, such as moments when one has muttered, "I hope one of these days that rotten kid (parent) (spouse) gets his (hers)!" Suddenly, s/he *has*. We all engage in a little magical thinking and at least fleeting moments of guilty terror—"Oh my God, my wish came true!"—are common. The rational mind says, "Don't be silly, of course that had nothing to do with it," but the gut still churns.

As if the self-blame were not problem enough, it is also far too common that guilt is inculcated in family members by others. Even more unfortunate, it is rehabilitation agency workers who, sometimes unwittingly and sometimes not so unwittingly, create this effect. Because of the enormous costs associated with catastrophic illness or injury, the family often is urged to assume as much as possible of the financial and care-giving burdens. However, when urged to carry an extent of the cost or aspects of care which seriously distress or overtax them, many feel ashamed and exposed when they refuse or try and fail.

Family members who appear to be more (or equally) concerned over the impact of their loved one's disability on their own lives may be subtly or not so subtly punished for this in a variety of ways. Direct remonstrances may be given, to the effect that the disabled individual needs all the help and attention the family can muster—with the clear implication that the latter should tuck away their own needs until the crisis is past. This overlooks the fact that the family is also in crisis and is in need of help, too.

The Family Is Not the Enemy

Much is said among the various professions working with disabled people about the problems posed by family members who "sabotage" their rehabilitative efforts. Criticism is sometimes harsh, as in the commonly heard phrase, "That parent (or spouse) will undo everything we've tried to accomplish during the week when we send the patient home for the weekend." Even when conscientious efforts are made to understand and help the family with *its* problems, an attitude is frequently evident that family members are obstacles to goal achievement with their disabled relative, rather than people who need and deserve help themselves. The following language from a brochure on family counseling, prepared by a person sincerely concerned with just this problem, still reveals the bias described.

> The rehabilitation enterprise can be facilitated or impaired by the attitudes and behavior of the family within which a disabled person lives. Sometimes a rehabilitation worker's consultation with a client's family can help this family process become less of an obstacle and/or more of a help to the rehabilitation process.

This statement shows the writer's concern with the problem and mirrors it at the same time. The family does not just affect the rehabilitation enterprise, it is an integral part of it; the family *is* the client. In other words, just as rehabilitation professionals criticize medical specialists for focusing on the object of their specialty (bones, nerves, various organs) to the exclusion of "the whole person," so do they, themselves, tend to focus on the "patient" to the exclusion of the family of which s/he is a part. Psychologists are amused when surgeons regard psychodynamics as alien factors muddying up what would otherwise be a clean job, but their own narrowness of perspective is little different. As a result, far more people than will ever come to them as patients are left to fend for themselves in handling the shock, disappointments, disruptions, fears, and suddenly imposed requirements that they cope with a vast array of totally new stimuli and demands—if they are to go on loving, working, playing, and transcending whatever fate deals them. The hospitalized patient may be fairly well insulated from the difficult and frightening adjustments the family must make in order to stay economically and emotionally afloat.

Ironically, the failure to extend genuine empathy and the sense of professional responsibility to the whole family can result in overlooking ways in which family members can serve as rehabilitation allies. This was dramatically illustrated in the case of an educational consultant who sustained a head injury. The man's wife was viewed rather unabashedly as "an aggressive bitch" who was highly opinionated and who intended to "dump" the patient in a couple of years. An outside consultant who participated in a discharge-planning conference listened to lengthy, emotional descriptions of the wife's interferences and unpleasant ways and pointed out that what he had heard was that she was a remarkably responsible, capable, aggressive person who wanted to and would move moutains to make her husband's life as pleasant and uncomplicated as possible before she divorced him; that she was willing to use her time and considerable skills as an airplane pilot, among other things, to help him get vocationally reestablished; that she wanted out of the marriage but was a highly principled person who had made a conscious decision to give him the next two years of her life; that she had trusted the staff enough to share that fact with them; and that, in short, she was "one hell of a resource that is being not only wasted but mistreated."

Rehabilitation workers often feel constrained from acknowledging negative feelings about their patients or clients; thus, dislikes, frustrations, and disappointments may be ejected from consciousness as inappropriate or unprofessional lapses from the ideal image for which they strive. Suppression of such natural feelings may serve to magnify any antipathies felt toward family members and reduce motivation to help them build the resources they need for coping. Moreover, the family may be scapegoated by frustrated rehabilitation workers just as readily as the latter are scapegoated by frustrated family members. The rehabilitation job is a difficult one, and when another member of the team—whether a professional, the disabled person, or a relative—fails to perform in line with the others' wishes and expectations, blame placing is likely to follow. Family members are particularly vulnerable because they are seldom integrated into the cohesive work group and are only sporadically present in the rehabilitation facility, at least during the professionals' work hours. The disabled person is less likely to be scapegoated by the professionals, who sometimes feel they must rehabilitate people in spite of themselves if that appears necessary.

With or without support, the family must progress through essentially the same stages of adjustment as the person who is disabled. Also in parallel, the question arises: when tragedy strikes, who copes? Once again, the answer is: those with the right combination of resources.

Family Coping Resources

Family members need many of the same kinds of resources as the disabled person, plus a few that differ. The required inner resources fall roughly into four groups: emotional, intellectual, personality, and physical. Emotional stability is the prime requisite for coping with any catastrophic change, in order to neutralize adverse reactions and facilitate the adjustment process. A loving nature, the ability to accept "what is" and proceed from there, and belief in one's own power to influence the future are crucial aspects of the emotional armamentarium needed. Families with such characteristics of emotional stability can rebound from catastrophe whether or not their intellectual resources are high. Unquestionably, however, possession of good intellectual resources will further aid the coping process and permit a richer style of adjustment to be reached. The ability to grasp the medical and other facts of the situation, to foresee and prepare for problems that may arise in the future, and to creatively devise and implement solutions to them, plus a working knowledge of the outer resources that exist in the community are exceedingly important intellectual resources to draw upon, both in times of crisis and later when the crisis stage has passed.

Complexly interwoven with the emotional and intellectual resources are personality resources, such as assertiveness, persuasiveness, diplomacy, and emotional supportiveness. The combination of strengths in these three areas (emotional, intellectual, and personality resources) will determine such practical matters as the family's skill in social management, both in general and under conditions of unusual need and stress. Many families lack, under ordinary conditions, adequate skills for procuring goods and services, managing money, and other family management activities. When disability affects a member of the family, these skills may be taxed to the maximum.

The list of personality resources that bear upon coping with disability in a family is endless. Some are primarily important in dealing with practical exigencies (for example, assertiveness, persuasiveness, and diplomacy in dealing with agencies), and some relate to helping the disabled individual and other family members deal with the changes imposed on their lives (for example, emotional supportiveness). Although emotional and intellectual resources are paid considerable attention in the literature, very little has been directed toward the role of personality or temperament factors. To cite again the traits of succorance and nurturance as illustrative, family adjustment will probably be easier—all else being equal—if it is a succorant individual who becomes disabled and a nurturant one who is thrust into the role of caregiver. The reverse situation would be expected to create far more dissonance.

An additional resource area that may be highly important for family members is that of their own physical strength. Good general health, stamina, endurance, and an ability to marshal extra strength in times of crisis are essential ingredients when one is called upon to continue doing all one has done in the past, plus take over the duties formerly assumed by the disabled family member, plus—in cases of severe disablement—provide physical care for that individual. Family members with high energy levels will be at a considerable advantage in coping with the sequelae of disability compared with those whose ordinary level of energy tends to be low or even average.

In addition to the varieties of inner resources just described, there are two major types of outer resources that can make a significant difference in how effectively and easily a family deals with disability. These two are money and contacts. Having the financial resources to procure needed medical, nursing, and attendant care; equipment and supplies; and other illness/disability-related goods and services—without having to worry about impending bankruptcy or suffer the frustrations and anxieties associated with reliance on public agency funds—can reduce greatly the stress entailed. Similarly, having contacts with people who can help solve the problems can reduce the psychic wear and tear of coping. As an example, Doris relates that her family's friendship with the county medical officer was the reason her mother was allowed to stay with her in the hospital—despite regulations to the contrary—during the acute stage of what proved to be a permanently disabling illness. Of this she says,

> It may not be democratic, using contacts with influential people to get special consideration, but that doesn't mean I'm sorry we used them. I never needed my mother more, and I'm convinced that having her there during that time had very far-reaching, positive effects on my adjustment to disability. In sum, it avoided having to undo unnecessary damage done by being forcefully separated from the person who symbolized security when I needed it most. I think it's damn near criminal that it's not the rule instead of the exception whenever it's requested by the patient and family—especially when the patient is young.
>
> The only reason I'm sorry we had to pull strings is that that means people who don't happen to know the right people don't get the same treatment. . . . I know many people have been in even worse situations and they've not had such help to turn to. A lot of them have ended up as casualties of the *system* far more than as casualties of disability . . . especially parents of kids with disabilities.

The concept that parents or other family members also can be "casualties" of either the disability or the system is an important one. It happens when bureaucratic obstacles create more stresses than an agency's services resolve and when the family's needs for practical and emotional support are ignored. Both are related to changes that have come about in family structure. In the extended-family household of a previous era, there usually were relatives available to perform many of the special services needed when a member of the household became disabled. The disappearance of the maiden aunt and other extended-family personages willing and able to fulfill these functions has created increased needs for public and private agencies and sundry practitioners to fill the gap. At the same time as the extended family is being replaced by the nuclear-family household, socioeconomic changes have made it necessary or desirable for both spouses to work outside of the home. For one of the only two wage-earning adults in a household to remain at home to provide needed care could be an economic disaster for the family and be psychologically devastating to the person forced to interrupt a valued career.

Progressive Disability: Impact on Family

When the disability is progressive, family coping resources are taxed to the maximum. An active disease process exists here, one that progressively is eroding tissue: bone, nerve, muscle, or other. Many deteriorative conditions are characterized by remissions and exacerbations of symptoms and by the presence of pain. Often, there also is the specter of a downhill course and a hastened death to be reckoned with by the disabled individuals and their loved ones. These are the primary aspects that make individual and familial adjustment to a progressive disorder different, and potentially more difficult, than adjustment to a stabilized disability.

Living around someone who is in pain can be difficult for several reasons. The helplessness of knowing that someone you love is hurting and there is nothing you can do to relieve it is mentioned more often in literary than professional works, but it is not a fictional matter. The experience of helplessness, when control or power are desperately needed or wanted, has been shown to be one of the most destructive mood states known to humankind and to other animals as well. Curt Richter (1958) found that laboratory animals (rats), convinced of their own helplessness in a swimming situation, literally committed suicide by plunging to the bottom of a water tank to drown. He likened his finding to the phenomenon of voodoo death (wherein individuals convinced of another's power to kill them may actually die on cue) and to the reluctance of modern surgeons to operate on patients who are excessively fearful or pessimistic about the outcome because their chances of dying on the table are known to be elevated.

The loved ones of people in pain face not only the stress associated with helplessness itself, they are in triple jeopardy. As noted earlier, people who hurt may not have jolly dispositions, or they may have unpredictable moments of volatile emotionality. This puts wear and tear on the loved ones, too, who may get indignant when a minor infraction is met with a major response. Then comes the guilt: "I'd overreact, too, if I hurt all the time." Triple jeopardy exists because there is little support or understanding available for anyone but the one who is in pain. Those who self-protectively harden their hearts are apt to be perceived and treated as monsters.

Remissions and exacerbations can put the disabled person and all loved ones on an emotional roller coaster. When a deteriorative condition plateaus or improves, hopes abound and often exceed reasonable expectations. With many progressive disorders, there may be day-to-day variations that will necessitate changing degrees of assistance from family members who, accordingly, never know what to expect with respect to care-giving responsibilities or demands for emotional support.

When a downhill course is predicted, the family is faced with the double prospect of increasing responsibility and the eventual loss of someone they count on and/or love. When stress is considered an important determinant of the disease, guilt arises again as an issue for the family to deal with. If they grow fearful that expression of their own emotions will add to the stress of the disabled individual, they may begin to suppress their cathartic needs lest they become the trigger to accelerated deterioration or a fatal, acute attack. This, obviously, will lead to increased tension and stress for all concerned.

Regardless of whether the disability is progressive or stable, certain preexistent patterns of family interaction, or unmet needs on the part of family members, can create additional sources of strain. Not infrequently, a form of collusion develops between the disabled person needing help and a family member whose needs to provide it are partly neurotic.

The Neurotic Tie That Binds

Just as Stephen found that his disability "paid off" by removing him from the threat of negative evaluation by his athletically-oriented father, so some families find equilibrium in a way that requires the continuance of the disabled member in a dependent, needful role. Somehow, having such a person in the family "pays off." A recently divorced mother of a young man with cerebral palsy described one such situation with remarkable non-defensiveness and humor:

> For years, having Teddy around was a great way of avoiding the fact that Jack and I didn't have a damn thing in common except three kids. We could pretend that all of our anger, depression, or whatever we were showing related to *him*, not ourselves. It was kind of like the way some people use a television set: they're

together in a room, so they feel quite comfortable that they're big on togetherness, but each is attending to something else. They don't have to relate to each other, and, if they did, they'd get in a fight because they basically can't stand each other. Teddy was our television set. We watched him together for hours on end and our only conversation was to pick apart the last program.

I had planned on going back to work after getting two babies into school, but Jack didn't want me to. So I got pregnant again to have something to do. When number three turned out to have cerebral palsy, it was clear that I would never have any other career. Teddy made it legitimate for me to stay home without acknowledging that I was selling out to Jack just to keep from rocking the boat. And he became the stability point of the family, as well as my reason for being. I was a professional C.P. mother and oh! how cleverly I bludgeoned Jack with that! Greatest weapon a woman ever had!

Then all of a sudden, Teddy wants to leave home. He wants to go away to finish college and he has a roommate lined up to help him out. And the roommate's a young woman! He doesn't need me anymore, not to take care of him, and not to be the only woman who'll ever love him. What in the hell am I going to talk to Jack about now?

The next two years were awful. I bounced from one encounter group to another, getting told off for being a possessive mother and using a disabled kid's life to meet my own needs on a regular basis. Jack thought encounter groups were dumb and when he finally said so, we had the fight that should have ended our marriage twenty years earlier. The last two years have been okay, though. Life for a 52-year-old divorcee isn't half as bad as I imagined.

The most unusual aspect of this story is the fact that the neurotic pattern was dissolved successfully, at least for the disabled man and his mother. Far more instances exist in which the regressive symbiosis is not resolved, and no party to it could describe it with the insight displayed here. She alludes to two major issues involved in familial exploitation of a disabled individual: (1) the need for a stabilizing influence to keep the family together or maintain a familiar, comfortable status quo; and (2) the provision of a *raison d'être* for another family member who feels otherwise bereft of purpose and direction.

A third issue encountered is the need for a scapegoat to explain and absorb the hostility stemming from the family's general dissatisfaction with life. A grisly illustration of the extreme to which this can go is reflected in the case of a childhood burn victim who provided a "whipping boy" to his impoverished, angry, and disturbed family for many years. Nearly every evening at home ended with the severe drunkenness of his parents, two siblings, and two cousins who also occupied the large, deteriorating house. When they became drunk, they made vicious fun of his disfigurement, ordering him to bring more drinks for them so that he would have "some earthly purpose in life." When they were sober, they either ignored him or blamed him, in crisper speech, for the family's squalor. One evening when the group had been more abusive than usual, he systematically lured each inebriated individual into a different room of the house and bludgeoned them to death. After fifteen years in prison, he was released to work in a sheltered workshop, where he is considered a "highly religious, gentle, spiritual sort of person who almost surely would never harm another living being."

Most disabled people scapegoated by their families never strike back at the true objects of their hurt or hatred; they are more likely to take it out on others—or themselves—later on. Usually, the scapegoating is far more subtle than in this case; for that reason, it is more difficult to identify and resolve in either a socially acceptable or unacceptable way. The martyred care-giver who "sacrifices" a way of life to serve a disabled child, spouse, or parent is a frequent example. Kevin describes with unresolved bitterness his experience with this form of scapegoating:

> From the time I got injured, mother was right there to help me, and I am grateful for that. E.c* some funny stuff went down that I still can't sort out completely. She always found ways to kind of remind me that she was sacrificing everything for me; and, somehow, the implication was there that she was "buying" me forever. She was never so crass as to say, "After all I've done for you . . . ," but she mentioned, from time to time, that she had given up the chance to remarry after my father died in order to take care of me, and that she had virtually given up any kind of social life for the same reason.
>
> The fact is, she had been widowed for fifteen years before I got hurt, and she only dated a couple of times as far as I know. She had also complained, as long as I can remember, that her social life was terrible because "Everything fun is for couples." I just gave her an excuse to grab onto; somehow, pretending that she had no husband and few friends because of sacrificing for me made it more respectable to her.
>
> What still drives me crazy is that, now that I'm grown and have a home and family of my own, she feels I'm responsible for giving *her* life meaning. Half of the time I feel like, "Wow! I do! After all she did for me." The other half, I know I can't. Sometimes I get really angry and tell myself, "She made those choices and it's not fair for her to feel I should be signed, sealed, and delivered to her because she can't figure out other ways to make her life meaningful." Then I feel ashamed of being so cold . . . and around and around I go.

This last example illustrates all three of the issues cited: the need for a stabilizing influence to maintain the status quo, the need for a *raison d'être*, and the need for a scapegoat to "explain" dissatisfaction and absorb anger—whether directly or indirectly expressed. (A martyred air can be a more effective way to "get" somebody than hollering.) The feelings experienced by all concerned may never be confronted and acknowledged in ways leading to growth unless outside help is proffered. Kevin ventured the opinion that he had received sufficient emotional nourishment from his mother (in spite of the neurotic aspects of her giving) to allow him to grow up strong enough to break away and be an independent adult when the time came, whereas she had not fared so well.

> She needed help to get some balance in her life, if she was going to withstand what was in store for her. Someone who could see what she was doing to herself should have given her some counseling. Her so-called friends just kept reinforcing her self-sacrifice trip by telling her how wonderful she was. She *was*, but she needed honest confrontation about where she'd end up if she didn't make some kind of life for herself that didn't revolve around me. I sensed it, but I had a vested interest in seeing her go on giving, giving, giving. Someone should have been there to protect her from me!

The mother is elderly now, and her mental processes are impaired. For her, it is probably too late, but clearly she is not the only one to suffer for her lack of help. Kevin has been left with a tangle of conflicting emotions that he is only beginning to sort out.

Age of Onset: Impact on the Family

When disablement occurs during childhood, both parents and siblings face numerous problems related to child-rearing practices. A tortuous process at best, such issues as the appropriate degree of protectiveness to offer become incalculably more difficult. A primary issue that influences all others is the extent to which parents can accept—emotionally and intellectually—the facts associated with a child's disability. Their acceptance (or lack of it) will be an important determinant of the reactions of other children in the family. Also, the match between the mother's and father's acceptance levels is important in determining how their relationship with each other will be affected and the type and consistency of messages they transmit to all of their children.

Many divorces have been attributed to differing levels of acceptance; sometimes this is manifested by jealousy or disenchantment when one parent is viewed by the other as turning all attention toward a disabled youngster and withdrawing it from the marriage partner or the other children. Erich Fromm postulated, in his popular work *The Art of Loving* (Fromm, 1956), that the mother's role is one of loving unconditionally, in order to provide a base of security for the growing child; and the father's role is to love conditionally, thus to motivate striving for socialization and betterment. The clinical observation that mothers frequently are more accepting of disabled children coincides with Fromm's hypothesis.

Acceptance is not a straightforward matter. It can become especially convoluted when intellectual acceptance exceeds emotional acceptance. This situation can generate double messages to all other family members, breeding confusion and distrust. The overt message may be one of loving concern, solicitude, or acknowledgment of "hard realities," yet be accompanied by covert expressions of anger, disappointment, or desperate longing to be out of the situation. As for the disabled children themselves, the quality of acceptance in a family is contingent on the members' self-esteem. Parents and siblings unsure of their own self-worth are likely to be more disturbed by the prospect of being objects of pity or disdain from their peers than are those who are more secure and self-confident. Some families also simply have higher degrees of tolerance for disruptions and perturbations than others; those low in tolerance will find acceptance more difficult.

Such factors as these play determining roles in the soundness of child-rearing practices used with both disabled and nondisabled children. As cited earlier, the issue of protectiveness is one that is critically affected by the presence of a disability. At one extreme, overt rejections may lead to neglect or underprotectiveness, if not to institutionalization. Clinically, however, the more frequently observed problem is overprotection, excessive shelter, and disallowance of normal risk taking for the age level of the child—the "a scorched child fears the fire" reaction. This tends to add increased dependency and experiential gaps to the list of handicaps the child one day must overcome and, in true vicious-circle fashion, creates additional burdens for the parents.

They don't need any more. If they have other children, they probably are facing problems of sibling jealousy because attention to the disabled child appears to be given at their expense. Just as a newborn baby sometimes is met by an older child's return to infantile behavior, so may siblings of disabled youngsters vie for parental time by exaggerating their own helplessness. When the child reaches school age, the parents face the problem of securing an adequate education, not an easy task regardless of whether the disability affects the child's ability to learn. (Educational issues will be treated in detail in Chapter 6.)

If disablement occurs after the individual reaches adulthood, it may be the marital family—a spouse and offspring of one's own—that will be most critically affected and visible to rehabilitation workers. The impact of disability on marriage relationships and parenting will be discussed next.

The Marital Family: Maintaining an Established Marriage

Disablement impacts differently on marriages that began before it occurred from those that begin afterward. In the former case, the disablement of a spouse may materially alter the basis of the partnership both parties made commitments to. In the latter, both have more realistic views of what to expect. In either case, spousal disability will critically influence family striving toward a homeostatic balance that facilitates the pursuit of happiness.

Herbert Rigoni, who directed the psychological services program at a major rehabilitation hospital for nearly a decade, indicates that a necessary, recurrent duty was to reassure spouses of recently disabled patients that it was "okay" for them to contemplate getting out of the marriages (personal communication). He points out that general population statistics show that a high proportion of marriages are failing at any given time; therefore, when a married person becomes disabled, a high probability exists that the marriage was in trouble already. Clearly, the additional stresses placed upon it by the sequelae of disability easily could be the "last straws."

As is true of shared tragedy in general, the disability experience sometimes strengthens the bonds of a relationship. This appears to be most likely, however, when the bonds were fairly strong in the first place. In other cases, the marriage bond may be tightened rather than strengthened, as when a dissatisfied partner feels, "Now I *can't* leave her/him because s/he needs me." These are the cases to which Rigoni referred and in which he attempted to help the individuals see that they had the freedom to go, so that staying could be a positive choice.

If a marriage survives the intial shock, the marital family will face essentially the same disruptions and adjustments described earlier in this chapter, and they will need to call on the same kinds of inner and outer resources. Their richness will determine whether the marriage will survive in the long run. In addition, the degree of genuine intimacy that existed in the predisability relationship is of paramount importance because, as several people quoted in this volume have repeated, "Disability is one hell of a test of love!"

Numerous observers have pointed out that a significant proportion of marriage relationships are reminiscent of "independent/parallel play." The term emanates from child psychology and describes very young children who play together at identical games—scooping sand, pounding blocks—but do not, in this process, relate in any meaningful way to each other. The stability of such marriages is founded on shared activity interests: sex, skiing, the theater, political activism, or whatever it may be. The partners may have fewer than average problems in "getting along" and may even be viewed as a model couple. Their harmony is only skin deep, however; it is a façade born of conflict avoidance through suppression and diversion of attention. The lack of genuine intimacy between them may remain unrecognized until disablement occurs. If there is no hope for resumption of shared activites, the marriage is likely to end.

This instance reflects the general principle that the survival of a marriage after disablement occurs depends largely on its prior solidity and the nature of the relationship. One important question is whether the couple was in the process of growing closer together or whether they already were growing apart. Regardless of the previous status of the marriage, however, the disability experience can create a dramatic disjuncture in the individual growth rates of the partners. For example, the disabled partner's emotional growth may accelerate or decelerate in comparison with the nondisabled partner. (The phenomenon of accelerated psychological growth among people with disabilities will be discussed further in Chapter 8.)

In addition to intimate and parallel play relationships, other possibilities exist. Symbiotic relationships are fairly frequent, and these are expectably thrown out of homeostatic balance when disability weakens or destroys the contribution of the affected partner. For example, the hostess–wife may lose her value if a disability precludes continued entertaining and/or appearing to her husband's business associates to be an enviable prize. On the other hand, if sufficient latent resources are present, positive outcomes can ensue—as when a dependent wife learns that she can work and support a family in a time of crisis. If the husband needed her dependency to stabilize his own psychic economy, his problems of adjustment, and therefore *theirs*, will face other complications.

A companionship marriage could be less adversely affected, unless economic strains prove unbearable. Such relationships are most common among advanced-age marriages; often, the specter of future disablement already has been acknowledged and some psychological preparation made. Nonetheless, no elderly couple is really prepared for the nightmares that accompany the serious disablement of one of them, especially those who want to stay in their own homes. A single, disabled, elderly person is apt to be placed in a care-giving facility; and while the pain of such change may be great, a measure of security is gained. When a spouse is present, however, the couple may fight to stay in familiar surrounds despite poverty, extreme hardship, and almost total inability to procure even the few supportive services that are available. All over the country, frail, elderly husbands and wives, who themselves are eligible for attendant care, are struggling to provide it to even more disabled spouses. In cases such as these, it is not the love relationship that is in jeopardy, it is survival itself.

A specific aspect of the relationship to consider is the nature of the experienced, expressed love between the two partners. Holistic health spokespeople remind us that we are tripartite in nature: we are body/mind/spirit. So, too, can love be conceptualized, and each love relationship may stress one or two of these aspects over the other(s). This pattern will affect a couple's postdisability adjustment, but not in uniformly predictable ways. It simply must be contemplated in putting the pieces back together, in understanding what actually has been lost due to disability, what has not, and what will require attention in rebuilding.

Whether or not sexuality was a central or peripheral part of a relationship prior to disablement, it almost certainly will become an important adjustment area afterward if significant changes are entailed. Sexual arousal is highly vulnerable to stress (such as changed physical or emotional circumstance), and sexual behavior patterns that have yielded satisfaction in the past are very reluctantly relinquished. Since sexuality is a major topic of the following chapter, this aspect of the marital family's adjustment to disability is only mentioned here.

Equally important is whether love is experienced as either possessive or enabling; that is, whether the partners are motivated to ensnare each other and maintain the psychological and "political" (power-base) status quo, or to facilitate each others' growth through mutual support, caring, and sharing. Obviously, the prognosis for possessive love relationships is poor under any kind of stress, while that for enabling love relationships is favorable.

In addition to the couple's relationship with one another, the impact of disability—in one or both of them—on parenting practices and success in child rearing creates still another important set of issues that must be examined.

Child Rearing

Many questions are asked on this topic, but few answers are given. According to Buck & Hohmann (in press), the literature is impoverished in this area, and what little exists is preponderantly speculative exposition, purporting to answer such questions as: should disabled individuals attempt to raise children? how can discipline be maintained? can a disabled parent serve as an appropriate role model? what if a father can't play ball with his son? The fact that such questions are asked may be part of the problem. Buck & Hohmann's own research on parenting found no support for the foreboding speculations found in the prior literature on these and related issues. The questions seem to reflect proclivities for stereotyping disabled people and their lifestyles.

If children are part of a family when parental disablement occurs, it usually is expected that they will manage to grow up relatively unscathed. Nonetheless, disabled individuals confront strong social pressures against having children if they have not done so yet; occasionally, they are urged to relinquish children they already have. The questions listed previously, and many others, are posed as challenges. No negative answers can be supplied, but the absence of positive data is treated as if that should be sufficient deterrent. The field of rehabilitation psychology has only begun to do research designed to explode the myths and provide factual data. In the current absence of scientific findings, clinicians must rely on observations of child-rearing styles among parents with disabilities, and their apparent results.

Buck & Hohmann's discussion (in press) suggests that while emotional disabilities may pose serious problems for effective child rearing, physical disabilities do not necessarily do so. It is the parents' general emotional health and attitudes about their disabilities—not the disabilities per se—that can create problems. For example, if a man believes his inability to play ball with his son is a problem, or if his wife does, then the child–parent relationship may suffer. Another man with an identical disability, who believes the verbal guidance he offers compensates for any physical incapacities, can be a better-than-average father regardless of the severity of his disability.

There appears to be virtually nothing in the research literature on the impact of parental mental retardation on child-rearing effectiveness. It appears the presumption is made that mentally retarded people cannot possibly serve as adequate parents; however, one occasionally observes or hears of an "exception" to this "rule," so the need for research exists here, too. It may be difficult to implement, in view of what appears to be the intellectual elitists' disdain of encouraging reproduction among retarded individuals.

A rehabilitation psychologist interviewed by the author quoted the famous eight-word maxim on correct parenting—"Have 'em, love 'em, and leave 'em alone!"—and added, "There's no reason a disabled parent can't do *that* as well as anyone else." Additional interview material from rehabilitation psychologists tended to agree with Buck & Hohmann's findings (in press) that the children of reasonably well-adjusted disabled parents differ from children of nondisabled parents mainly in that they are more affectionate and apprecia-tive toward their parents and more responsible or mature than the typical child of the same age. This probably results from being assigned household and other responsiblities out of necessity, and is reminiscent of earlier times when children were a needed, valued part of the family work force. (The loss of a role of economic importance to the family is suggested frequently as a causal factor in today's serious behavioral/emotional problems among chil-dren and adolescents.) The child of a blind father was described as follows:

> At 3 years old, Christin could guide her father anywhere and she loved it. Whenver she was along, that was her job and she guarded it jealously. Once, she inadver-tently walked *under* a barrier that laid her father out cold. She was mortified but was finally consoled that it was an understandable error and she still had her job.

In some cases, children of disabled parents are thought to be old beyond their years, but this is attributed more to the emotional health of the parents than to the existence of a bodily disability.

When a disabled individual can produce children, and especially when a coparent is present, the opinions of others as to suitability for parenthood are of little practical consequence. Criticizing the child-rearing practices of others is a very popular indoor sport, hardly limited to people with disabilities. However, there are several circumstances in which an individual's *right* to be a parent arises as an issue: when nonvoluntary sterilization is considered (for retarded women usually); when a social agency or estranged spouse attempts to remove a child from a disabled parent's custody, on the grounds that disability renders her/him unfit for parenting; and when a disabled individual is unable to produce children and seeks—often fruitlessly—to adopt. These and other issues relating to parental rights will be treated in Chapter 9.

5 Pairing

Sexuality and Intimacy

The urge for pairing is almost ubiquitous, and, despite long-lasting rumors to the contrary, it does not disappear when disability intervenes. In fact, as will be seen, it sometimes grows stronger. Part of the urge is biological; we seem to be preprogrammed with a drive to continue our own particular gene pool. Too, the process of procreating feels good and even before the television show "Laugh-In" so advised us, we had strong proclivities to act on the principle, "If it feels good, do it."

Throughout recorded human history, social pressures have been exerted toward sanctioned patterns of pairing, and our immediate forebears endorsed one as permanent as the ravages of child bearing would allow. That is, in earlier times, males could be expected to wear out a wife or two, then avail themselves of another, creating a pattern of serial monogamy. As medical advances made child bearing less lethal, however, single, lifetime pairings became the social ideal in what is referred to as "the civilized world."

With monogamous pairings the accepted standard, sanctions against other patterns developed. Individuals electing not to conform were regarded as suspect, and those unable to procure mates were treated with contempt (tough) or pity (tender). For both biological and social reasons, individuals with functional defects were not prized as mating candidates and could expect to be rejected. The social order saw no earthly purpose in perpetuating what might have been defective gene pools, and survival requirements placed negative value on mates who could not pull their own weight. Happily, as survival has become less contingent on physical abilities to secure food and shelter, the rejection of disabled mates has lessened.

Next enters ego. With developing self-awareness, the urge for pairing became not only a matter of biological and social survival, but survival of the ego as well. To be mateless became a public humiliation, a clear message that one was regarded as inferior stuff. On the other hand, to have a mate of your own offered proof of your being worthwhile to *someone* and, therefore,

70

salvation from ignominy. As a greeting card once proclaimed, "Who cares if the world rejects us? We have each other! Happy Anniversary."

Last, but assuredly not least, and true to the topic of this chapter, pairing offers a convenient, effective means for gratifying the human needs to give and receive love. Love seems to evolve in such a way that much of its power to gratify takes time to develop, and this can occur only in an extended relationship. Moreover, considerable attention to one's object of love is required.

Thus, many forces converge to reinforce the urge toward pairing, and with some degree of exclusivity. None of them are neutralized by the advent of disability, and some are enhanced. If you are disabled, your peers may prefer that you not reproduce, but you are likely to have the same desire as everyone else to do exactly that. When the sensual pleasures associated with sexual contact occupy a high proportion of public media space and time as well as private conversation, the chances are that you'll want to get in on that, too.

When it comes to social and ego survival, a disabled person may have stronger-than-ordinary motivation to pair off on a long-term basis. Having someone who has promised to be there, for better or worse, can allay many anxieties about being able to fend for yourself. You may know that a quasi-welfare state will not let you starve, but it will not provide a very desirable lifestyle. As for your ego, it already has taken a beating and it doesn't want any more. For some, the ability to attract lovers becomes an excessively important proof of continuing worth in the face of self-rejection due to disablement. Although disability can be one of many factors that contribute indirectly to impaired ability to love, in the main, it does not neutralize this desire either; and it virtually never extinguishes the need to be on the receiving end of love.

Not all nondisabled people are interested in pairing, and this obviously holds true for disabled people as well. Some people can't stand children; others can't stand sex; and still others may have enjoyed either or both in the past, yet transcended beyond them through spiritual aspiration. Countless examples of less extreme reasons for the avoidance/neglect of pairing exist, and they apply equally well to the disabled and nondisabled. But, given that for most the urge is strong, the process of pairing is problematical enough under ordinary circumstances to have generated billions of dollars worth of business enterprise to aid or exploit it. The cosmetic and fashion industries; the entertainment industry, especially records and films; the preponderance of self-help publications; and body-building gymnasiums and spas are among the most obvious of such applications.

In addition, an overwhelming proportion of people who seek counseling, psychotherapy, or human potential development offerings do so because their love lives aren't satisfactory. When a disability is present, "normal" problems are apt to be exaggerated and new ones almost surely will emerge. Unfortunately, those with special needs are not only deprived of the extra attention they require, they are altogether ignored by mainstream "pairing industries."

The first area in which help may be needed is that of developing readiness to attempt pairing behavior; this is because of the vulnerability such a commitment creates.

Readiness: Self-Confidence plus Know-How

Many grown men can recall the courage it took to ask for their first dates. "What if she laughs?" Or worse yet, "What if she tries to be nice but can't hide the fact that she'd rather be dead than be seen with a creep like me?" Similarly, many adult women can recapture the agony of wishing *he* would call—*anyone* would call—when a dates-only party was but a week away. The vulnerability of being (exposed as) unselected in the game of pairing is a fearsome one for both sexes. Adjectives fail when individuals have disabilities that the objects of their desires may reject. In a society that venerates beautiful people, serious flaws seem intolerable.

Harnessing the confidence to confront a challenge for which one feels ill equipped is no easy matter. The necessary preparation can be divided into (1) making the most of what you have and (2) developing a philosophy of life that places more value on the achievable and less on the unachievable. The "up front" resource in pairing is physical attractiveness, and frequently this is impaired by disability. The clutter of wheelchairs, braces, and crutches; the appearance of disuse atrophy, joint and bone deformities, absent appendages, sunken eyes, and scarring; and the bodily irregularities that may accompany mental retardation are harder to camouflage than a flat chest, a receding hairline, or thick ankles.

Maximizing Physical Attractiveness

Sometimes, physically disabled people feel embarrassed about making the effort. They are so convinced that the end result will fall short of even modest success that they prefer not to advertise that they've tried and failed. Imagined success usually involves idealized images of what they might have been had disability not intervened—or of other unattainable standards of comparison. On the other hand, mentally retarded people may lack a conceptual grasp of attractiveness, being without concrete experiences of seeing themselves with improved appearance. Robert Shushan (1974) conducted an exciting doctoral dissertation on this subject. The project was initiated by his preschool-aged daughter. Riding in their car one day, she observed a child in a passing car and asked, "Daddy, is that little girl retarded?" Shushan responded that she appeared to be, and then he began to question this event. "No wonder mentally retarded people are put at a distance by others, if their differentness can be 'diagnosed' by a 4-year-old in a passing car! If concerted efforts were made to help them look more 'normal,' would they be accepted more?"

In the project that ensued, he took "before" pictures and then spent approximately twenty minutes with each subject, applying corrective grooming and coaching them to adopt facial expressions that maximized their good features and minimized their flaws. (For example, if they had good teeth, they were encouraged to show them when they smiled. If the teeth were bad, they were encouraged to do the opposite.) Wigs, cosmetic eyeglass frames, and everyday makeup were the only props he used. Then, "after" pictures were taken, and the resulting album is a dramatic presentation of the difference twenty minutes can make. On the left, one sees pitifully unattractive mentally retarded individuals; on the right is a collection of average to outstandingly appealing people. The panel of judges was unable to correctly identify the "after" pictures as those of retarded people when they were interspersed with pictures of nonretarded individuals. Shushan (personal communication) indicates that seeing themselves looking attractive had some lasting effects on the subjects, shown in efforts to maintain themselves in the more attractive mode; however, these would deteriorate over time without "booster shots" to keep the improved images fresh in their minds.

Obviously, the subjects of this study can't go on forever keeping a lock of hair over a sunken jaw, not smiling, or doing whatever was required to get a "normal looking" snapshot. However, if looking better has a positive impact on how they are regarded by themselves and others, the appropriate dental work or plastic surgery to make the improvements permanent would seem to be worthy investments. At least as much should be done as would be done if the person weren't retarded.

The appearance of mentally retarded people has been neglected for a number of reasons, some not altogether a tribute to those who care for them. At the most benign level, the neglect reflects an attitude that, if they aren't aware of their own appearance, there is no reason to create a source of concern for them. In addition, however, the neglect is sometimes an intentional effort to discourage pairing behavior. Operators of residential facilities for retarded people find that management of their charges becomes more difficult when romantic or sexual alliances are formed, and they hope that utility haircuts and nonattention to dental and grooming needs will be deterrents to such unwelcome complications. Moreover, the prospect of sexual activity among retarded people is disturbing to some individuals, similar to the discomfort experienced by adults over the sexual drives and experimentation of children.

With the exceptions noted, disabled people generally are more attuned to the importance of maximizing their attractiveness today than was true only a few years ago. The improved consciousness issuing from the civil rights movement has affected nearly every realm of being. As a result, many disabled people are trying consciously and conscientiously to make the best of what they've got, not only with respect to looks, but in exploiting in positive ways the unusual aspects of their experience. Once pairing efforts are made, they find that having successfully combatted adversity has given them qualities of character that are valued by potential lovers and mates; and that, although what they have to offer is different from what the ordinary person regards as requisite, it is no less worthy of appreciation.

Attention is paid to both the inner and outer determinants of beauty. Such encompassing "figure flaws" as total-body disuse atrophy accompanied by full-time use of a motorized wheelchair are dealt with as matter-of-factly and effectively as possible. What can't be changed can be compensated for, and the human-potential/holistic-health movement has contributed materially to helping everyone understand that beauty has more to do with what comes from within than the perfection of physical attributes. Part of what comes from within is the message that "I care about this body enough to make it as aesthetically pleasing as possible (without pouring excessive time and energy into it)." That message of self-respect helps to generate respect flowing from others, and an expectancy that "This person likes who s/he is so maybe I would, too."

Although such a level of self-acceptance is reached by a sizable proportion of disabled people today, it does not come quickly or automatically. Each individual seems to follow the entire phylogeny, which begins with self-loathing that becomes neutralized and, hopefully, finally transforms into a positive view of self. Dana, for example, says she burst into tears when she first saw her thin, lower legs after six months in bed. She wore ankle-length dresses during the fifties—counter to fashion—to hide their awful truth from view. Fifteen years later, she joyfully showed as much of them as possible during the miniskirt era because,

> Miniskirts were so easy to cope with in a wheelchair, and by that time, skinny legs didn't seem so bad. No guy ever rated my legs as one of my better features, but at least I got "ho hums" instead of the "yecchs" I had expected. I figure if your ego can't take a few "ho hums," you're in deep trouble!

Personality Resources

Maximizing physical attractiveness seems to be one of the few areas of "resource development" that can be accomplished through direct striving. The others, which fall under the general rubric of "personality," are more likely to develop as by-products of less specifically goal-directed efforts to mature and grow as a human being. For example, a self-conscious effort to become a good listener is apt to end in a manipulative façade where inattentiveness to what is being said is masked while the "listener" busily checks out whether the performance is having its desired effect of entrancing the speaker. The genuinely good listener, on the other hand, is such because of sincere caring about the other persons, not because of skillful use of a technique. The speaker almost surely will sense the difference and will find the latter more attractive, whether or not s/he can articulate why.

What is important for disabled people (or others who are/feel handicapped in the pairing process) is to be aware of the personality resources they do possess and place appropriate value on them; to know that "This is what I have to offer and that's not bad!" Even more important is to recognize that this is precisely what everyone needs, too, in order to approach pairing with confidence. Having a disability does not, in this way, create a unique or peculiar situation.

Courtship

Bach & Deutsch (1970) introduced the term "pairing" as an alternative to the term "courtship" in an effort to distinguish the traditional "put your best foot forward" approach (courtship) from a more honest and open style of "being yourself" (pairing). They point out that traditional courtship rituals often lead to rude surprises because flaws, foibles, and inconsistencies are hidden until after a commitment is made. "All's fair in love and war" is the slogan of such old-fashioned trickery. Because romantic duplicity has been idealized throughout a long span of history, both parties willingly collude in the deception. Unfortunately, both parties also pay.

People with disabilities have the usually unwelcome advantage of being less able than most to play courtship games. In this context the well-worn phrase, "What you see is what you get," has a poignant ring. To illustrate, it's hard to feign fascination with the art galleries your intended adores if you're blind. Or, if you're deaf, how do you display a rewarding response to sweet nothings whispered in your ear? Also, it's definitely not easy to stage a sexy entrance in a wheelchair. More basic than this, if you have a disability, a sizable proportion of the field of potential lovers will classify you peremptorily as noneligible for courtship consideration because of the functional and/or aesthetic liabilities you present. Being confronted with this form of dehumanization while you're trying to maintain confidence and hope can stimulate insight and growth in the strong, but it can virtually destroy those whose egos are weak.

As Nan pointed out, a normal degree of boldness must be tempered lest advances by a disabled person be viewed with alarm. It takes time and experience for one to develop the inner surety to accept, philosophically, a rejection so automatic that it is barely recognized as such by the rejecter—without, at the same time, accepting the rejecter's opinion of oneself. Once such assuredness is gained, however, automatic rejections can be dismissed in the knowledge that others exist who will look beyond the disability to decide whether they like whatever else is there.

More authentic sharing may take place when one or both courters has a disability, but this is not always so. It may be necessary to tell a prospective lover that you use a leg bag, yet cover up completely how wretched you feel about that fact. However, if anything is going to destroy the relationship later on, it will not be the leg bag, it will be the wearer's failure to integrate it into a positive self-image. As usual, it is lesions in self-acceptance that disrupt long-term love relationships.

Some of the problems arising are less philosophical than practical, such as fitting two wheelchairs into a car, or one into a sports car. In addition, a frequent complaint of people who find themselves attracted to individuals using wheelchairs is that the chairs make it impossible to "accidentally" get physically close. Also, so much of the courtship process centers about looking, talking, and doing together that impairments in any of these functions can damage spontaneity and require adjustments to be made. The dimly lit restaurant, so important in traditional courtship rituals, can be devastating to someone who needs good light to lip read, barely discern the writing on a menu, or avoid bumping into other diners' chairs.

Assuming the necessary adjustments are made and an alliance survives the tragicomic buffeting it has in store, the disabled lover may be in for a new set of tests and surprises. As Dana put it,

> If you think Tracy and Hepburn looked astonished when their white, middle-class daughter brought Sidney Poitier home to dinner, wait until Mr. America brings home a crip! One guy said his mother went into a diatribe about how girls like me should be locked up in institutions where they can't get out to try to marry people's perfectly normal sons. Hell, I hadn't even planned to ask him to go steady!
>
> It's not easy to be objective when a guy wants you to reassure him that he's not somehow abnormal for having fallen for you—and variations of that happened several times—but it's even harder to stay cool when he asks for advice on how to deal with parents who've dismissed you from the human race.

Courtship isn't solely a time for convincing someone you'd be a good partner for fun, sex, or maybe even marriage; it is also a time for screening out those willing candidates who might not be good for you. As illustrated by Dana's experiences, disabled people may have a particularly difficult task in this regard. People who are attracted to persons who are dependent on others for basic life functions may need to be needed in ways and for reasons they themselves don't fully understand. Sensing an unwholesome flavor to a lover's solicitousness, and rejecting it when it is found, are two equally difficult challenges, especially when the field of choices is limited. Developing the inner strength and emotional independence to say, "I'd rather be alone than used, controlled, or exploited," is likely to evolve from a sequence of valuable mistakes.

In addition, people who think poorly of themselves also may tend to seek out visible underdogs with whom to form romantic alliances. In relationships with physically disabled individuals, they may feel more worthy simply because they are physically intact. People with such tenuous self-respect may prove difficult to be close to, and this can be particularly troublesome to a partner who is not fully self-reliant. From the other's point of view, to choose a mate or lover who seems like a pussycat because of a disability and then find oneself linked to an emotionally stronger, more independent tiger can feel like a disaster.

Dana claims that if you are disabled, the ideal is to search for someone who wants you *in spite of* your disability, not *because of* it. She points out, however, that this requires you to have the emotional stamina to withstand a period of indecision and torment on your lover's part while s/he decides whether you're worth the various sacrifices that must be made. Others disagree. Max counters that he and his wife got married because

> We felt sorry for each other. I was a quad and she was tall, gangly, and no one else even looked at her. It has all worked out, though. We gave each other the love and support we needed and we've built a good life. As a matter of fact, Joy's become quite attractive as she's matured. I'm still a quad, but I *have* gotten rich, so I'm not such a bad catch either!

The Sexual Encounter

When the relationship either evolves or catapults into sexual activity, still another set of tests and surprises awaits. There are the usual concerns that generate a continuous market for the publishers of sex manuals and less didactically oriented erotica. Since most people seem to have at least a few "hangups" with respect to sexual functioning, there is no reason to believe that people with disabilities would have been free of them had disablement not intervened. Thus, one generally can assume the presence of doubts, fears, and confusions that bear no particular relationship to disability. In addition to this base of "normal" perplexity, disabilities frequently create further complications of attitude and action in the sexual role.

Body Image

Attitudinally, a central issue is body image. If a disability has altered one's appearance and/or mobility away from an accepted norm, antipathy toward the body may assume interfering proportions. Fears that a prospective lover may find it grotesque or uninviting are heaped upon the normative baseline of anxieties about a pending sexual encounter. Disability-related body aberrations that can be masked somewhat by carefully selected clothing will be revealed when the couple retires to the bedchamber. Moreover, limited mobility may threaten to render one the unpardonable in these days of sexual liberation and preoccupation: a lousy lay. If urinary or fecal collection devices are added to the equation, positive regard for the body requiring them may plunge precipitously. At the root, if you hate the way your body looks and behaves, it will not be easy to offer it joyfully to a lover.

Learning to love your body, no matter how far it falls short of the cinema-induced ideal (or even a more reasonable standard) takes time and is part of a larger process of self-acceptance. As this process advances, ideals can be relinquished for the apparitions they are and reality, of whatever sort, can become beautiful simply because it *is*. All over the world, disabled people and the rehabilitation workers who serve them are paying attention to such matters, and many have come forward to testify that they know such attitudinal transitions are possible because they have made them. They have found their bodies are loved because *they* are loved, spasms, deformities, collection devices, and all. A surprising number of both men and women who have severe disabilities report being told by nondisabled lovers that they "look better with their clothes off." This may be partly a function of eliminating fear of the unknown and partly due to the simple fact that some figures just don't wear clothes as well as others. Newly disabled people aren't likely to believe such hopeful messages right away, but, given time, most can learn. This is a relatively new awareness, and it has grown out of conscious, concerted efforts to retrain attitudinal tendencies and to make room for a wider range of differences that are not only accepted but appreciated and loved.

Interestingly, some disabled people have come to be in the vanguard of the sexual revolution, opening doors to self-exploration for people in general. Sexuality is seen as a right that has been denied to people with disabilities; as a result, the problems are being discussed openly and exhaustively today, not only in rehabilitation settings, but even on televison. Perhaps because the surface problems are related to politically important attitudinal barriers and practical issues that are somewhat distinct from the more usual psychodynamic factors that frighten people into silence, they are somehow easier to approach and examine than the typical problems of sexual dysfunction. Rehabilitaton workers and others thus observe increasing numbers of disabled people modeling what seems to be an extraordinary degree of openness about their sexuality and related concerns. This gives them permission and encouragement to be more open and less fearful about their own.

Many of the problems discussed relate to sexual action as well as attitudes: the practical problems that arise when one or both lovers are paralyzed, deaf, or otherwise impaired. The sexual performance and enjoyment problems of people with motoric disabilities receive most of the attention, but people who are blind or deaf have their share of problems, too. Harris, for example, points out that as a result of losing his hearing he still has occasional trouble "diagnosing" whether some of his wife's physical movements during intercourse are the sequelae of her passion or efforts to let him know that he is hurting her.

The list of practical problems that can ensue when one or both lovers has a physical disability is virtually endless. Paralysis creates one set of problems, pain another, amputations yet another, and neurological impairments affecting erotic sensation and bowel and bladder control produce still more. When an individual is very severely disabled, even masturbation may be impossible without assistance; or, if both lovers are severely disabled, an attendant's help may be necessary to make sexual contact possible. Fortunately, this new era of sexual liberation has brought with it at least a few good-quality guidebooks that disabled people can profit from reading, both for technical advice on solving specific problems and for their overall message that, as far as the need for and right to sexual expression and enjoyment are concerned, however you are is all right (for example, Shaul, et al., 1978). More often, the problem for disabled people is gaining access to such enlightened perspectives. A couple may be unaware that hundreds of other severely disabled couples are asking their attendants—with varying degrees of comfort—to help position them for lovemaking. This couple, then, must make a far bolder move to broach the possibility with their own attendant(s) than an informed couple.

The long silence on the conjoint subject of sex and disability was, in part, an outgrowth of devaluative attitudes. (As for the other part, everyone in the "civilized world" has been sexually oppressed for a long time.) Overvaunted values placed on physical attractiveness led inexorably to the multilevel conclusions that disabled people are distorted and/or ugly; therefore, no one will want or permit sexual contact with them; therefore, the kindest thing to do is help them keep their minds on other things. Moreover, the thought of disabled people wanting sexual involvement carries an implied threat that "If they want it at all, they might want it with *me*—and what would I say? I wouldn't want to hurt such a person's feelings." Disabled people held similar values and attitudes, and a conspiracy of silence ensued. But today is an era of massive attention to the acceptance, even celebration, of differences—whether related to race, nationality, gender, age, disability, or individual temperament. Although the silence currently is broken more by lip service than genuine clamor to embrace the unknown, such is a first step, and more palpable gains may follow.

Unfortunately, the embracement of differences sometimes takes unwholesome turns. The attraction of some men to women with amputations has long been considered as a form of sexual varietism that stems from emotional disturbance. As disabled people began to talk among themselves and go public with their experiences, it came to light that individuals of both sexes may be sexually drawn to a wide range of disabilities more than to the people who have them. Several disabled people who unknowingly formed alliances with such individuals describe as nightmares their dawning recognition of the source of their partner's titillation. Realizing that she had been sought out as a "freak" led Peggy to contemplate suicide. On the other hand, Naomi, after a period of time, was able to place the pathology where it belonged: not with herself, but with her former partner.

> He thought having sex with me would be kinky. When he first blurted that out, I was destroyed. Now I just think he was a little bit crazy, but I'm not going to get crazy, too. If I were "normal," I wouldn't blame myself for accidentally getting hooked up with a foot fetischist—as long as I got out when I realized he was a kinko, that is.

Another side of human acceptance is illustrated by a story told by Marya. A bilateral, above-knee amputee, she had been married to Emory for over three years when he confessed to her one night that he had, since early adolescence, entertained fantasies of having relations with women such as herself; and that her disability had been the prepotent source of his attraction to her initially. By then they had established a solid marital relationship and were viewed as an ideal couple by many of their friends. Marya recalled,

> I wanted to die. I wanted to vomit. Actually, I wanted to kill him. But somehow, the next morning, when he begged me not to leave him, because he had grown to love me for many other reasons, I weakened. He had trusted me enough to tell me something that still bothered—no, terrified—him. He had given me love and support and now he was asking me to accept *his* disability—a psychological problem that he was repulsed by and didn't understand. I agreed to stay if he would go to a psychiatrist. That was ten years ago. I don't know that he has completely resolved all of his hangups, but our marriage is a good one . . . and whatever crazy thing he has for my stumps, he is a lovely guy I'm glad I hung onto.

The Mythology of Sexual Perfection

Several states have introduced legislation requiring specified health practitioners to acquire continuing education credits in human sexuality. These training sessions rather consistently attend to the matter of exploding myths surrounding sexual experience. Included among these is "the myth of the orgasm." It is yesterday's news that the fictional ideal of simultaneous orgasm seldom exists in reality. Somewhat more current are the considerations that the orgasm may not be essential to sexual fulfillment at all. As people have become free to tell the truth about their sexual experiences, it turns out that many couples—disabled and nondisabled alike—place a high value on sex lives that seldom if ever culminate in or otherwise include the phantasmagoric orgasm.

Again, people with disabilities have been in the forefront of myth exploding. Individuals with neurological impairments to genital sensation report both satisfying sensual/sexual expression that does not include orgasm and orgasmic experiences produced by fantasy and/or localized in nongenital areas. Hearing it said by people with sensory impairments has made it possible for numbers of nondisabled people to acknowledge that a similar pattern is familiar to them, too. It has become common practice in sex therapy clinics to deemphasize striving for orgasm among women and men who find that it does not flow naturally from them. Instead of focusing massive efforts upon bringing it about, as in earlier days, clients are encouraged to savor the other pleasurable sensations associated with sexual activity and avoid creating a climate of weary, frustrated negativity because a particular sensation is not readily forthcoming. Not surprisingly, a number of them find that when they cease their desperate striving, the orgasm occurs. Those who do not have this experience are likely to find that nonorgasmic pleasurable sensations are sufficient reward in themselves. For all, the sensual pleasures and spiritual fulfillments of physical intimacy with a lover are stressed.

Today's sexual freedom revolution at times takes on the character of a reaction formation against years of sexual censorship. Censored were both freedom of speech about sex and the freedom to engage in the sex acts of choice with the partners of choice. As the bans have been lifted, the new message has become, "Whatever with whomever is okay." As wholesome as this has been for both disabled and nondisabled people who were viewed or viewed themselves as desirous of activities and fulfillments that were somehow taboo, it has concomitantly produced a new mythology of sexual perfection. This, in turn, has created further barriers to self-esteem when the quantitative and qualitative ideals described in the sex manuals are not achieved or achievable. Moreover, now that sexuality has been legitimized, it is not so legitimate anymore to regard it as an inconsequential or a sometime thing. As a result, people with low levels of sex drive (and, like other human traits, sex drive is assumed to be distributed along the normal curve) are forcing themselves to become the sensuous man or woman regardless of their natural proclivities. Disabled people have been caught up in this just as much as nondisabled people and in some cases perhaps even more.

Certain people, whose disabilities so severely inhibit mobility and/or sensual gratification that they would just as soon leave sex alone, feel that they are not permitted to do so now. The message coming from every direction is that in order to be psychologically "whole" they must be, in the words of Ernie, "hornier than thou." Although this is most likely to be heard from people with phobic feelings about sexuality that are unrelated to their disabilities, such is not always the case. Ernie also provides a good example of a related problem that arises. He bitterly denounced the efforts of a psychologist at his rehabilitation hospital to help spinal-cord injured patients adjust, sexually.

> She came in there wearing her miniskirts and strutting around and using four letter words and I wouldn't have trusted her any farther than a quad like me could have thrown her. She was working out her own thing, not helping anyone else . . . and she didn't pay any attention to the women, just the men.

Ernie's wife indicates that their sexual adjustment was relatively uncomplicated; in fact, he became a better lover for her because much of his pleasure centered about satisfying her. Her view of the "help" he was offered was this:

> I think [the psychologist] glommed onto the big furor about sex and disability as a way of dealing with her own problems. She was some kind of zealot and that really turned Ernie off because sex was the one area he kind of had together. I wish someone had been that interested in helping him see that he could still do some kind of work. It's been seven years now, and our sex life is fine, but he's still not doing much of anything else. *That's* what's beginning to turn me off!

And thus the pendulum swings. An era in which the sexual needs of disabled people are ignored may be followed by an era in which at least a few must face having the sexual problems of others imposed upon them in ways insensitive to their values and needs. In the main, however, the current attention paid to sexuality among disabled people has been a positive influence, enhancing recognition of the breadth and depth of sexual expression possible. In this respect, the field of rehabilitation already has contributed significantly to filling the gap left by the mainstream "pairing industries," as the latter are only beginning to acknowledge and respond to their disabled markets.

Even rehabilitation has made little effort to help disabled people whose sexual orientation is gay. This reality is almost as blithely ignored today as was sexuality *in toto* a few years ago. Sexual preference statistics that have been touted in the public media indicate that as much as ten percent of the population may choose same-sex individuals as lovers—a significant minority to ignore. The need for counsel is great; disabled gays express more fears than nondisabled gays about "coming out of the closet" because of their dual-devaluated status. Believing rejection by the straight majority could threaten their very survival, many stay silent and their problems of establishing love relationships remain unresolved.

Why is it that sex is such a powerful subject? Probably in part because it is potentially a vehicle for manifesting nearly every facet of human consciousness and of meeting the demands of almost every level in the human hierarchy of needs. This is true not only for the most basic levels of consciousness reflected in the needs for security, sensation, and power, but also for the "higher" levels of consciousness reflected in the needs for self-esteem, love, self-actualization, and spiritual enlightenment. This aspect of sexuality is only mentioned here, but these concepts will be developed fully in Chapter 8 ("Transcending").

The fact is, the development of a truly intimate relationship may be far more difficult for many to achieve than an imitation of sexual perfection. It has become almost a cliché in sex therapy circles that failures of intimacy are the primary causes of sexual dysfunction. Perhaps contrary to expectation, this does not change with the advent of disability. There may be organic bases for certain aspects of sexual dysfunction, but these do not explain an unsatisfactory sex life or love life. When genuine intimacy exists, couples whose sex lives consist of lying quietly together may report more satisfying erotic experiences than sex-manual gymnasts who reach orgasm but feel strangely empty and displeased nonetheless.

Intimacy

Intimacy seldom, if ever, happens suddenly. A special rapport is sometimes almost instantaneous, but true intimacy takes time to develop. It may or may not incude the sense of being "*in* love," but it involves loving. Caring about the other person's needs and ways of being, and freely sharing one's own, are the hallmarks of intimacy. Several years ago, one of the popular psychology magazines carried an article that asserted that the sense of being "*in* love" had only two basic requisites: (1) the loved individual keeps one in a state of arousal and (2) that state of arousal is labeled "love". This was thought to explain such phenomena as possessive love and the renowned hairline difference between love and hate. If the state of arousal generated by another is confounded by possessiveness or unresolved resentments (hate), there is very little chance that a truly intimate relationship will evolve from it, however powerful the chemistry appears to be. All of this holds true regardless of whether disablement is a factor in the relationship. When it is, however, it is poignantly relevant because of the heightened likelihood of the emergence of both possessive and resentful feelings.

As they relate to disability, feelings of possessiveness are most apt to be experienced by disabled lovers who feel insecure about their ability to "hang on" to a lover or spouse. Whether or not it is true, they are likely to attribute their insecurity in this regard to their disabilities. Possessiveness is also an important issue with nondisabled people who choose disabled lovers/spouses partly in the belief that they will be less subject to being wooed away by someone else. Resentments can emerge for a thousand reasons. The disabled partner may resent over- or under-solicitude or simply be jealous of the other's freedom from disability-related constraints. Gratitude for care-giving is notoriously mixed with resentment over its necessity, and those feelings tend to be directed toward the care-giver. A nondisabled partner may resent what feels like a burden, yet be afraid of alienating or hurting the other and thus say nothing but continue to seethe.

If the couple finds that such feelings can be shared and thereby deenergized, a step toward greater intimacy has been taken. If not, it becomes more remote, and ultimate dissolution of the relationship looms likely. Because the building (or rebuilding) of an intimate relationship is so central to marriage and other unions involving formalized commitments, these concepts will be pursued further in the following sections dealing with marriage and alternative lifestyles.

Building a New Marriage

If a marriage takes place after disablement is a *fait accompli*, statistics show the chances for success are greater than for marriages established previously. There are two fairly obvious reasons for this: (1) the marriage will not have to endure the emotional weathering associated with the acute stage of illness or injury and (2) both partners make their commitments in the face of known disability-related conditions. Each makes a positive choice that acknowledges the reality of disability; it is not a seemingly unfair, fateful event that is thrust upon them. There will, nonetheless, be the usual needs for adjustments, some of which will center about the disability. The problem areas will be little different from those of couples whose marriages predated disability. A signal example is the temptation to view every conflict as a "disability issue." Naturally, an early order of business is learning to sort what is from what is not an issue related to disability.

A disabled partner may have projected fuller acknowledgment of disability during courtship than was true at a deeper level. S/he even may have expected that having someone to "love and honor 'til death do us part" would magically make the pain of disablement go away. In one way, this is little different from the usual images of bliss that surround romantic alliances, and it must be brought into line with reality as the marriage matures. However, when failure to accept part of oneself that is frequently in the forefront of consciousness is at issue, efforts to "force" the partner to make everything better may redouble. Frequently, people who feel they have had much taken away from them look to their closest family members—parents, children, spouse—for compensation. It is a hard but important lesson to learn that others cannot make up for one's losses.

Linked to this are the problems of jealousy and fears of spousal abandonment whenever a nondisabled or less disabled spouse becomes interested in activities that can't be shared. A woman executive with one paralyzed leg resulting from polio described the panic she felt when her husband first took an interest in skiing:

> I was miffed that he wanted to do something I couldn't do. I thought, "How insensitive can he be?" I was very threatened by the fact that even though I could succeed in business, I still couldn't join my husband in what he wanted to do. For awhile, I really got paranoid; I refused to go along and then tortured myself with fantasies of him falling in love with some winter Olympian who looked like Sophia Loren. I damaged our relationship by tryng to make him feel too guilty to go.
>
> Finally, one of our friends told me what a jerk I was being. He really laid it on. After the sting went away, I knew he was right. Why should I force Jed to be a cripple just because I'm one? That's real dog-in-the-manger stuff. Anyway, now I go and have a good time sitting around the lodge, visiting, knitting, enjoying the beauty of the setting, and watching Jed ski. It took him awhile to trust that I wasn't pulling some kind of martyr act or spying on him, but now even that's behind us. The good part was when he admitted it was nice to find out I had a scared side, because the supercompetent businesswoman had kind of scared him!

This couple did not have to deal with the issues that arise when a spouse is called on to provide all or part of such needed services as attendant care, interpreting, reading, and driving. When this is true, delicate problems can arise.

The care-giving spouse may come to feel "used," like a "servant"; and the recipient may feel dissatisfied and angry over untimely or inattentive care. Moreover, the effects of care-giving responsibilities on sexual attraction to the disabled spouse create highly fabled concerns for numerous couples. Nondisabled individuals contemplating marriage to disabled men or women regularly are counseled, by friends, family, and professionals, to reconsider: "You may think you are in love now, but you'll get turned off fast after you've had to take care of him/her like a baby for awhile." The disabled parties, especially those who have not yet integrated their dependency into a positive self-image, inwardly and fearfully agree with such pronouncements. When marriage takes place anyway, chronic dread that proof is imminent may follow.

If frank discussion of all such issues is inhibited by fears and resentments, alienation can only increase. Both parties must struggle to be fair and realistic, while at the same time protecting their own rights and needs. Sound marriages are generally the product of equivalent giving and taking, and understanding *equivalencies* (not equalities) of contribution requires very balanced perception when disability creates highly visible areas wherein one gives and the other receives.

Two examples illustrate compensatory patterns that can reduce the extent to which a couple feels an imbalance in giving and taking. Harris has found that work colleagues are so used to his bringing paid interpreters to meetings that on social occasions they may treat his wife as if that were her only role. At her request, he now points out beforehand that she will interpret for him, but will be present, first and foremost, for her own social pleasure. Carol, whose husband provides her morning and nightly attendant care, says she tries to "repay" him by pampering him with breakfast in bed on weekends, and dinner in bed during football season, where he likes to lounge while watching the games.

Roy, the nondisabled husband of a very severely paralyzed woman, lamented,

> I wish Toni could just realize that I married her because she made me happy . . . she was so tender and understanding when we were going together and that's all I wanted from her. Hell, I knew she was disabled! But now, all she does is brood about what she can't do . . . says she's afraid she's going to lose me because she can't cook and keep house and raise kids. If that was what I wanted, I would have married someone else. If she loses me, it will be because I can't take her constant gloom anymore.

Learning that the best you can offer to someone else is to be the best you can be for yourself—and the happiest—is a sophisticated human lesson to learn. People with severe disabilities have the seldom-envied advantage of a great incentive to learn it well, regardless of whether they adopt lifestyles of traditional marriage. The urge toward pairing also can be satisfied in other ways, including quasi-traditional marriage, living singly and dating, and forming committed unions with more than one other individual.

Alternative Lifestyles

The first to be considered is more an alternative to poverty than to marriage. Many couples, wherein one or both are recipients of Supplemental Security Income and/or Medicaid benefits, may wish to marry but find it would entail a devastating loss of income. Administering agencies are reluctant to pay spouses for providing attendant care, so many couples remain unmarried, living ostensibly as "recipient" and "provider" when, in fact, their lifestyle is one of common-law marriage. Other couples, both of whom are "recipients," meet similar disincentives to legal marriage. On the positive side, "living together" is no longer regarded with the social disdain it once was. People do still marry, however, so the ritual, the contract, and the commitment of marriage continue to have deep and widespread meaning. Many disabled people/couples want to sanctify their love relationships in this way and enjoy the sense of security a marriage commitment connotes, but, because of the economic disincentives built into the income system on which they rely, they feel unable to do so. Couples such as these and others who adopt nonlegalized marital lifestyles for other reasons (for example, previous marital ties undissolved, preference for avoiding long-term or legal commitments, or gay "marriages") experience essentially the same issues and problems as the married couples described in the previous section.

A truer alternative to marriage exists in communal living arrangements that both serve familial functions of mutual support and offer opportunities for love relationships. Some disabled people join established communes, others select from the extant range of independent living arrangements (ILAs) referred to in Chapter 3, and still others create communal or independent living situations for themselves. Group marriages, though generally rare, occasionally include one or more disabled partners. ILAs are likely choices for severely disabled individuals, who need their practical features as much as their opportunities for love relationships. However, some residents are married couples who enjoy the sense of a large extended family in addition to the special facilities and services available.

Finally, the alternative of living singly (with whatever attendant or other help might be needed) has become "respectable" in society at large. It now carries less connotation of having been unchosen, since many people, including increasing numbers of women with ample opportunities to marry, are making singledom their choice. Here, the women's movement has had a beneficial side effect for single disabled people, by reducing the sense of stigma associated with unmarried life. Nonetheless, Cathy, the disabled feminist cited earlier (see Chapter 2), expresses the opinion that,

> Being single and disabled is still a little bizarre, especially for women. It's true that the stigma is *reduced*, but it's still a problem. If you're single and disabled, other people assume it's because you have no choice, even if that's not true. And if you haven't gotten past being concerned about your image, or being pitied, that bothers you. Also, realistically, dates aren't all that easy to get for most of us, and it's easy to get caught up in the "one night stand" syndrome, just for the momentary proofs that someone wants you. Many people don't want the obligations of marriage, but few people want to be alone—and marriage or living together or even having a steady are ways to combat that. Also, when you're disabled and have trouble finding jobs, having a lifetime partner is very reassuring. Economic security is still one of the main reasons people team up in marriage . . . and disabled people want that even more than most.

As cited in several earlier contexts, a couple's or family's economic situation can have significant impact on their interrelationships. Severe financial hardships are notorious for eroding love, whether or not disablement is a factor. Obviously, the major cause of fiscal difficulty among disabled people is the problem Cathy alluded to: under- or unemployment. Job barriers abound for the disabled population, and they begin being erected at least as early as elementary school. The following chapter will examine the education and employment processes as they relate to disabled people's work lives.

6 Working

Getting Educated and Employed

People disabled in infancy or childhood may begin very early, and without knowing it, to experience what one day will prove to be serious hindrances in getting and keeping jobs and in advancing in careers. This is because all aspects of one's education—not just the formal, didactic schooling, but the experiential parts as well—have the power to shape or misshape people for their eventual work lives. The well-known studies of creative artists and scientists consistently show that enriched early life experience—from world travel to simply being read to a great deal—is a commonly found factor among those who are most successful. Compare this with the homogeneity and stultification potentially present in the life of a child who is sheltered, isolated, and perhaps institutionalized for long periods of time due to a disability. It is thus that the problems that will beset getting vocationally established in the practical world begin even earlier than the first day of school. They are apt to increase markedly when that day arrives, however.

Special Education versus Mainstreaming

Many people alive today have seen public education for disabled youngsters progress from no education at all, to "special" education in segregated settings, to a concerted effort to integrate disabled students into mainstream schools. The accompanying change of attitude from "Tough luck, Charlie" through "separate but equal" to the recognition that separate is as inherently unequal here as elsewhere reflects growth in a positive direction. This trend, like others cited earlier, is a product of civil rights concern and legislation at national and local levels.

The special education era—which has by no means ended, despite massive efforts to desegregate disabled students—itself came into being as a result of dire societal need. In its time, it reflected important social progress.

As other conditions changed, however, and the artifact of segregation was observed to create its own set of problems, further change was seen to be required. This has culminated in the passage of legislation requiring all young people with disabilities to be educated in the "least restrictive environment" appropriate to their condition. This means, in essence, maximal integration into mainstream schooling, with a minimum of segregated programs.

The wisdom of this trend is controversial. While its proponents are primarily dissatisfied with the slowness by which the mandated changes are taking place, dissent comes from several different quarters. One group points out that the cost of providing an equal education to certain extremely disabled youngsters exceeds the value of the objective. That is a heavy message for disabled people to receive. Others believe that the quality of education for all will suffer. Depending on their interests, they may lament a regular classroom teacher's time being overly directed toward a few disabled students, or they may stress that teacher's inability to do an effective job with disabled students. Many of the displeased are teachers. Some complain because they dread having disabled students in their classrooms; others protest because they envision their special-education expertise being wasted. All reactions reflect a mixture of fact and unreality laced with fears of change and the unknown. Many disabled youngsters who are aware of the controversy are hurt or angered by it, as are disabled adults who can assess the implications for their social status more fully.

For the purposes at hand, disabled students might be viewed as comprising three distinguishable groups: (1) those whose learning ability is impaired, (2) those whose communication ability is impaired, and (3) those whose disabilities affect neither learning nor communication abilities. The reasons differ for segregating the education of each of these groups from the mainstream.

Students whose ability to learn is impaired by intellectual limitation, emotional/behavioral disorder, or other neurological dysfunctions are segregated so that their slower learning pace does not retard the progress of more capable students, and to allow the extra time and attention needed for them to absorb material. Accommodating both the faster and slower learners may require some segregation by classroom, but it no longer is clear why it once seemed necessary for them to attend school in altogether separate facilities. Desire on the part of the nondisabled populace to avoid contact with people thus limited is the most logical explanation for society's having taken this extra step.

Students whose communication abilities (reception/transmission of visual/auditory data) are affected by vision, hearing, or speech disorders are segregated into settings that specialize in presenting educational material in modes they can "receive" adequately, and that provide the extra time and equipment needed for them to "transmit." By segregating their education, regular classroom teachers are freed from concern over students with unusual communication needs, and school systems find it cost effective to provide special services and equipment in a single location, rather than at each mainstream school.

Students with physical disabilities affecting neither their learning nor communication abilities frequently are segregated simply to avoid the architectural barriers characterizing mainstream schools. Also, when severe disabilities require attendant care during the school day, having it available at one rather than all schools seems cost effective.

The problem is, separating disabled from nondisabled people early in their lives will create other social costs to be paid for later, such as expensive programs designed to break down the attitude and job barriers early segregation fostered. It is no wonder that employers, most of whom are relatively nondisabled, find it difficult to imagine that disabled job applicants could function in their work settings when, as children, they were led to believe that disabled people couldn't even function in the same elementary schools. It also is not surprising that disabled and nondisabled people have trouble simply relating to one another when they had no opportunities for contact from their earliest years. After schooling is over, they hardly can be expected to come together at last with ready-made mutual understanding.

The artifact of segregation is not the only problem cited with respect to special education. Nan, and many other disabled people who attended "special" schools, state the conviction that they did not get an education equal to what they would have obtained in a mainstream school. They say both academic and socialization standards were relaxed far beyond the levels needed for many of the students, and that orientation toward college preparation was virtually absent. Mindy, a rehabilitation counselor whose disability is leg weakness secondary to polio, states,

> There was no reason for me to be sent to a school for the handicapped except that my parents didn't know how to say "No." My disability in no way affected my scholarship, and I could even climb stairs. At the school, everything was geared to the slow learners, who were in the majority, and those of us needing challenge were out of luck. No one talked to me about college, so I never considered it until I found my way to the "voc rehab" bureau. This was four years after I finished high school . . . for four years I hung around home with no idea of what to do with myself. I'll never forget how amazed I was when my rehab counselor said she thought I'd be good at her kind of job. That compliment clinched my career choice . . . I never considered anything else. It's a good thing it was a good choice because I would have accepted anything she suggested. Ignorance makes you very, very vulnerable.

This brings us to the matter of vocational decision making.

Occupational Choice

In this society, most people grow up expecting—and wanting—to work. A few people, born into families that have been recipients of welfare programs for several generations, may not share this expectancy, but most others have primary role models (parents, usually) who work, and they intend to follow suit. Thus, occupational choice is not generally a matter of deciding whether to work; it is deciding what kind of work to do. Depending on the prepotency of geographic and familial occupational tradition, this may entail a simple or complex process of decision making. For example, if you live in a "textile town" and your parents, grandfather, and great-grandfather all worked at the mill, your occupational choice may appear automatic, a simple conformation to local custom. At the other extreme, if you live in a megalopolis and your father's people are professionals and your mother's are in business, you may confront a dizzying array of options to choose among.

When significant disablement is entered into the equation, the simple becomes complex and the complex, overwhelming. A job planned for or performed in the past suddenly may be precluded; or a disability may be so severe that no one can envision any suitable job. In such cases, because reasonably adequate welfare programs exist for people with vocationally handicapping disabilities, a serious decision process on *whether* to work may arise in a family with no prior history of welfare recipiency.

Why Work? Incentives and Disincentives

With the existence of welfare programs for unemployed people, work is no longer necessary for survival. Nonetheless, the incentives for working anyway are strong. Although one can survive on a welfare income, the lifestyle it affords is marginal and stigmatized. Moreover, work is a vehicle for acquiring such socially revered external rewards as money, prestige, and power, as well as the inner rewards associated with self-esteem, belongingness, and self-actualization. Unemployment generates sociopolitical and economic powerlessness, and powerlessness is the basis of learned helplessness—a form of depression. A vicious cycle can develop in which these, in turn, lead to a reduction in one's actual powers to influence the course of events in one's life.

The demise of the work ethic has been predicted for several decades now. Automation was expected to usher it in, as were more recent spiritually oriented shifts in human values. So far, however, the reports of its death have been highly exaggerated; consequently, people with disabilities are still under pressure, from within and without, to establish themselves vocationally, to have an occupational identity, to reap the materialistic rewards that accrue to wage earning, and to luxuriate in the good feelings that accompany being "a productive, contributing member of society." These are the incentives.

Disincentives also abound and are rooted in the welfare system. The Supplemental Security Income (SSI) program provides more realistic cash allowances to disabled recipients than general relief programs do for the nondisabled unemployed. Moreover, it is complemented by Medicaid coverage of sometimes extremely costly health-related needs, including a regular, monthly outlay for attendant care when required. Frequently, severely disabled recipients are unable to earn anything approximating an equivalent income, and certainly not from an entry-level job.

When individuals drawing (and needing) large total benefit amounts move into employment (thereby relinquishing eligibility for SSI and Medicaid), they place themselves in serious financial jeopardy. Work may offer no additional income and may even entail a reduction. This is especially true when attendant salaries have been paid, as group medical policies available through work will not cover this expense. Even more demotivating, the threat of failure or delay in reestablishing eligibility for benefits following an abortive job attempt generates fears of catastrophic life disruption or even institutionalization. Under such circumstances, the decision not to work and to opt instead for a life on welfare hardly can be viewed as social irresponsibility. It simply may be a very sensible decision.

The problem stems partly from a carryover of earlier thinking regarding the employment capabilities of severely disabled individuals. Predecessor programs were labeled "aid to the *totally* disabled," on the presumption that severe disablement rendered one totally unfunctional in the labor market. We now know that even extremely severe disability may not entail being vocationally handicapped at all, as blind, deaf, and completely paralyzed persons secure increasing numbers of high-level positions. But today's SSI system is premised on these older conceptions, and its lack of incentives for making a transition to financial independence reflects bygone beliefs that no such transitions are possible.

This is not true for the Social Security Disability Insurance (SSDI) program, but it creates another set of problems for recipients. Negative incentives have been introduced in an effort to abate no-work decisions, however sensible they might be for the recipient, because they are viewed as unfair to the taxpayers. Beneficiaries of these public monies are strongly encouraged to seek rehabilitation through the state–federal vocational rehabilitation program and thus vacate the benefit rolls. Failure to make efforts in this direction carries the threat of punitive benefit termination.

In short, disabled individuals are faced with a confusing, disturbing array of incentives and disincentives for both working and declining to do so. Those who decide that they want to try, like anyone in the throes of making an occupational commitment, immediately face three major questions: what are the options? how does one learn about them? and how does one decide which option to choose? When a significant disability must be incorporated into the decision making, a difficult process becomes even more convoluted.

The Perception of Vocational Choices

Clearly, disabilities do not limit vocational options to the extent people have been led to believe. Nonethless, the functional limitations associated with disabling conditions do eliminate certain jobs from consideration and surround others with impaired probability of success. This still leaves a vast assortment of options available for most disabled people, who then must try to sort the good-chance options from the risky, and the risky from the foolish.

When no role models can be found who demonstrate concretely that a blind or deaf or paralyzed or retarded person can land a given job and perform in it well, it is easy to conclude that the job in question must be among the impossible. However, because of prejudicial hiring practices in the past, this is not necessarily the case. Therefore, many disabled people entering fields uncharted with respect to track records of disabled workers must make subjectively high-risk decisions in choosing what, objectively, may be sure things vis-à-vis the interaction of functional limitations with job demands. Happily, with the advent of protective legislation regarding employment opportunities for disabled workers, role models are becoming easier to find.

Some disabled people go through many iterations of choosing vocational goals, only to be told, time after time, that their choices are unrealistic and they should choose something more in line with their capabilities. Sometimes this is accurate. Tim, a totally paralyzed youngster who insisted he wanted to be a carpenter like his father provides an unarguable example. In other cases, such advice reveals the limited imagination of the advisor. This was true for Carol, a triplegic psychologist whose undergraduate advisor said she should not pursue psychology because she could not operate a stopwatch and record IQ test responses simultaneously with only one functional arm and hand. Later, her rehabilitation counselor suggested that clerical work would be a more realistic level of aspiration. Tim went through a painfully disappointing series of confrontations before acceding to external opinion. Carol suffered needless anxiety before gaining enough experience to discredit faulty advice and pursue her chosen career.

Others may be unable to formulate even one vocational objective; everything seems beyond the range of feasibility. When a firm commitment has been made to a given job or field—through prior work involvement, highly developed interest or talent, or both—relinquishment may seem unbearable. Narrowing of vistas and refusal/inability to shift focus may obliterate the perception of other options, some of which might yield equivalent satisfaction if given the chance.

Any of these situations may call for professional assistance, in the form of testing and other evaluative procedures, and counseling and guidance to improve the person's chances for getting appropriate training. ("Appropriate" here means that the job objective and therefore the *type* of training are in accord with both the person's and the labor market's realities and that the *quality* of training, given the objective, is good.) Some disabled people claim the professional help they got was heaven sent. Others describe it as an additional handicap they had to overcome.

Professional Assistance

Vocational counseling is a service most people would find beneficial, but few get it. Oddly enough, disabled individuals have a better chance than most to get more than cursory guidance, because of the barriers to employment they face. In response to such, far more extensive services have been made available to them, through federal legislation, than are obtainable by the general public through the state–federal employment service plus private-sector programs. Most people consider this a dubious advantage, but it is a potentially valuable opportunity nonetheless.

Some are able to utilize these services with little ado. They understand or are helped to understand the reasons for esoteric-seeming evaluation procedures; they know how to participate or are coached to participate actively in drawing conclusions from the findings to formulate a vocational goal and a plan leading to it. From there, they know how to proceed on their own or are given the help they need when they need it. They have moral/emotional support from their own family and friends or find it available from the counselor and other professional helpers.

Many others, however, find that the vocational rehabilitation system is an extremely complex and confusing, multilevel stress test that is one more trial to adjust to. You are forced to go to doctors and psychologists whose inputs seem unrelated to your desires to learn a trade. You are forced to take tests that seem embarrassingly silly, or embarrassingly difficult. Your counselor doesn't seem to have time to see you and when s/he does, s/he has other ideas about what you should do. Nobody ever tells you how you did on all those tests and you have a feeling you must have blown it. Your counselor finally agrees with what you want to do, but the supervisor says, "No." Or your counselor never agrees but you're afraid to complain to the supervisor. Or the counselor goes along with what you want, the supervisor agrees, and after two years of training it turns out that the job market has dried up or that a person with your disability simply couldn't function in that field.

Most of the procedures and interim outcomes that vex and perplex clients actually have good basis; they just aren't explained comprehensibly. The counselor may play "doctor," in the negative sense, by expecting the client, uninformed, to follow advice without questioning. However, sanctioning the placement of a client in inappropriate training has no justification (except when done consciously to enhance reality testing). Too many disabled people have "lost" years of their lives in recovery processes or hospitalization. To lose still more because a presumed job expert understood neither the job nor the market is a gratuitous blow.

In most vocational rehabilitation plans, some form of training or education will be called for. This ushers in a new phase of adjustment to new settings, people, and demands.

Accommodation in Education

A few highly specialized training programs are available at home; video computer programming training for home-based workers serves as a familiar example. However, most people whose vocational rehabilitation plans involve some form of education will have to go to a campus somewhere to get it. Whether for reasons relating to the nature and/or severity of disability, financial inability to obtain a car, the lack or inaccessibility of public transportation, or all three, many people in all categories of disability will find their first problem to be, "How do I get my body there?"

Severely physically disabled students also may need to resolve attendant-care problems in order to get to class on time. Attendants who are accustomed to getting their employers out of bed, dressed, and ready to function in their own good time may resent and resist having to meet an earlier deadline. Vision- and hearing-impaired students will be confronted with serious barriers to learning once they arrive on campus because lecture (for deaf) and written (for blind) materials will be inaccessible to them without extraordinary measures of accommodation. Physically disabled students also will confront barriers in long distances between classrooms and in architectural design.

Some of the needed accommodations are being made on the campuses, and the state–federal vocational rehabilitation program is footing the bill for additional needs. For example, on-campus "enabler" programs for disabled students dispense information, advice, advocacy, and other valuable services. School libraries stock taped and Brailled materials for vision-impaired students and, occasionally, amplification devices that allow hearing-impaired students better access to lecture presentations. Still more occasionally, schools provide reader services for blind students and interpreter services for deaf students; but these more costly accommodations are most likely to be provided through the state–federal vocational rehabilitation program. The latter provides many additional types of adaptive equipment and personal services to students with all types of disabilities.

The last few years have seen rapid progress in the accommodations offered by both the schools and the vocational rehabilitation service system. This is, in large measure, an outgrowth of recent legislation relating to the rights of disabled people to equal educational opportunities (to be discussed in Chapter 9). At the same time, consumer-run independent living programs have appeared on the scene and begun to multiply; they offer help to students needing to tighten their off-campus support systems to allow reliable school—and, one day, work—attendance.

Once the major problems have been resolved and the student is matriculated safely and regular in attendance, other problems arise. These relate to "other people." Some instructors are reluctant to flex their teaching styles to accommodate disabled students. If they don't use ample handouts ordinarily, they are unwilling to adopt the practice for the sake of current and future deaf students. If they *do* use ample handouts, it is the responsibility of blind students to get them read. Although it may be illegal, some teachers still refuse to allow students unable to take notes to tape-record their lectures. Students physically unable to participate in laboratory activities may find instructors unwilling to allow them to play a modified role in meeting laboratory requirements. These problems, obviously, are felt most acutely by disabled students lacking in social presence and assertiveness. As a veteran rehabilitation counselor with a college student caseload once remarked, "I've never seen a client who was gracious and poised get hassled by teachers who didn't want to make allowances. And they'll fall all over themselves to help a pretty girl in a wheelchair!" Thus, physical attractiveness and assertiveness again arise as critical resource variables in the adjustment process. Both on-campus enabler programs and off-campus independent living programs are directing some attention to helping people who do not have these traits naturally to develop them to a level that will contribute positively to their school (and life) success.

School is a legitimate part of one's career. It is, in a sense, a full-time job, a time- and energy-absorbing endeavor that also becomes one's center for social relationships and recreation, as well as a place in which to prepare for future economic stability. Just as life can't be all work and no play, it can't be all scholarship and no socializing. Making friends and getting dates are avowed goals of many students, but they may be harder to accomplish when one has a disability. Deaf students may find others' desires to include them in social discourse waning as the effort required becomes evident; blind students may be as unseen as they are unseeing. Physically disabled students may fare better in the long run, but only if they are able to reduce others' anxiety over someone who looks markedly different.

A tendency exists for disabled students—like ethnic minority students—to group together, focusing on their visible core of shared experience. Special service programs may inadvertently or intentionally reinforce this by establishing social functions that prove to be of interest only to disabled students. This is especially true in schools that have set aside special housing for disabled students needing attendant care. A tight in-group camaraderie may develop, but social intercourse outside of the group may be inhibited. Although facilitation of relationships with other disabled students is a positive contribution, the lack of impetus toward building social contact with the nondisabled majority seems to detract from the overall social gains that could be made in school.

Thus, segregation of disabled from nondisabled students sometimes develops even in an integrated setting. Other disabled individuals do all or part of their vocational training in explicitly segregated settings established for the purpose of preparing disabled workers for jobs. These settings are referred to generically as "work preparation programs," and they exist primarily in rehabilitation hospitals and centers and in work-oriented rehabilitation facilities.

Work Preparation Programs

This genre of training does far more than impart the skills and knowledge necessary for performing jobs. Work evaluation, work adjustment, and job placement are as integral to these programs as skill training per se, and oftentimes moreso. They are oriented to disabled people with serious and multiple barriers to employment that stem not only from the nature and severity of their disabilities but from other factors as well. Some of these include histories of being overprotected or neglected, lack of prior work experience, educational deprivation, and behavioral aberrations that could make it difficult for them to succeed on a mainstream trade-school or college campus or in the world of work. As ample testimonials by grateful clients attest, some of these programs do excellent jobs of preparing their multiply handicapped clients for work. Individuals who have failed in mainstream work settings or to qualify as feasible for service by the state-federal vocational rehabilitation program have obtained the remedial help they needed to take the next step from private sector workshops. Such facilities are used extensively by counselors in the state programs when work evaluation, work adjustment, and specialized job placement measures are needed.

At the same time, the very nature of these settings creates certain problems for both the clients who use them and referring counselors as well. Many work preparation programs exist within "sheltered workshop" settings, using actual contract work as the vehicle for work evaluation, work adjustment, and training. Ten Broek (Nelson, 1971) labeled this practice a "dubious duality," and both he and others question whether clients' rehabilitation needs take first or second place compared with the workshop's business needs to meet production demands.

The differing missions of a workshop's production and rehabilitation staffs sometimes create additional problems for clients, especially when communication between the two is less than ideal. An example is drawn from a hospital-based workshop that was the subject of an evaluation research project (Kemp, 1973). Analysis of client surveys taken during their program participation revealed that the longer they stayed in the workshop the less they perceived the production staff as liking and respecting them. When this finding was shared with the production staff, it was discovered that they viewed their job as ending with the initial work evaluation. They did not conceptually grasp the longer-term process of work adjustment; thus, they did not understand why the rehabilitation staff left the clients in the program after their initial reports were completed. Moreover, they never really had "heard" what the rehabilitation staff wanted when they prescribed specific behavior modification strategies.

As a result of the clarification that the research project stimulated, a reevaluation several months later showed that client perceptions of production staff caring and esteem for them no longer declined over time. There probably is no way to circumvent trial-and-error learning in the human service arts; however, it is important to stay attuned to the effects error phases can have on disabled clients.

Referring counselors who use work preparation programs lament that the level of work available is so low as to be "dehumanizing." They question whether their clients' motivation for work can be realistically tested on work that is, to them, intrinsically boring. Naturally, their opinions on this issue have been shaped, in part, by complaints from their clients about the repetitive and unchallenging nature of the work they perform during work evaluation and adjustment, and its apparent irrelevance to their vocational goals. Reassurance that work habits can be assessed and improved regardless of the type of work used in the process does not satisfy either the clients or their referring counselors.

Finally, problems emerge from the fact that workshops generally serve a dual function. They offer work preparation services for clients who will go on to complete their training, and eventually to work, in different settings. They also offer long-term employment opportunities for people whose vocational handicaps are severe enough to preclude their getting jobs outside of sheltered workshop environments. More capable clients sometimes are frightened or angered at being placed alongside such extremely limited workers. They wonder if they are seen as like individuals by the professionals who referred both to the same setting, and they want to escape quickly from such an unwelcome confrontation. Those who are more philosophically mature can come to understand how a single facility could serve disparate populations. Those with less self-confidence may refuse to return.

An Answer: Workshops without Walls

On-the-job training is a well-established concept; "workshops without walls" extends it to more fundamental rehabilitation processes. The term refers to the growing trend to use mainstream industry as the setting for work evaluation and adjustment as well as training, instead of using rehabilitation facilities. The reasons are several. First, greater diversity of both types and levels of work can be secured. Second, it eliminates some of the guesswork in predicting how clients will fare in mainstream jobs after being tested and trained in settings that are, at best, simulations of the ordinary world of work. Third, just as well-publicized findings have shown that standardized tests predict job performance poorly for ethnic minority job applicants, experience suggests this is also the case for disabled employment seekers. Consequently, actual job performance sampling has been cited as the best predictor for both groups, and the workshops-without-walls approach is becoming an important means for obtaining it. Fourth, it aids placement efforts because employers get to know disabled workers through the relatively nonthreatening, noncommitted evaluation and training processes, thereby becoming less resistant to hiring them.

This trend yields an additional boon for disabled people: the opportunity to enter into the mainstream of occupational life at a much earlier point in time. Months or even years of segregated rehabilitation and work preparation may be eliminated, and social relationships with nondisabled coworkers can begin. The trauma of leaving the protective school or rehabilitation environment and facing the proverbial "cold cruel world" is lessened by a process that allows it to happen more gradually. Realistically, though, it will be somewhat traumatizing nonetheless. Relatively few will be so fortunate as to be hired by the same firm that provided work preparation. New decisions will have to be made and actions taken, touching such "old" issues as occupational choice and the risking of welfare security, plus new issues such as high unemployment rates.

Getting a Job

When the work evaluation, work adjustment, and skill training or college all are completed, many disabled workers will have to face again the important question of whether it makes economic sense to take a job. Individuals requiring full-time attendant care know that even a small salary will disqualify them for both their cash grant and attendant-care benefits after a short trial work period, yet it will not provide enough income to supplant these losses. Elsa describes the situation in which she found herself:

I've been on SSI since it came into being, and was on ATD [Aid to the Totally Disabled] before that. I need a live-in attendant and a weekend relief person, and their salaries mount right up. I went off to college and got a bachelor's degree in "human services" and was offered a job at a hospital where I used to be a patient. The starting salary was $14,000. That sounds okay to most people, but over $10,000 of that has to go to my attendants! My annual "income" from SSI and Medicaid was over $18,000. I couldn't afford to take a job that paid less because there's no way I can cut my expenses.

For me, the solution was to stay on SSI and go ahead and do the job as a volunteer. I still work a 40 hour week, it's just that I get paid by welfare instead of the hospital. I don't like it—getting off welfare really was a big thing for me—but I have no choice. It's better than sitting around doing nothing, which a lot of people in the same situation end up doing.

The matter of occupational choice also may arise again for the distressing reason cited earlier: the training selected proves to have been ill-chosen. A new vocational goal must be decided upon, requiring reevaluation of work-related strengths and experiences and grasping at whatever the labor market offers. When nothing is found, the decision may be to go back to school and get trained in a more appropriate area.

Support and survival systems may have to be reevaluated, too, especially for those who are severely disabled. Arising time may be even earlier than it was during training, and new transportation arrangements may have to be made. Transportation may be particularly difficult during job search, when times and destinations vary daily. Whether or not the individual needs help with basic functions, the process of job search promises to be a taxing one.

Job Search

More often than it happens for nondisabled job seekers, people with disabilities may have one or more professional experts coaching them on effective methods of job search and encouraging them to follow through. This may be another "secondary gain" of disability, since having guidance and moral support during what is destined to include a series of failures is fully worthy of envy. These supports are needed more by disabled people because of the reluctance of many employers to hire qualified workers simply because disabilities are unknown quantities that somehow make them nervous.

The quality of support offered by job-placement programs varies. Counselors in state vocational rehabilitation agencies are renowned for their dislike of doing job placement. Accordingly, many offer impoverished services, enjoining their clients to conduct their own job searches and rationalizing that such is the correct way to foster client independence. Others may contract out the job-placement process to specialty programs offering it as part of a package deal including work evaluation, adjustment, and training. On occasion, placement may be the only service really wanted, but regulations bar contracting it out unless it happens to be included with other, purchasable services. The bemused client may sense that needed help is not being given, or that inordinate time is being spent in questionably useful procedures, but most will accept these conditions as part of a mystique they simply don't understand.

The quality of specialty programs also varies, and sometimes an approach that wins a favorable reputation with one group of clients will prove, too late, to be altogether wrong for another. For example, a highly stimulating group-placement technique was conducted by a charismatic leader imparting an evangelical quality to his exhortations before assemblies of job-seeking clients. His approach attracted wide attention for its success in getting "hard-core unemployed" men into jobs. "Digging for gold"—in their work histories, avocational histories, and personal life histories—was a key element. Equally important was the leader's energizing, motivating effect; clients became infused with enthusiasm for job search and held high expectations for success. When the technique was used with a group of severely disabled state vocational rehabilitation agency clients, it backfired. In over half of the participants, enthusiasm turned to disappointment and, for a few, to serious depression when the expectations were not met. These casualties resulted from two major factors: (1) the clients' limitations were far greater than those of the previous client groups served and (2) an essential ingredient—supportive group counseling to combat the draining effects of job-search failures—had inadvertently been overlooked by the agency.

In short, it seems that services rendered in the employment area are sometimes part of the problem from the disabled person's point of view. Quality is apt to vary more among individual providers within an agency than among the agencies themselves, rendering it highly unpredictable. Happily, recent social changes are easing the problem somewhat. The emergence of protective laws during the 1970s is proving to be a significant aid in the 1980s to disabled people and professionals who try to help them get jobs. Equal employment opportunity laws will be discussed in Chapter 9. Here, let us look at an extremely important area these laws have influenced: methods of employee selection used by hiring authorities in both the public and private sectors.

The Selection Process

Once a disabled worker has been evaluated, counseled, adjusted, trained, and put in touch with a prospective job, a new set of problems may begin. Individuals who are fully competent to meet the demands of a job may be less able, or *unable*, to complete the job-screening process successfully. For example, upper-extremity-impaired applicants may be unable to turn pages and mark answers rapidly on timed tests; deaf applicants may not understand oral instructions or be able to interview without an interpreter; blind applicants cannot take written tests if they are unavailable on tape or in Braille. In other words, certain artifacts of the testing procedure may call for performance capabilities that are not required by the target job. The frustration and anxiety generated by this can undermine test performance further.

With the advent of affirmative action programs for disabled workers, efforts are being made to increase the fairness of testing methods for affected populations. For example, the United States Civil Service Commission has waived, for a number of years, written testing for mentally retarded applicants for selected federal jobs. In addition, Section 501 of the 1973 Rehabilitation Act now requires them to make annual reports to Congress of their progress in hiring disabled workers. The 1975 report cited such specific accomplishments as (1) making tests for blind competitors available in large type, Braille, or tape; (2) granting the use of an abacus or arithmetic slate; (3) emphasizing clarity of expression in tests for deaf competitors; (4) encouraging the use of interpreters; and (5) deleting test content inappropriate to blind or deaf competitors.

Still almost universally neglected are dyslectics. At the time of this writing, no systematic efforts to resolve the problems written testing presents to this group are known. Selection-procedure barriers are beginning to come down for most other disability populations, however, giving them a far better chance to experience what it is like to *do* a job.

Doing a Job, Keeping It, and Advancing

From a psychological point of view, one of the most important aspects of doing a job is *where* you do it. What kind of work setting is it? Such issues as the industry; its size, location, personnel policies, and work conditions; its organizational climate; and other factors too numerous to mention all play roles in determining whether the quality of work life for employees will be good or bad and for whom. In addition to these usual variables, two others become critical when the workers in question have disabilities. These are (1) the extent to which the work setting is integrated into the mainstream world of work and (2) the extent to which disabled workers are sheltered, as opposed to accommodated.

"Shelter" is the word traditionally used to denote ways in which job situations are allowed to conform to the needs of workers with disabilities. However, the last decade has seen growing discussion about such phenomena as the four-day work week, flex-time, job sharing, and job-site child-care facilities. These are ways in which job situations can be altered to conform to worker needs not necessarily related to disability. Often, they relate to parental obligations. In such cases, we don't speak of shelter, we generally use the term "accommodation." This is an era in which many aspects of jobs are being modified to meet the needs of workers, rather than forcing them to make all of the necessary adjustments. Providing accommodations needed by disabled workers is only one facet of this. The term "shelter," then, is reserved for cases in which some degree of reduced production quantity or quality, or inappropriate work behavior, is tolerated. Thus, *accommodation* is something an employer offers selected employees to enable them to produce up to standard, whereas *shelter* is something the employer provides for selected employees who are unable to meet the standards.

Figure 1 depicts an ascending scale of increasing integration into the mainstream world of work, coupled with decreasing accommodation or shelter. The term "homebased" is used as an alternative to "homebound" because it has been found that when homebound individuals are given the opportunity to do work in their homes, this often enables them to break their former ties to home and enter the mainstream world of work, or at least a sheltered workshop. The opposite of mainstream employment is "segregated employment" in a separate, specialized, sheltered workshop where most of one's coworkers also are disabled. The exceptions are generally management and rehabilitation staff, plus a few nondisabled workers hired to do heavy or complex work that staff believe disabled workers could not do.

A step up from segregated employment is called "semi-integrated employment" here. The blind-operated food-service stands and cafeterias in

Figure 1.   *Levels of Employment*

V	Competitive employment: no disability-related accommodation
IV	Fully integrated employment in mainstream industry: some disability-related accommodation
III	Employment in semi-integrated units in mainstream industry: significant disability-related accommodation, some shelter
II	Employment in segregated workplace hiring predominantly disabled workers: the prototypic *sheltered workshop*
I	Homebound or homebased employment

Reprinted from Caroyn Vash, 1980. "Sheltered Industrial Employment," In Pan et al., eds., *Annual Review of Rehabilitation* (New York: Springer, 1980), p. 82.

public buildings offer a familiar example of this. The workers in these concessions come to work in the same plant as the mainstream of workers, allowing for familiarizing contact and socialization between them, even though they are not integrated into the same work force. Also, buffer-zone enclaves in manufacturing industries are becoming a more frequent example. In these, disabled workers may receive work evaluation, work adjustment, and training, as well as actual work supervision by rehabilitation and plant personnel. "Fully integrated employment" is close to what is referred to as "competitive employment," but accommodations, sometimes costly and extensive ones, may have been made to enable the disabled worker to function adequately.

It often turns out that certain accommodations are needed only initially, while a disabled worker resolves transportation, attendant care, and other survival system problems. Once these systems are in place, such accommodations as flex-time may no longer be needed. Unfortunately, job applicants needing flexibility in personnel policies are likely to get the gates slammed in their faces because hiring authorities cannot envision the temporariness of the special needs.

With some exceptions, disabled people prefer to work in mainstream settings and regard sheltered workshops as sorely lacking in prestige. In addition to the favorable new laws, regulations, and policies that currently are advancing such opportunities, a relatively new professional discipline is virtually working miracles. Rehabilitation engineering is opening up thousands of mainstream career possibilities for disabled workers, even when their functional limitations are very severe.

Job Performance Problems: Technological Solutions

Disabled people now are entering occupational fields heretofore undreamed of because technology has generated solutions to job-performance problems created by their disabilities. Moreover, this revolution appears to have only begun. Just as the widespread use of motorized wheelchairs inaugurated an era of increased independence and expectation for one group of disabled people (see Chapter 3), other applications of technology have vastly improved the functional capabilities and quality of life for people with nearly every type of bodily disability. Many serious problems, encountered in activities of daily living, communication, transportation, homemaking, recreation, and, of course, meeting the demands of jobs, are melting under the torch of twentieth-century technology. We now have calculators that speak answers to blind users, machines that use air currents to separate materials for people with poor coordination, miniaturized teletypewriters for deaf individuals, and a seemingly endless array of both more and less esoteric devices. Disabled people are reaping spin-off gains from the space and defense industries; in fact, they are becoming, in the opinion of some, their primary beneficiaries.

Sensory aids for the visually- and hearing-impaired and mobility aids for motorically-impaired workers are proliferating under the relatively generous federal funding of rehabilitation engineering centers, and information about their accomplishments is beginning to be disseminated systematically to consumers and professionals. As a result, the psychological well-being of multitudes of disabled people is being enhanced, not by psychological methods, but by sophisticated modifications of their physical world and capabilities. In effect, technological substitutions for absent sensory and motor capacities are restoring occupational options previously considered lost to those with given disabilities. This allows them access to higher-level and more interesting kinds of work.

Quality of Work Life

Until fairly recently, disabled people were considered lucky to get any job at all. Intrinsically interesting work offering opportunities for career advancement was beyond expectation. Rather than focusing on resolving this dilemma, the more frequent course taken was to cite work-life research findings that the same is true for many nondisabled workers as well. In the past decade, however, grant funding has been directed toward research on the quality of work life. With the concurrent impetus of the civil rights movement for people with disabilities, attention finally is being paid to work as a source of life satisfaction for disabled people, as well as a means for reducing the size of the welfare rolls.

Welfare recipients of any kind seldom find agency workers highly motivated to help them locate gratifying work. The workers appear to reflect the taxpayers' attitude that recipients are obligated to accept any available job and have little right to be choosy. In some agencies, the workers themselves have not found satisfying work and cannot envision it for their clients. In others, it may be an outgrowth of pressures to accumulate high numbers of job placements with little official concern for their quality. Whatever the reasons, it has required social pressure from consumers and other advocates to initiate changes in entrenched operating philosophy. The technological developments described previously also have contributed significantly by making more intrinsically rewarding fields feasible.

Increasing numbers of special projects are being funded to encourage disabled people to enter the fields of technology and science. A few even encourage disabled artists to pursue their painting, acting, writing, or other creative expression, but artists are not as generously supported in this country as scientists are. The emergence of consumer-run independent living programs and affirmative hiring of disabled people in rehabilitation organizations is opening up professional and management options. Service agencies are developing better methods for helping clients with entrepreneurial interests and talent to establish independent businesses. Since time immemorial, the secondary labor market has been the primary work resource for disabled people. (The secondary labor market consists of undesirable jobs that no one but the desperate want. They disappear in times of economic crisis and when they exist they offer minimal salary, no fringe benefits, no security, poor working conditions, no inherent rewards, and no opportunities for advancement.) Now, at last, its mindless use is going out of style.

Since work occupies fully half of our waking lives, it seems only reasonable to expect it to be an important avenue through which we learn to be, do, and get what we want from life. Most of us have these three types of goals. We want to *get* specific materialistic rewards, such as homes, cars, adult play toys, and so forth. We also want to *do* identified activities, either for the pleasure of the process, the outcome, or both. And we want to *be* a certain way, viewed by ourselves or others as good or honest or tough or whatever characteristics are deemed desirable. Disabled workers have little chance of reaching these goals through their work, or at all, if they are relegated to traditional or conveniently available jobs. They may eat, pay the rent, buy a few clothes, and successfully avoid returning to the welfare office, but a quality work life entails much, much more.

As the theoretical basis for the Strong-Campbell Vocational Interest Inventory reveals, a crucial part of job satisfaction is working with and around compatible people. More than this, work provides the major avenue for many people to form friendships; thus, people working in areas suited to their temperaments are more likely to find coworkers with whom they will want off-the-job social and recreational contacts. Friendship and recreation are the subjects of the following chapter, but before turning to them, there is a last, brief point about employment opportunities for disabled people to be made.

The Last Discrimination

As reported earlier (Vash, 1980), the fact that disabled people are unabashedly discriminated against with respect to participating in the federally funded military services has long been an irritant to the author's system. Consumer groups are not clamoring for their rights to be inducted for both obvious and not-so-obvious reasons. Some disabled people, specifically young men during wartime, figure being 4-F is one of the few benefits of disability. Most, however, don't realize the magnitude of benefits they are giving up by maintaining this protected status.

The author recalls an abortive attempt to discuss this issue with a recruiting officer during a television program on which they both were guests. The officer nearly exploded and the moderator quickly changed the subject, since the author obviously had lost her reason by suggesting that severely disabled people may have not only a responsibility but an inalienable right to serve their country. Recalling this, she asked Dean Phillips, then President of Goodwill Industries of America, what he thought about the issue. For a moment he was silent. Then he cocked his head to one side and spoke:

> Well, you kind of got me there. I just hadn't thought of it. Why of course disabled people should have the opportunities military service provides! The Marine Corps is the only branch that requires everyone to be combat-ready at all times, so disabled people ought to be inductible into every other branch. The opportunities for trade training and the many benefits of veteran status should certainly be available to disabled citizens. The Peace Corps and VISTA are alternatives, but they don't offer anything comparable to the fringe benefits of military service . . . complete health care for self and family, lodging, meals for self, cheap/convenient supplies for self and family, experience, and salary, plus the whole host of benefits that accrue to the veteran, whether from peace or wartime. [Vash, 1980, P. 116]

Most military occupational specialties have civilian counterparts, and most civilian jobs can be done by people with disabilities. If a paraplegic, say, can do a clerical job in the civilian sector, there is no reason why s/he cannot do it in the military; therefore, s/he should have the opportunity to reap the benefits like anyone else. So far, the efforts of Phillips and others to meet with the Vice-President of the United States on this issue have proved fruitless.

7 Playing

Friendship and Recreation

In view of the fact that almost no one claims to know exactly what "play" is, there is remarkable agreement that it is necessary for optimal human functioning and happiness. Such well-worn clichés as "All work and no play makes Jack a dull boy" attest to its importance in the psychic economy. John Nesbitt (1979) delineates "four R's" that he believes play fulfills in the lives of both children and adults: *recovery* from the rigors of working and learning; *relaxation*; *reward* for work (school) performance; and *renewal* for returning to such responsibilities. He points out that the reward function also may be seen as the satisfaction and fulfillment that issue directly from one's chosen play activities. Very simply, play may be what you choose to do because it feels good rather than what you have to do to survive. At the same time, Nesbitt and others observe that it also can make survival-related activities less arduous and more effective.

This dual nature of play—as a source of primary gratification and an enhancer of success in survival-related activities—means that it serves different functions for different individuals. People devoted to their work, domestic, or scholastic pursuits may use it primarily for recovery, relaxation, and/or renewal; whereas those who are bored with their jobs may use it as their primary source of reward in life. Either way, because of social and economic changes that are occurring, play—or leisure time—is becoming more sharply focused in the thinking of today's society than has been true in the past. The work day and the work week are shortening; retired workers are living longer; automation and high unemployment rates thrust leisure time on some whether or not they want it; television displays exotic forms of play in which others engage; and affluence makes emulation possible.

As usual, the disabled population has been largely left out of the social planning for use of leisure time, at least until recently. Museums, parks, and other recreation areas have been built for years with no regard to their usability by people with disabilities. Now, with the advent of disability-related civil rights laws and improved social consciousness about disability, efforts are being made to correct the errors in physical facility and program design. Recreation therapy has emerged as a new rehabilitation discipline; and both the primary and spin-off values of avocational pursuits are receiving rapidly escalating attention. Some of the developments, as well as remaining gaps, in recreational opportunities for people with disabilities will be described in this chapter. First, however, let us look at a topic concerning play that is still receiving almost no attention.

Friendship

Friendship ties receive very little emphasis in this culture, compared with others. To cite an extreme example, certain African tribes have ceremonies as elaborate as marriage rituals to solemnize primary friendship bonds. In Mexico, the ties to one's chosen compadre or comadre are enduring and strong. History tells us that Native Americans have long ritualized "brotherhood" bonding by an exchange of blood; it is a deeply felt friendship commitment made with solemn reserve. Today, the formal celebration of friendship ties in the dominant culture grows ever less frequent. Antique jewelry stores display the "friendship links" of a bygone era; friendship rings are exchanged still, but primarily during fads of decreasing frequency and duration. It is not just the ritualization that is passing; with increasing geographic mobility, friendships become as disposable as consumer products. At the same time, the honorifics "brother" or "sister" are bestowed casually on strangers with little part in the users' lives. Many people enjoy remarkable friendships, but the trend described is nonetheless real. Acquaintanceships proliferate with increased social and physical mobility, but committed friendships may not survive socioeconomic or geographic separation.

This trend is particularly disadvantageous to disabled people for several reasons. First, friendship bonds are often more important to unmarried people than those with spouses and children to fulfill their needs for companionship, love, and interpersonal interaction; and a large segment of disabled people spend a significant part of their adult lives unmarried. Second, people who are not socially or physically mobile miss opportunities to form acquaintanceships that meet some interpersonal needs; and disabled people often lack mobility. Third, friendship ties are particularly important to people who might be termed "social underdogs" because of the extraordinary practical and moral-support needs their devalued status generates; and disabled people are unquestionably social underdogs.

The foregoing illustrates several different functions that friendships fulfill. Friends are more than partners in play; they also figure importantly in meeting one's needs to love and be loved and to have practical and emotional support. Thus, friendships, like marriages, can be characterized or "typed" according to the needs being met and the interactive styles used to meet them. Let us next look at some of the effects of disablement on friendship patterns and satisfactions.

Old Friendships; New Disability

Here we will consider the interaction between disablement and friendships established prior to its occurrence. Naturally, the viability of such relationships will depend largely on their nature and solidity before being subjected to such a test. This is important because friends can be crucial to the adjustment process, lending—or failing to lend—practical and emotional support during the acute, postacute, and rehabilitation phases.

It is difficult to assess the importance of popularity. An individual's ability to develop a wide circle of friends and admirers may prove to be invaluable in some instances; whereas only one or two devoted friends may be equally helpful in others. Clearly, however, an attractive, magnetic personality will elicit more concern and desire to help. An individual's involvement in a large friendship group (usually tied to organizational affiliation, such as a church, school, or club) may have especially positive implications for group-motivated support efforts.

Despite the reported trend away from the centrality of friendship in many people's lives, instances are known wherein friends have given heroic aid to recently disabled individuals. One such case was described by a rehabilitation nurse as follows:

> Ed had just passed the bar exam when he became a C-4 quadriplegic in a car accident. He and his wife had many friends, but one couple was particularly close. They left their jobs, moved to [the town where the rehabilitation hospital is located] and rented a house nearby so Ed's wife could stay with them and Ed would have a place to go home to on weekends.

Far less extreme measures of friendship than this can also be vitally important. It is amazing how many disabled people would not part with their collections of get-well cards, years or even decades after their illnesses or injuries. Families need help and support from their friends, too. Kevin pointed out that his mother particularly needed a friend who could confront her with the pitfalls of "self-sacrifice." Others simply need help with the shopping, a small loan, or a shoulder to cry on. Hayman (1975; see Chapter 1) described the demoralizing effect that the gradual disappearance of hospital visitors can have on a newly disabled person.

This raises the specter of the impact of institutionalization on existing friendships. Unquestionably, people who are catastrophically ill or injured must be hospitalized while their conditions are acute. After that, controversy exists with respect to the wisdom of extended hospitalization for long-term rehabilitation in centers remote from home, family, and friends. The disabled rehabilitation hospital staff member quoted earlier had this to say:

> The medical director here once announced at a teaching conference that I was a sterling example of what rehabilitation could do, and then asked me where I got my rehabilitation. I said I was sent home as soon as I could leave the communicable disease ward (I had polio) and was never sent away for rehabilitation. The county health department sent a physical therapist to my house daily, then weekly, then monthly, for over a year, and that's all the rehab I got. I feel I was lucky there was no rehab center I could be sent to, because I never got out of the social swing with the kids at school. They simply moved all club meetings to my house and dropped by every day on their way home from school. As soon as I could be up in a wheelchair, I got pushed to all the extracurricular functions, and when I could go out in a car, I was dated up right away. I felt "unique" and "special," not "different" in a devaluated sort of way. True, I didn't learn to be as physically independent as I would have in a rehab center, but I learned that later when the need arose. If I am a "sterling example," I think a lot of it is due to the fact that I wasn't wrenched away from my friends at that critical stage in my social development.

This puts into new perspective the relative importance of gaining functional skills versus maintaining emotional and psychosocial equilibrium at different stages of the rehabilitation process. Resolving the problem is not easy. The major effort has been to create more, smaller rehabilitation centers located nearer to residential communities as an alternative to large ones serving widespread geographic regions. The cost today of the amount and quality of home care this staff member enjoyed probably precludes returning to her ideal solution.

After the newness of the disability experience wears off, both for the disabled person and his or her friends, what is likely to happen to friendships formed before one party became functionally impaired? The answer depends largely on the nature of the relationships and their potential for adapting to changed circumstance.

"Being" versus "Doing" Relationships

As it is true for marriages, friendships can be characterized as based on intimacy or parallel play. An intimate friendship is a form of "being" relationship; a parallel-play friendship is a form of "doing" relationship. The terms are almost self-explanatory, but some elaboration may be useful. People involved in "doing" relationships simply enjoy doing the same activities together. Not all "doing" relationships are parallel play; there may be central and considerable interaction between the friends. People involved in "being" relationships enjoy being together, communing or communicating, sharing feelings and ideas, or simply feeling good because of the presence of the other. The degree of intimacy may vary. "Being" and "doing" relationships are in no way mutually exclusive; in fact, most relationships combine both aspects but have one that is predominant.

A friendship that is predominantly a "being" relationship is apt to be little affected by the functional losses resulting from disability. Poor tolerance, on the part of either friend, of emotions stimulated by the disability may strain or disrupt it, but seldom will the disability itself. A friendship that is predominantly a "doing" relationship may be in serious jeopardy no matter how well disability-related emotions are handled, if the shared activities cannot be resumed or replaced by new or modified ones. Sometimes a friendship that entails a great deal of conjoint playing actually has a strong basis for intimacy and sharing on a feeling or ideational level that was masked or overridden by activity. Such relationships have good potential for enduring and deepening after their active play aspect is interrupted. Just as work can be play for people who enjoy the process as much as the outcome, so can feeling and idea sharing be relaxing, renewing, and rewarding. Naturally, many "doing" relationships endure simply because the modality impaired has little relevance to the shared activities. For example, concert goers can continue to enjoy each other after one becomes blind; chess players can go on with their games whether or not one begins to use a wheelchair.

Friendships help people avoid loneliness, whether by connecting with another at an intimate level or by filling time and consciousness with activities and absorptions. The styles differ, but the goals may be much the same. For anyone, the dread of being alone may stem partly from a failure to distinguish solitude—which can be richly rewarding—from that state of deprivation labeled "loneliness." But whatever the genesis, people with disabilities, like people who have grown old, frequently express dismay over the extent to which they find themselves alone.

Either kind of friendship can alleviate the immediate need for human interaction, but certain types of "being" relationships can help people learn to enjoy their solitude, themselves *by* themselves, as well. Friends such as these may be thought of as teachers, guides, counselors, or gurus, or their beneficent influence may go consciously unnoticed. At other times, both friends see these qualities in each other. Such friendships may be "made in heaven" and as rare as the individuals who reach high levels of personal development. Nonetheless, numerous disabled people report life-changing experiences facilitated by friendships with highly evolved personalities. Carol, for example, declares of her friend Kate,

> She helped me see that it's okay to just *be*; I didn't have to do, accomplish, act, achieve all the time. At first, when she talked about how she treasures her

alone time, I didn't even know what the devil she was talking about. But somehow, I learned from her all about just being, enjoying solitude, and enjoying the time I *do* spend with others even more . . . they are all interrelated. My block was fearing to be alone because of my physical dependency, yet longing for it and not recognizing that fact. She saw it all right away. Actually, the best thing she did for me was like me. I thought she was so fantastic that if she picked me for a friend, I had to be okay . . . any friend of hers is a friend of mine . . . even me!

This last remark may encapsulate the core meaning of friendship, but the description also shows that friendships can assume the quality of a counseling relationship that supercedes commonplace supportive listening, validation of ideas and feelings, and advice giving. A friendship that stresses mutual counseling support (cocounseling) is one form of symbiotic relationship.

Symbiotic Relationships

Such friendships (or marriages) are sometimes considered alternatives to intimacy—which may be accurate—but symbiosis also can coexist with intimacy. All that is required is for the relationship to serve certain practical purposes as well as provide pleasurable human exchange. When friends serve as each others' confidants, sounding boards, advisors, or counselors, this can reasonably be viewed as a form of symbiosis. Without such informal "services," either or both might find it necessary to seek, and pay for, professional help.

Cocounseling is a method used by numerous professional counselors (psychologists, psychiatrists, social workers, and others) who need or want professional assistance or "training therapy" but are unwilling or unable to pay for it. Therefore, they team up for cocounseling, each serving as counselor to the other in separately designated time periods. They "pay" for the counseling they receive by providing counseling to the other—a uniquely modern sort of barter system. Many friendships, whether or not they involve professional counselors, entail at least a component of cocounseling. The techniques used may lack sophistication, and the time separation between providing and receiving may be less formalized, but the counseling function is central to the relationship nonetheless.

Along with growing awareness of the value of "peer counseling" for people with disabilities, the counseling role of friendships is becoming more salient among disabled people. Informal friendships may begin as a result of formal peer counseling contacts, and established relationships may take on counseling aspects as their benefits come to be more widely advertised, legitimized, and personally experienced. It is important to keep in mind that symbiosis implies roughly equivalent give and take on both sides, but not necessarily identical. It is quite as likely that one friend will offer counseling in exchange for a different kind of support that is needed.

Programs designed to train paraprofessionals to work with disabled (or other service-needing) populations sometimes refer to their work as training students to form *helping friendships*. Perhaps when the public grows weary of sex manuals, the next interpersonal how-to-do-it fashion could focus on how to become a truly helpful friend who fosters growth and avoids reinforcing maladaptive tendencies. Disabled people who have been associated with independent living programs might be in the vanguard of such a movement. Because of the peer counseling emphasis in these programs, they now have headstarts in a direction that could benefit everyone, whether or not they have disabilities.

The "using" aspects of relationships are often overtly disdained, but nonetheless constitute a benefit of many friendships. Friends may have contacts useful for anything from quick, cheap appliance repair to landing prestigious jobs. Disabled people find it particularly desirable to develop friendships with their neighbors, people who will be close by in times of crisis. There is nothing inherently selfish about using friendships in such ways, assuming the friendly caring is authentic and the giving and taking are more or less balanced. When they are not, the friend with the deficit is likely to end the relationship.

Because it is not always obvious to the external observer who is getting what out of a relationship, it may be the apparent "taker" who ends up feeling drained. For example, nondisabled people with strong needs to be needed not infrequently attach themselves to disabled people who are, at first, grateful for their help. After awhile, however, the latter may find themselves emotionally exhausted by the subtle exaction of a price for all services—in such forms as patronization, solicitation of gratitude, and reminders of dependency. As was discussed relative to pairing (see Chapter 5), disabled people sometimes must be wary of friendship candidates who would help too much.

New Friendships; Old Disability

After one has grown used to having a disability, an eventual consideration is making new friends. "Will people still want to be friends with me now that I can't do many things or 'keep up' with them?" "Will they be uncomfortable around me?" Even apart from such deliberations, it is easy for people with disabilities—especially severe ones—to narrow their experiential worlds to the close and familiar. This is a fairly natural reaction to "stimulus overload," which is the prevailing condition when much of life is seen as new, unusual, demanding, or depressing. Such narrowing may include limiting one's associations and seeking to meet all interpersonal needs through parents, spouse, or children who will be part of one's world anyway. This avoids the addition of more sources of unwelcome stimulation. When disability is so severe as to inhibit mobility away from home, associations may be limited still further. The result is friendless individuals who place enormous demands on the family members they live with to meet all of their needs for companionship, needs that usually are distributed among a larger constellation of relatives and friends. A spouse, parent, or child may become virtually the person's only friend—a heavy burden for those who feel trapped by responsibility already.

Some disabled people resolve to associate only with other disabled individuals "who will understand." As indicated earlier (see Chapter 2), this may issue from self-derogation, a belief that one will not prove worthy to nondisabled friends. The act of making a resolution suggests a self-defensive maneuver, and this is most likely to be the case when it happens early in the adjustment process. Others, who have found themselves fully able to attract friends regardless of disability, simply may find that their firmest ties are to those who have shared the disability experience. This is more likely to be the result of need evolvement through learning, and reflects a positive choice, not a defense.

The kinds of people sought as friends always depend on where they are found, whether through school or work, at church, in clubs, or around the neighborhood. For the high proportion of disabled adults who are unemployed, a major source of friendship contacts is eliminated, even for those who have no desire to limit their associations. Fortunately, the consumer movement among disabled people has opened up alternative opportunities in recent years, through the burgeoning independent living centers and organizations "by and for the disabled." Although most of these have service and political action missions, they are proving to be a better resource for friendships than the "social clubs for the disabled" of an earlier era.

Now that rehabilitation and independent living programs are beginning to train disabled people in how to select and supervise their personal employees (attendants, interpreters, readers, and drivers), an issue that frequently arises is whether the relationship should remain strictly that of employer and employee, or if it also should be one of friendship. There is no simplistic answer. In every kind of work setting, people can be found who prefer to keep their work and social lives separate, as can others whose friends are almost solely work colleagues. Many employers socialize with peers, but believe it unwise to spend time with subordinates outside of work. Others forcefully disagree. In all cases, individual predilection is the key.

Some people can learn to play the dual roles of "boss" and "friend" effectively; others can't. Some fear the practice will lead to exploitation by the subordinate; others simply say they would be careful not to choose an exploitative person as a friend (or employee, if they have that choice). With respect to disabled people's personal employees, the issue is most salient with live-in attendants. Because the employment relationship is so much more intimate than with the typical live-in domestic worker, social distancing is less feasible. It seems the most satisfactory and enduring relationships do not lose the primacy of the employee–employer responsibilities, but are leavened with mutual caring and concern for the other's needs that could only be termed "friendship." Moreover, compatibility was usually given conscious consideration at the time of hiring.

There is an old saying: "From friendship to love, maybe; but from love to friendship, never!" Although modernized thinking is changing the accuracy of both clauses of this homily, disabled people especially find that the likelihood of "friendship to love" is more than a hesitant "maybe." Many report that most of their romances begin as friendships, contrary to their predisability patterns. The explanation appears simple. Visibly disabled individuals, no matter how physically attractive, are unlikely targets for the random dating efforts that go on in the singles community. They may, in fact, be seen by the nondisabled majority as sexless and therefore perhaps less threatening. While this might not be flattering to the disabled person thus regarded, it does facilitate cross-sex friendships. Once the individuals get to know each other, and the strangeness of the disability wears off, the "sexless" image is recognized as inaccurate and the spark of romance may ignite.

Regardless of the way in which a friendship develops, friends are widely thought of as people to do things with and who can share one's recreational interests. Let us next explore the topic of recreation—refreshment of body or mind through some form of play, whether pursued with friends, strangers, or alone—as it relates to people with disabilities.

Recreation

Almost every conceivable activity or pursuit can be construed as play or recreation by *someone*, however dull or terrifying or otherwise unpleasant it might seem to someone else. Nowhere is the cliché that "One man's dish is another man's poison" more descriptive. The person who relaxes, renews, and gains rewards from engraving the Lord's Prayer on the heads of pins is unlikely to enjoy a deep rapport with the one who prefers driving in demolition derbies. This is an important reason why friendship is such an integral aspect of the topic "playing."

To understand why certain recreational activities are attractive or unattractive to given individuals, it may be helpful to look at them in terms of the processes involved and their outcomes. With respect to process, such polarities as active–passive, physical–mental, delicate–expansive, formalized–spontaneous, and creative–fixed can be used to characterize them. The first two are self-explanatory. The engraver and derby driver just cited reflect the delicate–expansive polarity. Bridge is formalized; so is football. Fifty-two pick-up and catch are spontaneous. (Irrepressibly spontaneous players in formalized games are apt to be unappreciated by serious devotees to the rules in question.) The disco dancing of the 1970s ranged from highly creative to firmly fixed in the routines performed.

Outcomes can be described in terms of such qualities as their relative benefit to the individual or society, their potential for becoming vocations as well as avocations, and their "therapeutic" value. Perhaps, if the use of leisure time becomes a more critical societal concern, such process and outcome variables will be used for an "avocational interest inventory" to help people discern, with less trial and error, the types of recreations that will meet their needs best. This, of course, would overlook the possibility that the trial-and-error process is itself recreational. However, such an inventory might offer a different kind of help to disabled people needing information and guidance regarding feasible alternatives, particularly if it took into account the demands of various recreational activities for physical, sensory, and mental capabilities.

Few conclusions can be drawn, *prima facie*, about the kinds of recreations appropriate for disabled people. True, a high-level quadriplegic may lack options among "active, physical, expansive" activities, but paraplegic, spastic, blind, and other individuals who also are considered severely disabled can and do pursue vigorous and potentially dangerous pastimes. It is not unusual for those whose diversions seem incredible to the general public to appear in the news as inspirational examples to others. Ironically, this can have the opposite effect on disabled people whose motivation levels are more nearly normal but who nonetheless would like to identify hobbies or other leisure activities within grasp. At the other extreme, severely disabled people are apt to be encouraged to *try* to enjoy such "passive, mental, individual" recreations as art, music appreciation, or reading, despite protestations that they meet none of the person's felt needs.

Failing to find other sources of recreational gratification, some choose pastimes held in social disdain, such as the recreational use of alcohol and drugs, or television viewing taken to extreme. Both are renowned favorites among people with disabilities and are viewed as escape rather than renewal activity. This is an important reason for current efforts to open up more salutary outlets. This thrust combines advocacy with efforts to discover and educate disabled people about both traditional and new recreational possibilities.

Recreational Advocacy

In recreation, as in education and employment, mainstreaming has become an important issue. Activist groups all over the country are turning some of their attention to the wide range of indoor and outdoor recreational accommodations: museums, galleries, parks, amusement centers, beaches, forests, sports arenas, hiking trails, theaters, skating pavilions, boat harbors—the list is endless. They are requesting, sometimes demanding, that all public recreational accommodations be designed or modified so that artificial barriers to their use by disabled citizens will not eliminate recreational outlets that otherwise could be enjoyed.

The base-level demands are for (1) buildings and grounds that are accessible and safe for all disabled users and (2) user information available in forms accessible to communicatively-impaired users. Stairs, and failures to have guidebooks on tape as well as print medium, for example, are *artificial* barriers to the use of available programs. The next level of advocacy is for programmatic change toward inclusion of more recreational activities feasible for disabled people. If none of the planned activities can be done by a person who can't see or hear or walk or think quickly, accessible/safe facilities will be of little import. The third level of advocacy involves the reduction of *natural* barriers for designated populations. Tactile replica exhibits for blind people wishing to experience ancient artifacts that cannot be touched provides a prime example.

Changes are occurring slowly. As Sally's experience with the ice revue illustrated (see Chapter 2), some efforts to make mainstream recreational facilities accessible have resulted in intramural segregation, with disabled viewers being seated together, apart from their companions. Experience of this sort often leads to refinements, but the interim can be filled with disappointments and embarrassments. Now that government entities are creating advisory commissions of disabled citizens, recreation-related need information is reaching public policy setters, planners, and implementers through these channels. Thus, changes are coming about somewhat more quickly in the public than private sector. When an amusement area has historical significance, however, disabled citizens are apt to find themselves in political combat with the local historical society, which oftentimes values authenticity of style more than the rights of disabled people.

Not all recreational advocacy is aimed toward mainstreaming. Oddly enough, just as the concept of "special education" was losing favor, the parallel term "special recreation" was coming into vogue. The best-known examples of special recreation are the Paralympics, for physically disabled athletes, and the Special Olympics, for mentally retarded athletes. Despite the protestations of some who believe both should be integrated with the Olympics, most see these programs as offering invaluable experiences to disabled people with outstanding athletic prowess.

For others, special recreation centers are beginning to appear in which facility design and programming are specifically tailored to accommodate disabled participants. A pioneering example is the DC Therapeutic Recreation Center in Washington, D.C. Henderson (1979) describes it as "a thoughtfully designed complex constructed to be fully accessible for participants with many types of disabilities" (p. 20). He explains the architectural design features that accommodate without conflict wheelchair users and blind, mentally retarded, epileptic, and other disabled participants; and the varied programs, including physical recreation, arts and crafts, manual arts, home arts, performing arts, library, and leisure counseling. The role of the center in aiding transition to mainstream recreation is consistently stressed.

Perhaps, with time and experience, special recreation can go the way of special education: limited to an ever narrowing band of the population. It might even be that the Special Olympics and Paralympics one day will be integrated—or at least more closely combined—with the Olympics. Further advocacy will be required for any of this to occur. In addition, preparation for recreation is needed by many disabled people at various stages in the rehabilitation process.

Recreational Preparation

Because sports and recreation are so strongly associated in the American consciousness, nonathletically inclined individuals may ignore programs labeled "recreation," expecting them to be comprised of wheelchair basketball, bowling, archery, and little else. At one time, this was true of the author, who related to a recreation therapy symposium:

> Until I recognized the prevocational potential of recreation, I was never very interested in the field because I identified it with sports. When it comes to athletic prowess, disability helped me avoid a distressing source of embarrassment. In school, when team captains chose up sides, they fought over who was going to get stuck with me. The loser would tell me to go to the backfield and under no circumstances to touch the ball. I wouldn't have anyway. My unvarying reaction to having a ball thrown at me was to cringe and duck. I consider this a sensible reaction to this very day. Looking over the program for this symposium, however, one sees how much more than sports is entailed. There's music, dance, arts and crafts, drama, gourmet cooking, water play, puppetry—literally something for everyone. [Vash, 1978b]

Rehabilitation centers and hospitals have long included recreation programs for their patients, but their character has made a significant change in recent years. As recently as the 1960s, many still were oriented toward passive entertainment during institutionalization, the idea being to fill evening or weekend hours not taken up by medical, nursing, or therapy activities. By now, most programs have evolved into recreation preparation, emphasizing exposure to feasible alternatives and training in the constructive use of leisure time *after* returning to the community. "Recreation Departments" have become "Recreation *Therapy* Departments," reflecting the changed philosophy.

As noted earlier, recreational participation can serve as a powerful pre-vocational tool, especially for individuals whose vocational potential appears marginal to the evaluating professionals. Sometimes competencies can be discovered and developed in the less challenging milieu of a recreation program—from which there is no threat of "mustering out"—that later can be translated into a vocational plan. However, whether the intent of recreation is vocational or avocational, once the individual has returned to the community, there is likely to be little or no professional follow-up.

The initial physical rehabilitation stage is a little early for most newly disabled people to become seriously attuned to their recreational wants. They have higher priorities then, such as continuing relationships with their loved ones and, somewhat later, earning a living. When they *are* ready to explore recreational alternatives, there is seldom anyone around to help. Many will be involved with their state vocational rehabiitation (VR) agency during this stage, where, in the main, virtually no attention is paid to recreation. An outstanding exception exists in the state of Nevada, where the VR agency has an exemplary program centered on winter sports. Even there, however, the recreational development of clients lacking athletic interests is left largely to the unguided individual.

The primary mission of the consumer-run independent living programs can be construed as filling gaps created by the state–federal VR program in its efforts to move too directly toward the goal of vocational rehabilitation. When it became clear that vocational plans were being sabotaged by failures to attend to such "tangentially" related issues as community survival skills/resources and the psychological well-being of clients, funding support for the independent living centers began to flow. These centers are making some efforts to fill the recreation gap left by the VR agencies, but it is seldom a high priority for them, either. Issues more central to community survival (for example, financial advocacy, attendant recruitment, and transportation) tend to usurp the funds available. When a volunteer instructor is available, good recreational programs may take place. When the volunteer disappears, however, so does the program.

Sometimes what is needed is not so much preparation as instigation. This can be illustrated best by an additional passage from the author's previously-cited address to a recreation therapy symposium:

> Dance was an important part of my life before I became disabled. My sister was a dancer and tutored me from pre-school days. My unheroic career as an athlete became less painful in high school when modern dance was offered as a physical education option. When no one was throwing balls or hockey pucks at me, I did

okay. Since then, with two significant exceptions which I will share with you, the only "dancing" I've done is with men who are strong enough to carry me while leaping about a dance floor.

The first exception was at a party a dozen years ago where a woman instructed me, at inebriated length, on how to "dance" in a wheelchair by shaking my shoulders and torso to the music. I was having so much fun I almost missed seeing her march over to my date and beg to be carried, "like you do *her!*" Then her date asked me to dance. I make the usual gesture of someone expecting to be lifted, but instead he looped his belt through the arm rest of my chair and sent me spinning. Everyone got off the dance floor, including our respective dates. Mine almost dropped his. He had an uncanny knack for making a wheelchair with a ninety-pound load go where he wanted it to. This was purely passive on my part, but it was a lot of fun. The shoulder/torso dancing was active but, somehow, the disinhibition I needed for such a routine—and got from an instigator—hasn't happened again.

The second exception reinforced the important role of an instigator. While serving as a VR administrator, I visited an independent living center. A movement and dance group was going on and the director made clear that there would be no observers—only participants, including bureaucrats. The others had gait problems, poor coordination, or weakness, but I was the only wheelchair user present. Since it was motorized, I was the most mobile person there. I had a ball . . . creating routines that took advantage of both the chair's movement characteristics and my own. My lack of inhibition amazed even me, but, again, I had instigators: one said, "You must" and a dozen showed that *they* were game. [Vash, 1978b]

The motorized wheelchair is not the only rehabilitation engineering aid available for recreational purposes. The *Rehabilitation Engineering Sourcebook* (Institute for Information Studies, 1980) presents case examples illustrating the use of a broad range of recreation-related assistive devices and aids. Expositions of equipment for disabled individuals can be counted on to have large crowds around such items as the platform motorcycle for wheelchair users. In recreation, as in other aspects of life, technological advancement offers expanding means to enhance the quality of life, yielding more and more to discover.

Recreational Discovery

Most discovery of feasible and rewarding recreations comes about adventitiously. One hears about hobbies, sports, and games from associates and, occasionally, one of them "clicks." Recreational fads are common in the general population, and the same is true for specific disability groups, especially when popular pursuits prove feasible for people with given functional limitations. For example, ham-radio operation was a perennial favorite among people severely disabled by polio when that portended being homebound—as was frequently the case. Currently, trap/skeet shooting and radio-controlled model airplanes are enjoying prolonged vogues among wheelchair users with good arm function.

Not all recreations look like play on the surface. Volunteerism, for example, looks like work; however, if the individual is not being paid (and is not using volunteer work to expiate sins), the chances are that the intent is pleasure. It is very convenient for people with well-developed social consciences to be able to play and contribute to the social good at the same time. In addition to church, civic, political, and other traditional types of volunteer work, disabled people now have independent living programs and organizations "by and for the disabled" eager to receive their help. Membership in a group, and the opportunities for human contact and belongingness it provides, is often the prime motivator for doing volunteer work. Perhaps equally often, it offers a way to secure a sense of doing something worthwhile when one is not employed, or such satisfaction is not forthcoming from one's work. Because the unemployment rate for disabled adults continues to be exceedingly high, this is an especially important motivator for disabled volunteers. Disability-related advocacy also offers the promise of personal benefit.

Professional efforts to guide recreational discovery do not always happen within the confines of planned programs. A retired recreation therapist related to the author that his most rewarding venture in this respect occurred spontaneously, *after* a planned outing for severely disabled child-patients of a rehabilitation hospital. Passing a grassy slope on the return trip from an amusement park, one child murmured, "Wouldn't it be fun to roll down that hill?" On cue, the therapist stopped the bus and spent the next two hours wrapping disabled children in heavy sheets kept aboard the bus, rolling them down the hill, and returning them to the bus. A few weeks later, none of them had much to say about the official outing, but he reports that they never stopped talking about the hill rolling. He believes the rare opportunity for severely paralyzed youngsters to experience the kinesthetic pleasures of gross and rapid body movement was as therapeutic as it was enjoyable, and that such spontaneous adventures should be encouraged.

Sadly, he also reports that he "caught hell" from his supervisor for doing anything so risky, although not one child was hurt in any way. This brings to mind the well-known poster of a child wearing leg braces who is perched on the limb of a tree. The caption reads, "There is dignity in taking risks." This is an important reminder in general and is particularly applicable to recreation.

Guided discovery also is taking place within an exciting cluster of relative newcomers to the field of recreation: therapies based on the transcendental arts and a host of techniques imported from the Far East. Sometimes viewed as psychotherapy (or psychogogy, see Chapter 11) and at other times considered recreation, these approaches can be both, simultaneously. The transcendental arts therapies include such modalities as art therapy, music therapy, dance therapy, psychodrama, and poetry therapy. Their use is greatest with people who have emotional disabilities, but their potential for people with bodily disabilities is becoming appreciated. Dana illustrated the potential value of poetry therapy to her (see Chapter 1) and made the further observation that,

> Certain insights seem to fall out of your brain when you write poetry . . . as if the rhythm *pulls* them out, in a way that doesn't happen in reverie, conversation, or writing prose, however hard you are searching.

Yoga and the martial arts are being incorporated gradually into therapeutic recreation programs, too. Their practitioners cite their value as play, as well as their physical and mental health benefits. Martial-arts training for disabled people has the added value of reducing feelings of vulnerability. More will be said in Chapter 11 about this entire constellation of new techniques based on ancient arts, and their roles in psychological strengthening.

A number of disabled people who, by and large, did their own recreational discovery without professional guidance, are serving now as guides to others. Jim Brunotte is a familiar example: the horseman who lost both legs, an arm, and an eye in Vietnam and teaches equally disabled people to ride horses. Brunotte offers an outstanding example of instigation through role modeling. Less well-known is John Nelson (1975), who published a "guide and goad for the handicapped traveler" based on his own experience as a "wheelchair vagabond." These and other disabled people have found ways to have fun, as well as survive, and are sharing their methods with people newer to the process. They have, in a sense, *transcended* their disabilities—and this is the topic of the following chapter.

8 Transcending

Disability as Growth Experience

Acceptance of disability evolves gradually, for most people, over a span of years filled with instructive experience. It comes seldom, if ever, as a *coup de foudre* followed by getting on with life. Instead, the process of living teaches, little by little, that disablement needn't be viewed as an insurmountable tragedy. It may be only a complication or an irritant—and whose life is without those? As the struggles to survive, work, love, and play show evidence of some success, individuals find awareness of disablement slipping longer and oftener into the background of consciousness. Eventually, for some, it may come to be seen as a positive contributor to life in its totality—a catalyst to psychological growth. Since these changes take time, trial, error, and correction to unfold, forward movement does not always look like progress.

The initial chapters of this volume described the effects of devaluation on acceptance of disability and on reactions to disablement, especially in the early stages of adjustment. This chapter will augment those descriptions with a finer analysis of the lifelong process of acknowledging disability, physically, intellectually, emotionally, and spiritually. It also will pursue the process farther than usually is done, beyond the range of "normalization" to higher levels of self-actualization that are fostered by the disability experience.

Acknowledgment of Disability

Nancy Kerr, a psychologist who is paraplegic as a result of polio, describes five major stages in the process of adjusting to permanent disability: shock, expectancy of recovery, mourning, defense, and, finally, adjustment (Kerr, 1977). She hastens to point out that the stages are points on a continuum, not discrete categories, and that they describe common, but not inevitable, behavioral phases. During the shock stage, the individual has not really comprehended the fact that s/he is ill or disabled, so little anxiety is present. The realization that something is truly wrong is often accompanied by expectancy of recovery, including preoccupation with improvement of the disabling condition. There is no motivation for learning to live with the disability, however, since it is expected to vanish. When this does not transpire, mourning may follow. Acute distress, readiness to "give up," and thoughts of suicide are common. Reprimands for self-pity may engender hostility, and some resign themselves to their fates and remain at this stage indefinitely. Most others progress to the defense stage, characterized by coping efforts and interest in learning to be as normal as possible. Barriers are acknowledged and either conquered or circumvented. This is considered healthy defense. The defense stage is considered neurotic if the person employs defense mechanisms to deny that barriers exist. Kerr believes that reinforcement from others to "look on the bright side" and reprimands for sadness are conducive to the use of defensive denial. People who reach the adjustment stage no longer consider their disabilities as barriers to be fought, have found ways to satisfy their needs, and feel that they are adequate persons.

The Value of Denial

Different variants of denial are evident in the shock, expectancy of recovery, and defense stages. Traditionally, denial is viewed as maladaptive, but Kerr draws no such inferences respecting the shock and expectancy-of-recovery stages. Only when it appears later, in the defense stage, does she describe it as neurotic. Arnold Beisser, a psychiatrist who is quadriplegic as a result of polio, has discussed the adaptive value of denial in surviving myocardial infarction and other life-threatening conditions (Beisser, 1979). He indicates that the view of denial as a psychopathological sign of poor ego strength is fading as research supports its survival value, and he exhorts physicians to judiciously consider whether, when, and how to interrupt it. Most of his examples reflect the shock and expectancy-of-recovery stages; however, in all cases, the physician is enjoined to consider foremost the patient's psychic economy and at what expense to self s/he must adhere to a particular view.

The following account of personal experiences with denial illustrates its multiform nature as it evolves over time (Vash, 1977b).

> I became paralyzed over a matter of three or four hours. Until I finally collapsed, I simply refused to believe it was happening. I felt weak but not ill, and kept struggling out of bed to walk around and prove to myself that what seemed to be happening could not possibly be happening until I fell flat on my face—at which point I was more or less convinced, at least temporarily. That is plain, old-fashioned, *primitive denial*. The facts are there and you deny them admission to consciousness.

Wnen the doctor told me I'd had a slight case of polio, I breathed a sigh of relief. I'd read an article about how awful polio used to be until the Sister Kenny treatments, but now the main requirement was determination to do your exercises. As an erstwhile gymnast and dancer I wasn't afraid of exercises, so I figured in a few weeks I'd be fit as a fiddle again. That form of denial is called *selective attention*. You admit some of the data to consciousness, but not all of it—not the part that would be upsetting.

About three months later, when I'd gotten back some use of my left arm and hand but not much more, I hesitantly asked my physical therapist, "Hey! I don't mean to get worrisome about this but is there any chance that I might not get all better?" Her answer was classic: "Well, you hardly ever hear of a case that doesn't anymore." She belonged to the school that professed, "Give them an ambiguous answer that permits them to hear what they're ready to hear." I was ready to hear that recovery might take a few more months, and that I might have to settle for choreography instead of performing dance, to the extent that I continued dance as either vocation or avocation. I had heard a rule of thumb which stated, "If you don't get it back within a year, you won't get it back." I turned that around to mean, "Don't worry for a year." So I didn't. This goes beyond selective attention; I was working very hard to keep the facts out of consciousness.

The year went by. I was about to adopt an alternate rule of thumb. By then I had heard of cases taking up to two years for full return of function. It was beginning to look like I was one of those. The issue was forced by the school psychologist during a vocational counseling session. In the seventh grade I had decided that I was either going to major in psychology and minor in dance, when I went to college, or vice versa; but in the ensuing five years, I had never decided which. I told the psychologist it was looking like a forced choice but I wasn't ready to give up get. He suggested it was time to ask my doctor, since college was only a few months away. I did. He said, "Better prepare for a sedentary life." I said, "What's sedentary?" Now, I was known in school as a walking dictionary, but all of the sudden I didn't know what "sedentary" meant. Isn't denial fascinating?

He explained and I said, "Oh shit." Mother frowned but didn't chide. I cried on the way home, straightened up my act, called my two best friends, told them, swore them to secrecy because I feared the other kids couldn't handle it and might start avoiding me, and two weeks later I ran off and got married. Everyone knows what that one is called. It's called *acting out*. It's one of the niftier denial mechanisms; it drives other people crazy. They can't believe you are just ignoring the whole thing.

I wasn't ignoring it. I was relieved. It took much less energy than that damned two-year plan. And I was depressed. No Gloomy Gus on the outside, I smiled and smiled and smiled—another form of denial. But on the inside, such self-loathing, such world weariness, such cosmic depression as few are privileged to experience. I'd wake up and look across the room at my wheelchair and the hydraulic lift used to put me in it and say, "No. No human being was ever meant to be like this—a useless blob of protoplasm that has to be moved from one place to another with a crane."

I had moved through one level of acknowledgment—facing the facts—only to find myself immediately embroiled in a struggle with a second level—acceptance of the implications.

Reasons for Denial

Aside from practical reasons for wishing disability were not so, there are additional reasons, issuing from devaluated status in society. The social implications are either known or sensed by newly disabled people, and experience tends to confirm the worst expectations. Disability leads to devaluation, which in turn leads to segregation and its ubiquitous companion, oppression. The person is seen as outside the law, too aberrant to be included under constitutional or statutory protection. This leads to impoverished education and socialization, with resultant noncompetitive status. Poverty and powerlessness ensue, reinforcing both self-devaluation and devaluation by others. Efforts to accommodate the devaluated in jobs, laws, and architecture are meager, generating still further segregation and oppression. When the vicious cycle set in motion by disablement is examined thus, it is readily apparent why individuals would wish to deny being caught up in it. Conversely, as disabled people are able to escape this cycle, they become able to relinquish the "protection" that denial affords. They then can move into Kerr's (1977) adjustment stage and from there onward to higher levels of psychological development.

Models of Psychological Development

If we're lucky, we all experience the processes of birth, infancy, childhood, adolescence, young adulthood, mature adulthood, old age, and death. The early stages reflect changes in the direction of growth; the latter, decay. Theorists from many disciplines, ancient and modern, have been redividing and renaming the developmental stages with astounding regularity over the years. They also have debated the inevitability of psychological decay; whether psychological (spiritual) development ceases or progresses with death. To illustrate: Freud named his developmental stages after the psychosexual stages he believed we all go through: anal, oral, phallic, and genital (Hall & Lindzey, 1957). Like many Western theorists, he used these same labels for his personality typology; that is, he claimed that we do not all get to be "genital" characters just by virtue of growing older. Some of us, because of certain experiences, get fixated at certain levels and become or remain "anal," "oral," or "phallic" personalities. In this case, psychological growth lags behind physical development.

A very different approach comes from Hindu philosophy. In one system, life is divided into four twenty-year segments. The first twenty years are the time for learning. The second twenty years are the time for getting established in the practical world. The third twenty years are the time to search for oneself and God. The fourth twenty years are the time to renounce the material world and wander about teaching others what one has learned. (Isn't it odd? That is when we in the United States enforce mandatory retirement from our schools and universities.) According to the Hindus, psychological or spiritual growth continues and perhaps intensifies long after physical development has sloped downward toward decay.

Kerr's (1977) stages of adjustment to disability are a model of psychological development focused on a particular segment of the population in a limited aspect of their lives. It purports only to describe the developmental process of regaining or establishing a normative adjustment under nonnormative conditions. Following is another such model, one that offers a different emphasis.

Levels of Acknowledgment

The model put forward by the author (Vash, 1978b) condenses the five stages described by Kerr (1977) into two levels of acknowledgment of disability and adds a third level that goes beyond the resumption of normalcy to what might be construed as development into higher consciousness—catalyzed, in part, by experience with disability.

Level I: Recognition of the Facts.   Here the person understands the nature and the extent of the limitations, the probability of permanence, and the realities of social stigmatization, but detests every bit of it. Disability is seen as a tragedy and has negative valence.

Level II: Acceptance of the Implications.   Here the person acknowledges the realities of his or her condition without a sense of loss and shows acceptance of what is without recrimination. The facts and implications of the disability are integrated into a chosen lifestyle. Disability is seen as an inconvenience that can be mastered and has neutral valence.

Level III: Embracing of the Experience.   Here the person recognizes that without the disability s/he would be different from what s/he is, and there is no desire to be different. There is appreciation of the fact that disability has been, is, and will continue to be a growth catalyst if allowed to be so. Disability, like all other life experiences, is seen as an opportunity or gift and has positive valence.

Naturally, there is a period of time before Level I is reached when the person fails to acknowledge even the facts; and acknowledgment and denial alternate in and below consciousness throughout life for most disabled people. With varying degrees of difficulty, most people advance into the second level of acknowledgment. Individual differences in the degree to which most "old hands" have acknowledged their disabilities usually could be described in terms of how far *within* that level they have progressed. Few get stymied at the first level any more. This has not always been true, and the consciousness-raising going on of late regarding disability is largely responsible for this positive change. How far one has progressed within Level II could be defined in terms of the extent to which one accepts without rancor the conditions life presents, versus tendencies to lapse into moments or days of disappointment, rage, despondency, self-hatred, or other erosive emotions related to the facts and implications of disability.

At the same time, relatively few people even conceive of the third level—embracing the disability experience as a positively valued opportunity—and fewer still actually progress into that level. In part, this simply reflects the reduced numbers of people who progress into higher levels of consciousness generally, regardless of experience with disability. At Level III, one embraces disability as an opportunity for psychological growth and spiritual development which has few parallels in life; an opportunity that can be wasted or exploited, a gift in disguise. The individual arrives at a faith in the maxim, "You don't always get what you *want*, but you always get what you *need*" (for progressing toward spiritual goals). To the extent that we learn through pain, disability is an excellent chance for learning. It's a little like the proverbial two-by-four. If you're not strong enough, it may kill you. But if you survive and it gets your attention, it can be the beginning and the way of a great adventure.

One reason so few people aspire to this level of development is that it is not ingrained in Western culture. The biblical story of Job is as close as we get to it in our widely-read writings. It is integral, however, to Eastern psychology and philosophy, which are now being read eagerly in the West. The concept would strike most newly disabled people as a cruel hoax or sardonic joke, and may strike others as an example of "sweet lemon rationalization." Easier to accept is a related concept, reflected in the claims of numerous disabled people, that severe disability has made them strong. While there is little doubt about that, there also appears to be a level beyond strength, where such individualistic qualities are surmounted. People who have survived, accepted, and transcended painful loss—and disablement is but one example—may be uniquely enabled to grow beyond the limits Western thought has allowed for. They can move into a realm we are only beginning to appreciate and aspire to as the spiritual East and the technological West discover that each has ignored a vast part of life for centuries and if the human race is going to survive, they must begin to learn from each other.

Moving Forward

Rehabilitation: A Lifelong Process

A television interviewer once asked the author if she felt she were fully rehabilitated at that point in her life. She responded that she doubted she ever would be, and asked if he felt *he* were, although he had no discernible disability. He understood quickly what was meant and agreed that the term "rehabilitation" tends to be substituted for phrases connoting "human development" whenever a person has had such catastrophic life experiences as disablement or incarceration.

People working with disabled children assert that the concept of *rehabilitation* doesn't apply well to people who had not established themselves physically, socially, and vocationally at the time of disability onset. They self-consciously speak of *habilitation,* to stress the illogic of trying to restore a person to a previous level of functioning when applied to individuals disabled since childhood.

It may not make very good sense when applied to other disabled people, either. "Going back" to a previous state is not the natural direction of growth at any age, and language suggesting it as a goal may not be a wholesome influence. It has the weakness of any regressive effort: it is a growth retardant. It says, "The past was better, the present (and maybe the future) is (are) not so good; I was something then, I'm not much now." Worse, the concept of restoration to a previous state denies the validity and value of the disability experience as a potentially powerful stimulant to psychological growth. The following quote elaborates on this point of view:

> I have been disabled since I was sixteen, yet hardly a week goes by, nearly thirty years later, that I don't make some discovery or improvement that in one way or another makes my disability less handicapping. Since I hope that happy process never stops, I have to say that I hope I am never fully "rehabilitated." My physical abilities are still increasing. When, with age, they begin to decrease, I fully expect to continue or accelerate in the psychological and spiritual discoveries that make my disability not only less handicapping, but a matter or trivia compared with the nonphysical realms of discovery and improvement I am experiencing. Each in its own age, but all part of my own human growth . . . or psychological development . . . or rehabilitation . . . or whatever you prefer to call it. Sometimes I'm not sure what my disability is. Is it being paralyzed, or does that add a laughably small increment to the primordial handicap of being mortal human? The core of psychological development is realistic acceptance of one's limitations—be they physical, intellectual, spiritual, or of some other realm. We are not perfect; we are never what we would wish to be—however beautiful, good, gifted, serene, or strong we appear. These imperfections must be accepted without rancor before we can get on with the real and simple business of psychological development—doing the best we can with whatever we've got. [Vash, 1976, pp. 2, 3]

Thus, the continuity of the "rehabilitation" of disabled people with the "human development" of people-in-general is stressed. The developmental tasks are the same; the unique aspects and different situations created by disablement are of secondary importance. In the context of this chapter, growth relates to such tasks as achieving self-actualization, maximizing human potential, and developing total mind–body–spirit health.

Devaluation: Both Block and Catalyst to Growth

A sense of being devaluated is not unique to disabled people or even to minority-group members in general. At an individual level, it is probably the primal human "hang up." Feelings of worthlessness are central to nonorganically caused mental disorders, and self-esteem is a cornerstone of mental health. The issue has simply become highly salient to the psychology of disability because of the extreme self-devaluation that stems from inability to perform ordinary functions that others take for granted. Having to be led, fed, taken to the toilet, or helped in other ways associated with infancy highlights helplessness, which is conceptually linked with incompetence, and the individual feels (and often is) devaluated. The spiraling ramifications outlined previously can block growth severely for a period of time. However, those with the resources to break free from the spiral often find that the process has freed them from human hindrances to growth in a more encompassing way. Being forced to "put away childish things," such as needs for approbation and material comfort, and to do so successfully, constitutes a giant step toward the higher levels of psychological maturity and spiritual development.

Thus, current social and technological advances are making it possible for disability to catalyze rather than block growth for an increasing proportion of disabled people. When disability took away too much, it seemed to stultify growth for all but a few. But the Zeitgeist is right for change, and the civil/human rights movement, plus rehabilitation engineering technology, are rescuing seriously disabled people from being too overwhelmed to look upward. When they do, some find they have advanced beyond their peers and their own expectations, to a level of existence where more than disability is transcended.

Transcending Disability

Before disability can be transcended, first it must be acknowledged at the three designated levels: recognition of the facts, acceptance of the implications, and embracing of the experience. Here, keeping the distinction clear between "disability" and "handicap" is particularly important. If one is to function effectively in the world and enjoy life at the same time, it is necessary to accept without rancor the fact that one is blind, deaf, paralyzed, mentally retarded, or otherwise disabled. However, it is neither necessary nor desirable to accept such handicapping sequelae as no job, no friends, no sex life, no fun, and—most importantly—no job. It is not even reasonable to accept, unquestioningly, a secondary-labor-market job, a disappointing love life, and unreliable moments of pleasure that always happen at someone else's caprice. This occurs when external, stereotyped definitions of "handicap" are accepted instead of discovering through personal trial and error what is truly beyond the range of capability.

The author was once a member of a rehabilitation hospital team that defined a young man's disability (severe cerebral palsy) as an immutable handicap to driving a car. He wisely rejected that definition and independently obtained driver training from a private school. Five years later, he had an unmarred driving record and the author had the privilege of presenting an award to the driving school. From this, and countless other similar illustrations that could be given, it is clear that the handicapping effects of a disability must be accepted reluctantly, not only by disabled people themselves, but also by the professionals who work with them. Only when the actual limits for a given individual are determined from sufficient experience should the type and degree of handicapping associated with a person's disability be accepted. The next step, as for disability itself, is transcending the handicap.

"Transcendence" connotes rising above or beyond the limits imposed by certain conditions. With respect to the present topic, those conditions may be the disability itself, societal expectations related to it, or emotional reactions to either/both. Transcending disability requires one, first, to escape from the mind–body trap, the Cartesian duality that eliminated spirit from commonplace consideration. As indicated earlier (see Chapter 2), overlooking or denying a spiritual aspect of human life is particularly subtractive to people whose minds and/or bodies are disabled. Once a spiritual component has been admitted to consciousness, then the components vulnerable to disablement are placed in a less potent, more favorable perspective. It becomes progressively easier to say, and mean, that disability doesn't matter much most of the time. The accompanying perceptual mechanism is illustrated by a passage from Beisser (1979).

> The author of this paper is a postpoliomyelitis quadriplegic with severe respiratory paresis [who is] confined to a wheelchair. He is actively engaged in his profession, and when doing so, is absorbed with the tasks at hand. He is frequently asked questions such as, How do you bear spending your life in a wheelchair? When he is, he is aware that his attention is redirected from what he is doing in an affirmative way to what he is unable to do in accordance with the standards implied by the question. Thus, when what he cannot do becomes foreground, he is aware that he is disabled; while working or carrying out his social or family activities, his disability becomes background and his competence and health are foreground. [Pp. 1026–1030]

This reflects the basal level of transcending disability. Its reality is no longer either struggled against or denied. It simply fades, irrelevantly, into the background until rare, extreme circumstance, or someone else, calls it to the forefront of consciousness. Once there, it is experienced with neutrality or—as growth progresses—with positive regard.

Transcending Normalization

"Normalization" is an increasingly popular term used by professionals and consumer activists to describe the goal they envision for disabled people. It connotes having equal rights and opportunities, taking equal risks, assuming equal responsibilities, and expecting equal heartaches and disappointments. It is an unimpeachable goal for those whose lives might otherwise be deprived and disadvantaged, but for many others, striving for normalization is aiming too low. Jung (1929) captured the essence of this in a passage indicating that to be normal is a splendid ideal for the unsuccessful, for all those who have not yet found an adaptation; but for people who have more ability than the average, for whom it was never hard to accomplish their share of the world's work, for them, restriction to the normal signifies the bed of Procrustes, unbearable boredom, infernal sterility, and hopelessness.

Disabled people are present in the ranks of those gifted with "more ability than the average," and the experience of being nonordinary physically may catalyze acceptance of being nonordinary in other respects as well. We tend to forget that the normal curve has two tails, both of which are "abnormal." For example, it is not "normal" to be exceedingly beautiful and wise, or to abjure triviality and pettiness. Fred, a postpolio respiratory quadriplegic who heads an $80-million public agency, is abnormal in a number of highly desirable ways: he is brilliant; powerful; earns a large salary; and lives with a talented, beautiful wife. Although he values normalization as a goal of rehabilitation programs for many, it is doubtful that he would want to return to normality himself. Olivia, a double above-knee amputee, describes incisively the insight experience that led her to discard normality as a goal, having found it maladaptive:

> When Tom proposed to me I said, "Yes, I want to marry you, but there is something I must tell you first. I have decided not to try to use these damnable prostheses any more. I'm tired of falling down, and I've finally caught on that the rehab people only want me to use them because it's important to them that I *look* as normal as possible. They don't seem to tune into the fact that I'm totally unfunctional when I have them on. I look the way I look and if other people don't like it, that's their problem. I'm not making it mine any more. From now on, I plan to scoot around the house on my ass, because that's what *works* best, and I'll use a wheelchair when I go out; but I will never put on those dumb legs again. If you still want to marry me, I want that very much; but I won't change my mind just to meet any needs you might have for me to look more normal."

Olivia, obviously, is unusually confident about her own human worth. Tom proved to be fully in accord with her decision and has since developed some rather stringent opinions:

> I think you rehab people are really messing up by pushing so hard for disabled people to be and look "as normal as possible." What's so great about being normal? To me, that means being dull, drab, run-of-the-mill, and who needs it? You *ought* to be out there educating the general public to be more open and acceptant of differences. Then, when something happens to one of them, they won't be so apt to fall apart because they're not normal any more.

The first lines of the *Credo* of the Human Resources Center in Long Island, New York, reflect a goal that surpasses normalization: "I do not choose to be a common man. It is my right to be uncommon—if I can." Disabled people, like others who have been forced by usually unwelcome circumstance to recognize, accept, and then embrace their differentness in one respect, sometimes have a head start on acknowledging other nonordinary aspects of their being. An outstanding exemplification of this is Ken Keyes, Jr., a postpolio quadriplegic who has been a spiritual leader in this country for nearly two decades.

Ken Keyes, Jr.: Transcending Lower Consciousness

Keyes (personal communication) relates that despite being almost totally paralyzed, he was a successful real estate broker living on a yacht in the Florida Keys when he was introduced to the writings of Baba Ram Dass, John Lilly, and other significant figures of the still-current spiritual revolution. These stirred him to further studies, which culminated in his major work, the *Handbook to Higher Consciousness* (Keyes, 1975), and the establishment of a training center where students can learn to apply his living love methods to the science of happiness. His analysis of the human condition and methods for improving it (on an individual basis) draw notably from the ancient philosophical writings of India and the conceptions of modern biological, behavioral, and computer sciences—a remarkable melding.

Central to his system is the Indian paradigm of seven levels, or centers, of consciousness (chakras), which he describes in Western idiom. The consciousness of people operating at the first and lowest level is concerned with maintaining survival, safety, and security. It is usually referred to as the "security" level of consciousness. The second, slightly higher, level is called the "sensation" level of consciousness. Here, the individual is not solely preoccupied with matters of survival, but has opened his/her consciousness to sensual pleasures, such as sexual activity, gourmet foods, music, and the arts. Thus, "sensation" consciousness may run the gamut from the carnal to the lofty. The third, still higher, level is considered "power" consciousness. People operating at this level are motivated primarily to gain ascendance over others. Keyes (1975) indicates that most people operate within these three lower levels of consciousness most of the time.

He goes on to describe four higher levels of consciousness, associated with love, fulfillment, enlightenment, and cosmic consciousness. People living at the fourth level of consciousness are attuned to their lovingness toward others and others' lovingness in return. The fifth level Keyes refers to as "the cornucopia center of consciousness," in that one becomes aware that whatever is needed is available; whatever happens is what was needed; and one must only learn to appreciate these facts. Keyes believes that a significant proportion of the population can learn to live at the fourth and fifth levels of consciousness most of the time. On the other hand, the sixth and seventh levels, associated with enlightenment and cosmic consciousness, have been reached by only a few hundred individuals throughout history, and can be aspired to realistically by a very smalll number of totally devoted spiritual aspirants.

Keyes advocates advancing beyond security-, sensation-, and power-oriented consciousness and into love- and fulfillment-oriented consciousness because the lower three levels have a painful, addictive quality that virtually guarantees a high proportion of unhappy moments. When survival is at stake, needs become demands and are associated with intense emotions that are adaptive for jungle survival but become maladaptive after that stage has been passed. These emotion-backed demands are tantamount to *addictions* because you suffer when such demands are not met. Moreover, when they *are* met, they yield what Keyes calls a "yo-yo" or "roller coaster" type of enjoyment that necessarily entails at least as much suffering as pleasure. Table 1 summarizes the situation described.

Table 1

Level of Consciousness	Associated Emotions	Why Enjoyment Fluctuates
Security	Fear, worry, anxiety	Constant driving compulsiveness, fear of loss, projections of future worries
Sensation	Disappointment, frustration, boredom	Same as security, plus satiation and boredom
Power	Anger, resentment, irritation hate, hostility	Same as security and sensation, plus being caught up in defending from counterattack and trying to control

Adapted from Ken Keyes, Jr., *Handbook to Higher Consciousness.* (Berkeley, CA: Living Love, 1975), p. 59.

Keyes (1975) believes we are programmed by society and then continue to program ourselves to approach life addictively, with an attitude of "I must have/not have" instead of "I prefer to/not to." In a *tour de force* using simple probabilities, he shows why addictive programming is the mechanism for unhappiness. If you are addicted to having an event occur (for example, martini at five, lover always faithful), you may feel pleasure if it happens, but you will definitely suffer if it doesn't. If you are addicted to having an event *not* happen, (for example, charge account billing error, cockroach in the kitchen), you will suffer if it does but will probably not notice if it doesn't. Given equal probabilities for all outcomes, addictive programming yields half suffering and half either pleasure or no effect.

On the other hand, preferential programming virtually eliminates suffering. If you can say, "I would prefer to have such and such happen/not happen, but if it doesn't/does that is all right, too," you have only opportunities for pleasure or no effect and none for suffering. The higher levels of consciousness are associated with preferential programming, and much of the task of developing into these higher levels is reprogramming, that is, converting addictions into preferences. (Only at the highest level of consciousness do even preferences disappear.)

One reason disability is so difficult to adjust to is that it eliminates conditions to which people tend to be addicted. This is also why nondisabled people so often believe that "If it happened to me, I couldn't cope." Moreover, the presumption of similar addictions in others is an important basis for the attribution of mourning (see Chapter 2) to people who have experienced loss. Most presume they have *suffered* loss; however, to people who have transcended the three addictive, lower levels of consciousness, loss may not be accompanied by suffering. It simply may raise awareness that "whatever happened is what was needed" (for spiritual development or elevation of consciousness).

Readers probably can tune into their own pervasive acceptance of addictiveness by examining their reactions to the prospect of being unable to see, hear, or walk: "You'd better believe I'm addicted to seeing, hearing, and walking—who wouldn't be?" One answer is that some people have learned not to be in order to avoid chronic suffering. It is here that disability operates like the blow on the head by a two-by-four that can kill you or get your attention. Some react to it by becoming more tightly bound to security, sensation, and power preoccupations because survival and opportunities for pleasure have been threatened and powerlessness looms imminent. Others, however, in time may transcend not only disability-triggered, excessive preoccupations, but even an average degree of security-, sensation-, and power-oriented consciousness. Somehow, giving up such basic addictions as those to seeing, hearing, and walking can make relinquishment of lesser ones relatively easy, for individuals who have spent some time at the fourth and fifth levels of consciousness. An exerpt from a previous publication (Vash, 1975) illustrates several aspects of the process that takes place:

> I wasn't exactly happy and couldn't figure out why. It took a few months to realize that one reason was, I hadn't accepted my disability.
>
> When I did, it wasn't at all like [I had] envisioned; settling for second-rate goals and dreams. It wasn't even de-fusing the disappointment that I would never again hear whistles when I walked, or dance, or ride in a horse show, or walk alone in the rain, or go to the bathroom by myself. It sure as hell wasn't the much touted process of discovering substitute gratifications for the ones I had lost.
>
> It was more like those things not only didn't matter any more, they wouldn't have mattered even if I could still have done them. I didn't need to be able to do them—or to mourn their loss—in order to maintain some image of myself. I felt I understood the relinquishments that come with age. Joys of an earlier era are continuously "put away." Substitutions needn't be sought; new joys simply emerge, appropriate to the new era. I found myself no longer afraid of aging. Acceptance of disability was simply acceptance of myself; and there were parts of me that were harder to accept than my disability by far. I didn't have the language then, but from the personal studies I've done since, acceptance of disability was exactly the process Western interpreters of Eastern mystics speak of as "centering," "ridding oneself of ego," and "casting off attachments [addictions] so they become, at most, preferences." The fact that a few of these attachments were ego images and activities interfered with by disability was just one happenstance of a much larger process. [Pp. 152–153]

As a result of the spiritual renascence taking place in current times, more and more people are coming to value and seek the transcendence of lower consciousness, and this includes increasing numbers of disabled people. They are finding that the disability experience has been a powerful contributor to breaking through maladaptive societal programming. Being different and devaluated, knowing extreme loss and pain, facing poverty and even death, force one to adopt new perspectives that might otherwise never have been tried; and each new vantage point enhances growth and knowledge. Most important, however, is learning to give up addictions—which, without being "forced" by disability and an alternative of abject misery, one would be far less likely to do.

The disability experience can help one see that preoccupations with security, sensation, and power are "lose–lose" propositions. There *is* no security. No one can work, hoard, or plan enough to guarantee that nothing will ever go wrong. There is also no way to avoid the now-deprived, now-satiated yo-yo world of sensation-oriented consciousness. Finally, you can never achieve total power and until you do, whatever you have is threatened. This brings one to the obvious question: why not give them all up and start living in the higher levels of consciousness? Disability can catalyze this process. First, it instructs: it *can* happen here. Next, one learns: it *did,* and that's okay. This raises a number of growth-inducing questions: are things perhaps not exactly as they seem? do some things I thought mattered perhaps not matter? are there levels of reality I haven't yet comprehended? and what is "misfortune" anyway? Once people are in a mode of asking questions instead of imagining or pretending that they have answers, the most important step toward transcendence has been taken.

II
Interventions

9 Legislating

The Long Arm of the Law

The last chapter of Part I ("Transcending") and the first chapter of Part II ("Legislating"), though contiguous in this text, seem to represent opposite poles. "Transcending" suggested that benefits accrue when individuals can let go of personal power strivings. This chapter emphasizes the psychological benefits of belonging to a group with a solid, political power base. The apparent conflict is resolved only by apprehending the developmental and multifaceted nature of the coping process. Lawmaking is a basic power approach designed to give freedom and equity to groups of people. Transcendence of power approaches, as discussed in the previous chapter, is an individual's step toward liberation of a different kind. It becomes more attainable, it seems, after individuals have experienced the sense of being powerful in ways meaningful to them. Thus, while the previous chapter pointed out that excessive preoccupation with power may interfere with reaching the highest levels of self-actualization, this chapter unabashedly recounts the psychological values of having sufficient political influence to protect one's fundamental, self-evident, inalienable rights.

In earlier days of the civil rights movement, when desegregation of blacks was the prepotent issue, a conservative United States senator made the pronouncement that "You can't legislate morality." This gave a few people pause until it occurred to them that morality is just what we do legislate—or try to. The Constitution put forth a moral order, and statutory law attempts to maintain it. Ideally, the goals of the law are what's right, fair, and moral to the best of the lawmaker's ability to foresee and implement. Limitations on the ability to foresee have long created socioeconomic problems for disabled people; and these, in turn, generate difficulties in psychological adjustment. (This problem is not limited to issues relating to disabled citizens. It is sufficiently widespread that, in 1974, the House of Representatives passed, by an overwhelming majority, a resolution referred to as the "foresight provision." This stipulates that part of the process of drafting legislation must include an attempt to look ahead at the future implications if proposed legislation were to become law.)

As pointed out in the previous chapter, people with disabilities, especially severe ones, have been considered too aberrant to be included under the law, their hopes for pursuing happiness too unrealistic to be considered. The human and civil rights movements have brought greater clarity and improved the lawmakers' abilities to foresee in this respect. Once the process of mandating needed changes began in earnest, a snowballing effect occurred. A major role of federal laws is to serve as "enabling legislation," allowing and encouraging similar laws/ordinances to be enacted at state/local levels where enforcement can be accomplished more readily. (In many instances, the force of federal law can be applied only if interstate commerce is involved.) But the enabling effect has surpassed this. Jurisdictions and agencies not mandated to do so have jumped on the bandwagon and established rules and procedures thought to reflect the spirit of civil rights legislation. When efforts to help through legislation have created problems, it usually has been due to limited foresight, but backlash also is an omnipresent reality.

For the greater part, however, the long arm of the law, like rehabilitation engineering, has proved to be a nonpsychological tool for vastly improving the psychological status of disabled individuals. The remainder of this chapter will chronicle legislative changes that have come about in recent years, plus advances in regulatory, rulemaking, and procedural design that have been directly or indirectly stimulated by them. The psychological impact of these developments on disabled people are often self-evident, but some of the subtler aspects will be pointed out. The discussion will highlight needed changes yet to be accomplished, many of which can be brought about best by the team efforts of disabled individuals and rehabilitation professionals.

The Creation of Benefits and Services

The many laws that have been passed to ensure the rights to life, liberty, and the pursuit of happiness for disabled people can be viewed as belonging to two major clusters. The first creates needed benefits and services for the target group, and the second aims to protect them from abridgment of their rights under the Constitution. This section will discuss the first cluster; the second will be discussed in the succeeding section.

The benefits and services created by law can be arranged similarly in clusters designated "basic living needs" and "vocational preparation." Benefits may assume the forms of cash grants, loans, discounts, tax deductions, and goods; services may include virtually any known human service program plus special opportunities to acquire earnings. "Basic living needs" include such elements as food, shelter, transportation, and health; "vocational preparation" includes such elements as education, training, and the establishment of a business. Detailed information on sources of particular benefits is available in *A Guide to Financial Resources for Disabled Individuals* (Institute for Information Studies, 1980). The same document also offers a listing of other resource guides to benefits and services.

Early laws provided for the establishment of institutional programs for housing and, later, for treating people with disabilities construed as so severe that they precluded living in the larger society. Mentally retarded, mentally ill, and very severely physically disabled people were the primary occupants of such facilities. Still later, this philosophy was to be reversed and service and benefit programs would be created to allow many who were formerly destined for institutional living to remain in or return to the outside world. The basic survival programs for such individuals are contained in the Social Security Act. The Rehabilitation Act has been associated, historically, with vocational preparation, but recently added provisions for independent-living rehabilitation have expanded its coverage into the basic living needs arena. Legislative provisions for veterans cover both areas, and their far greater generosity, compared with available resources for nonveterans, has been a point of contention among the latter.

Workers' compensation laws also contain provisions in both areas for people who become disabled in the conduct of their work, and "mandatory rehabilitation" provisions in state workers' compensation laws (requiring employers to provide rehabilitation services rather than solely cash compensation to industrially injured workers) are becoming increasingly common. The insurance carriers and employers administering the funds are often willing to expend larger "up front" sums and take greater risks in rehabilitation programs than state rehabilitation programs, which are under taxpayer scrutiny, are willing to do. At the same time, they are less willing to support long-range rehabilitation programs entailing years of schooling. The state agencies may expend as much in the long run for their clients, but they spread it over a longer period of time. Each orientation is appropriate for some clients and inappropriate for others.

The states have a great deal of latitude in how much they enrich the basic federal programs' allowances. California and Massachusetts, for example, commit state/local funds to provide extensive in-home supportive services for people needing attendant care, and, at the time of this writing, eleven other states have programs providing some level of in-home attendant care. This has reduced significantly the threat of reinstitutionalization for severely disabled people in these states, a threat that still hangs heavily over similarly disabled people in the other thirty-seven states.

Numerous less comprehensive laws also have been enacted to create special programs, sometimes for specific disability groups. For example, the Vocational Education Act provides for this specific area of benefits to a wide range of disability subpopulations, and the Developmental Disabilities Act provides for a wide range of services to a delimited disability subpopulation. Even more specific, the Wagner O'Day Act has, since 1938, provided government work contracts for workshops employing predominantly blind individuals. In 1971, it was amended to offer similar opportunities to sighted but severely handicapped individuals, and now is known as the Javits Wagner O'Day Act. The Randolph-Sheppard Act of 1936 created the business enterprise program for the blind (BEP), commonly referred to as the "blind-operated vending-stand program." Although this act has not been amended to include sighted but disabled people, it provides an example of enabling effects. Over three decades later, the California rehabilitation agency became the first to attempt creating an analogous program for sighted clients. They sponsored a state bill enabling other state units and municipalities to enter into contracts with the Department of Rehabilitation to establish businesses to be operated by disabled individuals, which in 1978 was signed into law. It is expected that other states may follow this lead.

The psychological benefits of such legislative thrusts are enormous. Without them, the concept of "opportunity" is a vacuous hoax; with them, it can be a reality. Possibilities for partaking of the routines, risks, joys, sorrows, excitement, and tedium of ordinary human life begin to exist when such laws are enacted. When they are implemented and emulated, social participation by disabled people becomes increasingly probable. Nonetheless, limited abilities to foresee have plagued nearly all legislatively created means of helping disabled citizenry.

Benefit programs were created without cognizance of the future capabilities recipients would have for entering the labor market; thus, welfare-related work disincentives were to become serious problems for the recipients as well as society. Vocational rehabilitation services were created *before* independent living services were, guaranteeing painfully demoralizing failures for hundreds of thousands of vocational rehabilitation clients over the years. One reason for such backward planning is anxiety about accountability to the self-interested taxpayer. Services other than those aimed in a straight line toward "removal of the beneficiary from the welfare rolls and into the ranks of the taxpayers" were regarded as frivolous "handholding" that extant taxpayers would spurn. Only when the evidence that failure to attend to such "tangential" issues as independent living/survival systems was massive and incontrovertible did lawmakers and agency heads reverse their orientations and begin to plan for taking first steps first.

Benefits and services also were created before the basic rights of the affected groups were protected. Frustration, anger, and depression are the likely aftermaths when individuals are encouraged to partake of opportunities for education or vocational training only to find, at the end of it, that their rights to secure employment are being blatantly, callously, and systematically abridged. The following sections will address these issues.

The Protection of Disabled People's Rights

Laws protecting disabled people's rights to equal opportunity for employ-ment are among the statutory latecomers. Wage and hour laws designed to protect disabled workers from economic exploitation led the way as early as the 1930s, as did the first state statute advancing the unique right of blind people to be accompanied by dog guides in areas otherwise restricted to humans. Little more was done specific to the protection of rights—as distinct from the creation of benefits and services—until the 1950s. During this decade, concerns over disabled people's rights to use public accommodations began to be reflected in federal and scattered state legislation. Much of the impetus came from a small cadre of disabled people who had managed to become taxpayers and resented supporting facilities they could not use.

The legal statements were generally vague and unenforceable, proclaim-ing the right of blind or physically disabled people to use public facilities, but issuing no requirements for modifications making it physically possible for them to do so. The major accomplishment of this decade was the heightening of awareness among rehabilitation professionals that their efforts with dis-abled "patients" or "clients" would come to naught unless the social and physical world were altered to accommodate them. It was rehabilitation providers with political contacts who provided much of the early educating and prodding of legislators to mandate changes they now recognized as necessary. Parents of mentally retarded individuals were equally early advo-cates for political and legislative change, but disabled individuals themselves were not yet a potent force as their own advocates.

The Right to a Barrier-Free Environment

Near the end of the 1960s, the federal and several state legislatures passed laws requiring that public accommodations funded wholly or in part with federal (or state) monies must be "accessible to and useable by the elderly and handicapped." The laws were strictly proactive; only facilities to be con-structed in the future were required to be accessible. Shortly thereafter, a number of states began passing parallel laws requiring privately funded public accommodations to meet similar standards. This reflected responsiveness to local advocates who insisted it was only "right, fair, and moral" to go farther than the federal law had gone. The close of the 1970s saw regulations im-plementing the "civil rights" provisions of the 1973 Rehabilitation Act (sec-tions 501 through 504) widely interpreted as either requiring or strongly urging correction of obstructive design in certain public accommodations, regardless of when the facilities were constructed, if any federal funds were involved. Section 502 explicitly established the Architectural and Transporta-tion Barriers Compliance Board for oversight purposes, and sections 501, 503, and 504—which called for affirmative action and nondiscrimination—implied the necessity of barrier reduction.

By this time, disabled activists had taken the lead as their own advocates and were fighting hard to solidify and maintain this hard-line interpretation. Not even in the women's movement, where it began, has the slogan, "You've come a long way, baby," been more aptly descriptive. The advance guard was comprised mainly of gifted, disabled individuals who had broken into the Establishment without benefit of protective legislation or elevated public consciousness. (As was true for ethnic minorities and women, the early successes were "overqualified.") Their trail-blazing, plus the concomitant improvements in benefit/service programs, made it possible for more "average" disabled people to join the battle. Dedicated, driving, volunteer efforts on the parts of unemployed disabled people who joined the barrier-reduction campaign became the first steps out of the proverbial back bedrooms and into the mainstream of social politics for scores, then hundreds, now thousands of people who, not much earlier, might have led more passive, less fulfilling lives.

The Right to Participate in Society

Section 504 of the 1973 Rehabilitation Act rapidly became known as the "bill of rights for the disabled." Many were quick to point out that it was a very limited "civil rights act"; others claimed the regulations promulgated in 1977 by the (then) Department of Health, Education, and Welfare to implement the law went far beyond what Congress had intended. Both may be correct. Section 504 is a forty-five-word statement that says only this:

> No otherwise qualified handicapped individual in the United States, as defined in section 7(6), shall, solely by reason of his handicap, be excluded from the participation in, be denied the benefits of, or be subjected to discrimination under any program or activity receiving Federal financial assistance.

These forty-five words stimulated nearly twenty-seven pages of regulations with far-reaching implications for expenditures that would have to be made by programs receiving federal funds in order that they comply with the law; yet no appropriation was made to cover any part of such expenditures. The attitude of "liberals" on this subject was, "Why should the government appropriate money to pay for affected parties to do what they should have been doing all along?" "Conservatives" on this issue simply awaited the backlash and noncompliance they were sure would come. Nondiscrimination mandates relating to ethnic minorities cost virtually nothing to implement, but those for the disabled minority can engender massive costs, simply to render accessible the housing for the targeted programs. Thus, while the law addressed only *program* accessibility and did not purport to confront physical barrier problems, the regulations incorporated this other, costly issue. In some sectors, concerted compliance efforts began and are continuing still. In others, massive resistance was mounted, usually because of the projected costs of compliance but sometimes because of disagreement with the principles of integration. Examples will be cited later.

Despite pockets, and sometimes groundswells, of resistance, Section 504 has proved to be a strong card in the hands of disabled people and their advocates as they seek to redress discriminatory practices. Often, educating officials of programs receiving federal money is enough to stimulate voluntary efforts to make it possible for disabled people to participate. This effect appears not to have been diminished greatly by the fact that the first court case elevated to the United States Supreme Court yielded a negative finding (the Davis decision). The Supreme Court decided against a deaf woman who sought to enter nurses' training, indicating, in essence, that they did not view her as "otherwise qualified" and that the law did not require the school to make the extensive curriculum changes needed to make the nursing program accessible to her. They further opined that the DHEW regulations had attempted to create law rather than simply implement it (Southeastern Community College v. Frances B. Davis–US–, 60 L Ed 2d 980, 99 S Ct 2361 June 11, 1979).

For weeks, the activist disabled community was stunned, fearful, and angry over this decision. They were not only angry at the Supreme Court, they were angry at Davis and her attorneys for pursuing what they considered, at best, a "borderline" case, one with slim chances for producing the kind of precedent needed. Soon enough, "all is lost" turned to "the show must go on" and the slow but steady campaign to eliminate discriminatory practices against disabled people proceeded—sometimes with and sometimes without the leverage of Section 504.

Also in the mid 1970s, the United States Congress and several state legislatures enacted laws requiring that disabled students be educated in the least restrictive environments compatible with their special needs. Both the federal "education for all handicapped act" and parallel state statutes have "mainstreaming" (desegregation) as a prime goal. A great deal of controversy and backlash resulted, from school officials protesting the lack of appropriations to carry out the mandates, teachers fearing disabled students in regular classrooms would drain time and energy from the nondisabled majority, and teachers/parents fearing disabled students would not get the special attention and teaching skills needed. (See Chapter 6 for additional discussion.) Despite weak efforts toward full compliance, the existence of such laws continues to stimulate small, slow steps in the intended direction. For example, school plant accessibility is improving gradually, and semimainstream programs (wherein disabled students attend special programs on mainstream, rather than separate, campuses), though not yet frequent, are no longer rare.

Psychologically, this is among the most important of all legislative accomplishments. Devaluative attitudes, which are at the root of disabled people's adjustment travails, are potently shaped by the separation of disabled from nondisabled in the early, formative years when belief and value systems are being laid down.

The right to participate extends beyond such basic need areas as education. It also includes the pleasures of recreations and cultural activities and the satisfactions associated with making civic contributions. To illustrate, Section 504 and state statutes enunciating the right of disabled people to use public accommodations were cited in a lawsuit designed to force a theater receiving federal and local tax funds to install an elevator, after a disabled person was injured when being carried down a flight of stairs (Vash v. The Music Center Operating Company–LA Sup. Ct. C 76331, 2d-CIV No. 57519). The presiding judge chose to deny the applicability of "civil rights" laws; nonetheless, as a result of the educative process that accompanied the judicial proceedings, the defendant decided to install an elevator without being legally required to do so.

The Right to Equal Opportunity for Jobs

The most critical area in which disabled people want and need to participate is employment. A few states included disabled people as a protected population under their fair employment practice laws before federal "enabling" legislation was enacted. The 1973 Rehabilitation Act called for affirmative action efforts on the parts of the United States Civil Service Commission (Section 501) and firms receiving as much as $2500 annually in federal contracts (Section 503). Since these federal measures affect only a limited segment of the job market, their primary value is to enunciate the principle to be emulated by local governments. By the end of the 1970s, a survey indicated that at least fifteen states had laws that protect physically and mentally disabled workers, and eleven states had laws protecting physically disabled workers only (Vash, 1980).

Clients of rehabilitation programs are sometimes encouraged to seek redress through their state's fair employment practices enforcement agency when they believe hiring, promotional, or other personnel decisions have been discriminatory. Often, such efforts succeed in securing job opportunities previously denied, or reversing on-the-job assignments reflecting discriminatory bias. A frequently reported example is assignment to duties entailing no public contact. The message thus conveyed is difficult enough for disabled people who harbor lingering doubts about their self-worth, but a greater problem is the implication for promotional opportunity. Most jobs with advancement potential do involve public contact.

Caroline Connell, an employment discrimination investigator, described the psychological aspects of pursuing a fair employment practices complaint (personal communication). She indicates that most of the people come in either angry or almost hopeless.

> They have just enough hope left to give us a try. Most are unprepared for the fact that we are not a social service agency; we are more like a district attorney's office. This requires us to re-educate them as to what we can do and cannot do, and many can't accept this and simply abandon the charges. Most are very concerned about privacy, and can't understand why we require medical examinations.
>
> There is a great deal of fear about retaliation, which leads to increased tension, especially if they are still on the job. This can create real problems if the disability is tension-related in the first place. There is also a great deal of stress if they didn't get the jobs—not knowing whether to wait and hope or consider moving to take a job somewhere else. As the tension increases, their need for support again may cause them to misunderstand the legal rather than social service nature of the office. They usually don't get what they came in wanting, although many are pleased and, often, on-the-job relationships are improved for all concerned. Many want back wages, but it is difficult to obtain this remedy unless discrimination is provable . . . which is complicated by the fact that employers are becoming more sophisticated.
>
> Having their cases heard by a judge is very rewarding almost regardless of the outcome. When we feel the employer has offered an equitable remedy and recommend that the complainant accept it, they have to give up the hearing and that is very hard for them.
>
> In summary, I'd say the major psychological aspects of pursuing a complaint relate to frustration, tension, fear of exposure, and the system's lack of ways for dealing with feelings. Fear of exposure comes about because we all have little secrets and some might be brought out by the other side in their efforts to combat the charges. [Alcohol problems and psychiatric treatment histories, unrelated to the complaint situations, were cited as examples.] Whether or not any emotional support is given depends on the individual consultant and how humanistic she or he is. Many staff are strongly oriented that way, but this is not true of all. Some are very cold and want only the facts.*

Rehabilitation agencies report that their job placement efforts have been aided substantially by the enactment of the various federal and state laws addressing equal employment opportunity for disabled workers. All levels of government are trying to increase hiring of disabled workers through a variety of programs and modernized personnel selection procedures. Private employers are more willing to attend seminars on the subject, to follow through by developing affirmative action programs, and more frequently turn to rehabilitation agencies as sources of workers when they have job vacancies to fill. Legal provisions for offering tax savings to employers who will hire disabled workers and correct mobility barrier conditions in their work settings contribute to the improving trend.

*Reproduced by permission of the author.

The employment picture for disabled workers also has been improved by the 1978 amendments to the Rehabilitation Act, which added provisions for independent living rehabilitation. States and municipalities have made funding available since to consumer-run independent living programs, providing many jobs for disabled individuals.

Although civilian employment opportunities for disabled workers appear to be on the increase, as mentioned in Chapter 6, military opportunities are almost nonexistent still. This area needs legislation to enunciate the right of disabled individuals to serve in the military and reap the benefits it affords. The reasons given for excluding disabled people are largely without substantive basis. A sizable proportion of military occupational specialties entail job demands compatible with significant disabilities, and must be performed by someone during armed conflicts or combat training. What is resisted is change—and considerable system change would be required. It seems necessary, however, to eliminate this lingering area of needless discrimination.

The Right to Economic Protection

Related to, yet distinct from, employment opportunity is the matter of protection from economic exploitation. Wage and hour laws that require documented justification for paying disabled workers less than the minimum wage have the longest history. During the 1960s and 1970s, considerable attention was paid to potential and actual exploitation of institutionalized individuals whose work assignments were construed as part of their therapy programs and who therefore were paid token wages or nothing at all. Legal foreclosure on such practices benefited some, who truly were being exploited, and created harm for others. The loss of work responsibilities proved to be antitherapeutic for many mentally retarded or emotionally ill residents, and funds formerly devoted to services were diverted to facility maintenance. Compromise solutions (such as securing subminimum wage certificates for selected residents and paying them as prescribed) were devised in most affected institutions. However, some staff believe it is psychologically wholesome for their residents to expect to make a work contribution in exchange for tax-supported room, board, and services. They say it increases the sense of responsibility for their own lives and reduces feelings of helplessness and dependency.

Numerous other types of laws can be construed as providing economic protection to disabled people. The federal income tax exemption for legally blind individuals is one example that many deaf and physically disabled activists believe should be extended to severely disabled people in general. Antitrust laws are being used as the basis for efforts to deter manufacturers of durable medical equipment from charging what the traffic will bear in a captive market. Efforts continue, in the federal legislature, to formulate a workable law to provide for wage subsidization to disabled workers not capable of earning living wages, a law that will foresee correctly and circumvent future problems of abuse and work disincentives. All such legislative efforts and accomplishments provide a more stable, higher level, economic foundation for disabled individuals, reducing the emotional wear and tear of wondering how the costs of living can be managed.

The law also provides for workers to organize to improve their working conditions, rates of pay, and employee benefits. This includes workers in sheltered industries, many of whom are paid less than prevailing rates, ostensibly because of reduced production capacities. Situations are known in which disabled workers performing at or above ordinary standards have been paid below prevailing or even minimum-wage levels, simply because they were designated "handicapped." In such cases, unionization could offer needed protection from exploitation. In other instances, unionization of disabled workers unable to produce at levels commensurate with demanded wages has resulted in the actuality or threat of forcing the sheltered industry out of business. Most are fiscally marginal operations that cannot afford to be the sole source of subsidy to partially productive workers. Such failures of foresight on the parts of union organizers and of disabled workers to perceive correctly their production deficits have led to the loss of even low-paying jobs when sheltered industries either closed or transformed their missions. Several have ceased providing long-term job opportunities, turning instead to selling work evaluation services to state rehabilitation agencies.

Confidentiality and the Right to Know

Laws, agency regulations, and professional codes of ethics have long attempted to protect people's privacy by prohibiting improper disclosure of information contained in agency files. "Proper" disclosure meets two primary criteria: (1) the person's permission to disclose is obtained in writing and (2) the need to disclose can be justified in terms of benefit to the person. Two types of information thus are protected: (1) that provided by individuals in the processes of seeking and receiving human services (for example, health, education, welfare, employment, legal, and pastoral services) and (2) information generated by service providers (for example, medical diagnoses, treatment/service plans, nursing notes, welfare memoranda, counseling progress notes, and psychological reports). The first type of information offers few conceptual problems. It is deeply ingrained in the general culture that one should not gossip about confidences, however well one adheres to the principle in practice. On the other hand, for reasons relating to professional insecurity, fear of lawsuits or personal danger, and beliefs that people (especially "patients") could be harmed by facts/opinions about their own conditions/situations, the second type of information came to be held as confidential from the service recipients themselves! This meant that recorded opinions—to which they were not privy—about patients, clients, students, or otherwise designated service recipients would influence the opinions and decisions of all providers with access to the files. It also meant that when they signed release forms permitting information of record to be disclosed to other agencies, this situation would follow them.

People insistent on taking charge of their own lives traditionally have found ways to gain access to their medical charts, school records, and/or other agency file materials. Many have been surprised and angered by what they found: entries they considered inaccurate, prejudicial, or otherwise detrimental to them. An expanding volume of complaints led to the creation of "right-to-know" legislation: the federal Freedom of Information Act of 1966, the federal Privacy Act of 1975, and comparable state laws/executive orders and local ordinances. All of these now enunciate the right of individuals to know what has been written about them in agency records.

Initially, professionals from virtually every human service discipline had difficulty accepting this turn of events; and serious concern lingers, especially when psychological information is at issue. A psychologist lamented, "Our reports will be watered down and useless if we have to write them so the patient or client can read them." A psychiatrist added,

> We daren't say anything that might offend the patient. But how can you avoid offending patients who are denying that they have psychiatric disorders? If you say they have them, they're offended and might sue. Then some judge, who is not a qualified diagnostician and who'll be working from persuasive rather than objective information will end up deciding whether your diagnosis is correct!

Here, however, is a more positive view of the effects of writing psychological reports (or other reports containing psychological material) with the knowledge that the subjects may, sooner or later, read them:

> The psychology staff at a Veterans Administration Domiciliary learned quickly that certain Dom members made a regular practice of going into the chart rooms every evening to review entries made in their charts during the day. We knew the policing required to put a stop to the midnight chart review would be more damaging than permitting it, so we learned to write our reports so we felt comfortable with the fact that the subjects of those reports would probably read them sooner or later.
>
> It took little time to learn that we could say everything we needed to say to the colleagues to whom the reports were ostensibly addressed—deleting no concept of substance—when we wrote "as if" to the member whom they described. The rules were simple. Sadly, the first turned out to be "Don't get cute." When cleverly

sardonic or other witty ways of describing a patient or client occur to you, suppress them. Experience in dealing with legal representatives over this issue in programs I've administered shows the primary type of material clients object to falls in the category of "unkind witticisms and insulting broadsides."

The second rule was "Describe the subject in behavioral terms." We learned to avoid the use of high level abstractions, particularly those which have crept into lay usage with inflammatory overtones (such as "paranoia") and those controversial as to their meaningfulness within the psychological community (such as "schizophrenia"). This was a particularly good lesson. As a result of disciplining ourselves to think through the actual, behavioral substrates of a diagnostic label or trait name we had accepted as describing the person, we came to understand him better as a human being, and to make sharper distinctions about both his problems and strengths. We saw, for example, how damaging it is for people to be labelled "hostile" or "passive" as if those labels encompassed their total beings. Once such a label "sticks," others stop looking for, or seeing, the moments when the person is loving, not hostile, or assertive, not passive. If lovingness or assertiveness are the qualities you want the person to develop, you won't reinforce them if you fail to notice when they happen.

I began to write my reports as if they were summaries of progress to the Dom member himself. I recorded my views of where he was making gains and where he was resisting change and what I thought that was doing to him. It was within this climate of honesty—with members about members—that more effective counseling techniques for aiding their transitions to the outside were developed.

The third rule was "Make sure your own motivations/emotions toward the subject are helpful/caring before you start to write." If you are feeling angry or disrespectful toward the person, you will have to re-write twenty times to keep it from showing. If you take time to get yourself centered first, you can save nineteen re-writes. If you are motivated to caution other professionals about what a difficult son-of-a-gun this person can be, the first order of business is to deal with your feelings about that. Probably, if this rule were followed, there would be no need for rules one and two. A caring mode tends to block witticisms, broadsides, and jargonistic labels.

From more recent experience in a large bureaucracy comes a fourth rule. "Don't include undocumented, third party 'hearsay' material in reports or file notes"—especially if it could be construed as damaging to the person's reputation. To illustrate, drawing from an actual case, if a worker from a sister agency tells you by phone that a mutual client frightened her to the point that she felt her safety was endangered when he came to her office, don't put it in the record unless she is willing to put it in writing. You can't count on her being around later to testify if the client files a grievance. If she is, she might decide in retrospect that it wasn't so serious; and fail to recall feeling actually endangered. You, then, will have blemished the client's reputation by putting undocumented gossip in the chart. [Vash, 1977a, pp. 4–6]

Thus, while there are necessary rules to observe, the overall effect of writing reports to conform with realities such as those created by right-to-know legislation can be viewed in a favorable light. The potential for tightening clinical thinking, and the incentive for careful adherence to principles most professionals endorse anyway, combine to render this new type of demand more an opportunity than an imposition.

The Right to a Fair Trial

Two issues that have arisen in the wake of the civil rights movement are (1) the claimed rights of hearing-impaired individuals to interpreter services during court proceedings and (2) the rights of all disabled individuals to have their cases tried by juries of their peers. The first issue is clear cut and is directly analogous to the claimed rights of non-English speaking people generally to have adequate translation services in courts of law. The second is more convoluted and has come from disabled people wanting to serve on juries more than from disabled defendants/plaintiffs and their representatives. Blind and deaf individuals object strenuously to municipal, state, and federal court rules barring them from serving because they are not considered to be "in full possession of their faculties." Wheelchair users object to being excluded from the experience by reason of architectural barriers existing in juror facilities—conditions they believe the law requires to be remedied.

As of this writing, neither "right" is granted consistently. Although no statutes exist, many states have unwritten codes that, in criminal cases, the court provides interpreter services for the accused. Plaintiffs, however, must supply their own. No such provisions exist in civil cases. A few states are beginning to enact laws allowing disabled individuals to serve on juries (for example, California, as of 1980). In addition, a few courts have independently relaxed their rules against including disabled people on juries, but these are rare exceptions that usually admit only self-care independent, physically disabled individuals.

The Right to Appropriate Treatment by Police

Local elected officials are establishing with increasing frequency advisory bodies to keep them apprised of the needs of "the disabled community." It is becoming common experience for these groups to receive complaints from disabled individuals claiming mistreatment by law enforcement officers who did not recognize or refused to believe they were disabled. Countless stories are heard of deaf people being shot or nearly shot for failing to comply with "halt" commands, people with cerebral palsy or multiple sclerosis arrested for public drunkenness, paralyzed individuals pulled out of cars onto the ground, and retarded people physically abused for failing to respond correctly. These stories have been familiar sources of helpless outrage to disabled people and rehabilitation professionals for years, and the complaints of both were largely ignored by the police chiefs, sheriffs, and police commissioners who received them.

The disability-related advisory groups to mayors, city councils, and county governing bodies appear to be potentially helpful intermediaries in this respect. Their ability to draw both the elected officials' and the media's attention to such dramatic problems has led to some "self-policing," that is, attempts by scattered law enforcement agencies to provide their officers with needed education and attitudinal reshaping. In the main, however, the problems continue unabated.

Mistreatment by law enforcement officers—whether due to failures of discernment or angry assumptions that claims of disability are attempts to flout their authority—happens to a relatively small segment of the disabled population. To those to whom it happens, however, it can be devastating. The fear and anger or depression resulting from such episodes can take a long time to resolve. The opportunity to have one's experience and complaints aired before an official body with no vested interest in protecting the law enforcement agency, can ameliorate these aftereffects somewhat, whether or not correction/apologies can be secured.

The Right to Be a Parent

This issue was introduced in Chapter 4, where instances of nonvoluntary sterilization of disabled women and wresting of child custody from disabled parents were mentioned. Disabled activist groups all over the country are taking a keen interest in situations such as these. News accounts of litigation and other forms of protest appear ever more frequently in the press. Elected officials are being pressured for action to stop such practices as the sterilization of retarded women without evidence of genuinely informed consent. Disability-related legal programs have aided in restoring children to disabled parents when agencies/estranged spouses have attempted to wrest custody from them.

Historically, child-custody suits almost always have ended with custody being awarded to the nondisabled parent, regardless of whether affectional and socioeconomic advantages could have been offered by the disabled parent. A recent decision by the Supreme Court of the State of California in the case of Carney v. Carney (L.A. 31064, Superior Court Number SDD 68540, August 7, 1979) promises to reverse this trend, however. In a unanimous decision, Justice Mosk stated,

> We are called upon to resolve an apparent conflict between two strong public policies: the requirement that a custody award serve the best interests of the child, and the moral and legal obligations of society to respect the civil rights of its physically handicapped members, including their right not to be deprived of their

children because of their disability. As will appear, we hold that, upon a realistic appraisal of the present-day capabilities of the physically handicapped, these policies can both be accommodated. The trial court herein failed to make such an appraisal, and instead premised its ruling on outdated stereotypes of both the parental role and the ability of the handicapped to fill that role. Such stereotypes have no place in our law. [pp. 1–2]

To date, no comparable progress has been made toward facilitating adoption of children by people with significant disabilities. From all indications, this particular problem is getting worse, not better. As an illustration, Max and Joy adopted two children from their county adoption agency in the early 1960s. Max, you will recall from Chapter 5, is quadriplegic and Joy has no disability. They are well off financially and wanted to share what they have with a larger family of children. When they returned to the agency in the middle 1970s and applied for two more children, they were told, "Sorry, we have a *freeze* on giving children to parents with disabilities [emphasis added]." Clearly, disability had become a logical-sounding excuse for eliminating a group of would-be adoptive parents in the face of excessive demand and short supply of children. Max and Joy searched private agencies but were told the same thing. Their solution entailed a trip to Thailand—and they again found this restriction. Determined, however, they pretended Max was ill with "tourist complaint" and he stayed in the car, wheelchair covered by blankets, while his wife dealt with the officials. In three weeks' time, they had their two "new" children and came home. Unfortunately, most couples could not afford this extreme measure, although they could provide adequately for a child or two. This is an area still in need of civil rights attention and protective legislation.

The Right to Redress

The final type of legislation to be considered here takes us back to the topic of legislatively created benefits and services. Provisions for redress when applicants/recipients are dissatisfied with administering agencies' decisions sometimes are built into the original legislation and sometimes must be added later. The decisions grieved usually involve eligibility, amount of allowable benefits, or appropriateness of services. The grievance systems generally are comprised of an internal subsystem of administrative remedies—reviews and hearings at escalating levels of supervision—and an external appeals system to turn to if resolution cannot be achieved through administrative review.

In the main, such systems probably are well used and offer benefits to both aggrieved parties and agencies; however, problems exist at two extremes. For reasons of temperament and personality, a few people overuse such systems in ways that are costly and impair their credibility, not only with the involved agencies, but with the disinterested adjudicators as well. For the same reasons, many more are afraid to use the system at all. It takes a great deal of courage for most people to say to an agency worker, "I am dissatisfied with your decision and I want to talk with your supervisor." If the supervisor supports the worker, it takes even more courage to confront that person, too. For people who feel oppressed and hopeless, it takes a measure of courage that often simply doesn't exist.

For this reason, many agencies have developed ombudsman programs that allow greater anonymity to aggrieved parties and provide practical/ emotional support during redress procedures. A few such programs are provided for in the law; provisions for grant funds to agencies willing to establish "client assistance projects" in the 1973 Rehabilitation Act serve as an example. Most, however, are established at the agency's own behest, often as part of a larger effort toward self-policing.

Self-Policing

Since the 1960s, dozens of disabled people's "bills of rights" have been published, each specific to some particular group of consumers of rehabilitation services. Some of the better-known examples are "A Bill of Rights for the Handicapped," developed by the United Cerebral Palsy Association; "A Bill of Rights for the Rehabilitation Client," displayed in many offices of the state–federal rehabilitation program; the "Declaration of General and Special Rights of the Mentally Retarded," composed by the International League of Societies for the Mentally Handicapped; and the "Patient's Bill of Rights," put forward by the American Hospital Association.

Commonly included elements of these examples relate to the issues examined in the foregoing sections of this chapter, namely, rights to (1) timely and accurate eligibility determination, (2) knowledge of what is being said about one to other service providers, (3) information being used for decision making about one or needed to make intelligent decisions for oneself, (4) confidentiality of sensitive information, (5) timely and responsive services, (6) respect, (7) consideration, and (8) avenues of redress when reasonable expectations seem not to have been met. Most of these bills of rights avoid guaranteeing any right to expect effective or competent services. Those displaying them are divided with respect to whether that "goes without saying" or "would be impossible." Despite any shortcomings, however, consumers' bills of rights reflect good-conscience efforts on the parts of service providers to hold themselves accountable for correcting errors made in the past. The age of accountability also has created a new form of "market research."

Client Evaluations of Services

First, college professors had to get used to receiving report cards from their students at the end of each quarter/semester. Student evaluations of instructor effectiveness have by now become the rule rather than the exception and, in most places, are considered a valuable source of feedback by teaching staff. More recently, similar evaluations of service providers by agency clients have begun to be solicited. Their purpose is to help agency managers determine how agency effectiveness and methods are perceived by their "customers." The information from such *program evaluation* efforts is meant to be fed into *program planning*, where deficiencies would be corrected through policy or procedural changes, in-service training, or whatever seems to respond best to the kinds of criticisms received.

The path from such theory to actual correction is tortuous, partly because change tends to occur slowly and partly because the credibility of the client evaluators frequently is impugned. The threat to the evaluees is enormous, posing a sensitive test to the solidity of their outward attitudes toward service recipients. Thin veneers may be stripped away, exposing negative beliefs just under the surface, such as, "Clients can't realistically evaluate professionals, they don't understand the complexities we face"; or "If you give them the store you'll get a high rating, but if you deny them something they want, watch out." Instructors, as a group, went through a similar period of doubting whether they would be evaluated fairly, and, as the system matured, their fears leveled out. In time, the same probably will occur in this newer area. Regardless of whether corrections follow rapidly or slowly, the opportunity for clients to voice their frustrations and advice to agencies yields benefits similar to those observed by Connell (discussed previously above) in relation to fair-employment-practice hearings.

Voluntary Affirmative Action

Not only service agencies are involved in self-policing. The last form to be mentioned here concerns employers throughout the country who are going far beyond what any law requires in the way of affirmative action for disabled workers. Local government and private employers alike are responding to the spirit, not the letter, of the law by developing outreach programs to recruit disabled applicants for job vacancies. Some participate in Projects with Industry (see Chapter 6) to train and help secure job placements for vocational rehabilitation clients. Others are attending to matters of accommodating disabled workers through rehabilitation engineering and personnel policies designed to reduce job barriers.

An outstanding example has been set by the California State Department of Rehabilitation. This government agency employs over 2000 individuals. It has an explicit policy stating that it will provide the equipment and support services necessary to allow its employees to perform their duties satisfactorily, including special items needed to accommodate disabling conditions. This might include such equipment as electronic reading aids and motorized wheelchairs, or such assistance as interpreter, attendant, reader, or driver services. The underlying philosophy assumes that "If individuals offer sufficient potential to cause the agency to want to hire them, then adequate support must be given. If the projected extra expenses seem unwarranted by an individual's limited ability to contribute, s/he should not be hired in the first place."

The administration of this agency points out that it costs the taxpayers far less in the long run to provide even expensive equipment and support services permitting talented, severely disabled persons to make work contributions to society than it would to fund the likely alternative of paying for their total support through the SSI program and receiving no work in exchange for the much greater expenditure. Acknowledging that such operating principles apply only when both the employment and welfare costs are tax supported (pass-through costs in the free enterprise sector create, as yet, unresolved problems), this agency encourages other government agencies to adopt similar approaches.

One Step Beyond

In the spring of 1978, hordes of severely disabled individuals descended upon the federal office of the Secretary of the (then) Department of Health, Education, and Welfare (DHEW) in Washington, D.C. A smaller, still impressive number followed suit at the regional office in San Francisco. They were using their right to assemble in an effort to pressure the Secretary to sign the long-delayed regulations promulgated by his agency to implement Section 504 of the 1973 Rehabilitation Act.

Although they were the targets of the demonstrations, DHEW staff interviewed later reported staying long into the night to provide emergency attendant care and ensure sufficient food supplies for the demonstrators. One indicated that "It was a mess. We wish they could have found another way, but we were in sympathy with what they wanted and saw the demonstration as a big step toward the independence we've tried to help them achieve." This goes a step beyond "self-policing" to show the commitment rehabilitation officials can have to the spirit of "disabled civil rights" laws. It also demonstrates what many consider the most appropriate style of partnership between disabled people and nondisabled professionals/advocates: the former taking the lead to achieve their goals and the latter using their expertise/resources to help—not a reversal wherein the professionals try to do the job for their "constituents."

The following section will explore other aspects of the utilization of protective laws.

Utilization of the Law

Becoming Informed

For protective laws to be of practical consequence, the target populations must be informed of their existence, strengths, and limitations. For example, the utilization potential of the right to assemble came into sharpened focus during the antiwar demonstrations of the 1960s and has been employed regularly by protesters ever since. In the case at hand, disabled people, rehabilitation professionals, and other advocates must get, and stay, informed about a wide range of laws, plus court tests and precedents that affect their applicability. These same groups of people also are responsible for overseeing the enforcement of such laws, because they almost certainly will not be enforced without "watchdogging" by concerned citizens.

Overseeing Enforcement

In approximately a decade's time, the responsibility for enforcement oversight has expanded from being assumed by a few individuals and informal committees, through formalized organizations of disabled people and rehabilitation professionals, to lawyers in large bureaucracies and attorneys general. In the early 1970s, none of the state rehabilitation agencies had full-time attorneys on their staffs; now, many do, and some have two or more full-time equivalents. Some of these agencies also have succeeded in gaining active cooperation and commitments from their states' attorneys general in pursuing litigation arising out of failures to observe state laws relating primarily to accessibility of privately owned public accommodations. Cases handled at this level are usually "showcase" examples, selected in the hope that favorable outcomes will provide highly visible lessons to others tempted to ignore the same laws. Most of the work must go on at less auspicious levels, however, and both consumer and professional organizations have played major roles in identifying local offenders. From the infractions thus discovered, disability law programs and interested private attorneys are pursuing a great deal of additional litigation.

The field of law is attracting increasing numbers of disabled individuals, many of whom eventually devote some portion of their practices to disability law, often without expectation of compensation. Others establish or go to work for the similarly increasing number of disability law centers devoted to helping disabled people who can neither afford nor elsewhere find qualified attorneys to pursue their unique kinds of cases. The existence of such resources is both a practical and psychological boon to the many individuals who otherwise would be unable to use legal avenues of redress.

A Closing Note

As the foregoing illustrates, legislation has proved to be an important "psychological intervention strategy," by offering improved quality of life and access to opportunity. It becomes clear how Hohmann's words (see Chapter 2), "Disability isn't as depressing anymore," relate as much to the bettered politico-legal status of disabled people as to the advances in health science and technology. Also clear is the responsibility of rehabilitation professionals to be aware of such strategies, know how and when to use them, and help their clients know how and when to use them.

The next four chapters will examine intervention strategies more typically construed as psychological in nature. Such strategies use psychological research findings and clinical experience to help disabled people enhance their psychosocial functioning and, concomitantly, their subjective states of psychological well-being. The next chapter will discuss issues relating to psychological evaluation, and the following three chapters will turn to "treatment" or psychological service approaches.

10 Evaluating

Individual Differences

An implicit message of this chapter is that, contrary to the manifest attitudes of the general public, disabled people are not all alike. It is not possible to describe "the handicapped" or "the disabled" as a homogeneous group. As is true of people in general, the human traits of this subpopulation tend to be more-or-less normally distributed, and individual differences are marked. For reasons to be set forth in the following section, it becomes necessary to measure these differences from time to time. The process is called "assessment" or "evaluation." This chapter will discuss issues relating to psychosocial–vocational (PSV) evaluation in particular, and the psychological aspects of evaluative processes in general.

Although the terms "assessment" and "evaluation" often are used interchangeably, there is an important distinction that will be adhered to in this context. "Assessment" connotes measurement and nothing more, whereas "evaluation" connotes both a measuring and a judging process. Assessment yields data reflecting the presence, absence, or relative standing of a measured variable or set of variables. Evaluation includes the additional step of assigning value judgments to the findings, such as favorable/unfavorable or adequate/inadequate, always with respect to practical, functional criteria. (Neither term legitimizes the making of moral judgments.) For ease of expression, the term "evaluation" will be used to include assessment whenever a clinical judging process is entailed.

The ensuing pages will explore the fundamental issues associated with the evaluation process: why we evaluate, whom and what we evaluate, who does the evaluating, when and where it is done, and how it is done. In addition, certain ethical issues, problems, and pitfalls will be examined. The primary emphasis will be on the evaluation of psychological variables and others influencing psychological adjustment to disability. The general psychosocial impact of assessment procedures on those evaluated will constitute the secondary focus. Third, attention will be paid to the psychological aspects of serving in the evaluator role.

Why: Purposes and Uses of Evaluation

Interviews with an adventitious sampling of rehabilitation providers and service consumers revealed a startling degree of cynicism about the purposes of psychosocial–vocational (PSV) evaluation. Nearly half of each group expressed the opinion that a major purpose of PSV evaluation is to provide a sizable job market for rehabilitation professionals. Although many believe PSV evaluation has grown beyond its usefulness to clients because of its professional employment potential and appeal, most also acknowledged genuine benefit for clients, whether direct or indirect. The cited purposes of evaluation and uses of evaluative information include behavioral prediction, treatment planning, screening and adjudication, tool for counseling, stimulation of self-evaluation, and research. These categories concur with the author's experience and seem equally applicable to the wide range of rehabilitation-related evaluation procedures. It is worth noting that some are oriented toward rehabilitation providers or other professionals as the users of the information, while others assume the users to be the evaluees themselves.

Behavioral Prediction

This is the overriding theme common to all purposes and uses of evaluation. Assessment, coupled with knowledge of the findings' implications, enables one to predict such future behavior as responses to disability-related events, facts, and situations. According to Lewin (1935), behavior is a function of the person and the environment, thus, $B = f(P,E)$. Once the appropriate values of the relevant person and environment variables are inserted into the equation, and the nature of the mathematical relationship is known, the probability of occurrence of a given behavior (or set of behaviors—a behavior pattern) can be predicted. This is a simple statement of the basis of behavioral science research, and it is equally applicable to individual clinical prediction.

Person variables are all those descriptors used to identify/characterize individuals or groups of individuals: demographic data, traits, historic variables, and so forth. These person variables are the objects of most clinical assessment procedures. Lewin (1935) separated environment variables into "proximal" and "distal" subvarieties. Proximal (nearby) variables influence the person directly, and distal (remote) variables exert their influences indirectly. Examples of proximal environment variables, with relevance to rehabilitation, are family support and community service availability. Examples of distal environment variables that influence behavior are federal funding trends and the first lady's interest in rehabilitation. Measurement of environment variables is primarily a research activity; but certain proximal environment variables, whose importance has been demonstrated, also may be assessed in the clinical situation.

Some people find efforts to predict human behavior objectionable, in the mistaken belief that prediction always implies a corollary will to control the behavior predicted. Typically, two arguments are offered to counter this. The more frequently used one admits to a control corollary but justifies it on the basis of benefit to the individual and society. In other words, the control potential is seen as morally neutral, and its use for good or ill is regarded as a separate concern to be monitored by ethical and legal systems rather than science itself. The less frequently used argument seems more to the point: prediction does *not* always imply the potential for control. For example, our ability to predict planetary movement in our own solar system is virtually perfect, but no one fancies that we will ever alter or control it. The predictive knowledge is used in other ways to make our lives more comfortable.

The same is true for much of the information gathered during clinical assessment. While it is true that efforts to change (control) maladaptive behavior patterns are sometimes intended, in many other instances the information is used only to alert the person to pertinent environmental stress conditions s/he may wish to avoid, or to point out hitherto unrecognized inner resources s/he may wish to exploit, as through training or job choice.

Treatment Planning

Use of the information by professional helpers is frequently for purposes of planning treatment. "Treatment" is construed here as a generic term encompassing all varieties of rehabilitative intervention: medical, psychological, social, and vocational. Each type of treatment planning may require information about the individual's status in all areas. To illustrate, nonemergency surgery should be scheduled to minimize interference with the person's work responsibilities, potential harm from excessive fears must be assessed, and adequate posthospitalization care assured. Similarly, vocational goal setting cannot overlook pertinent medical issues, nor can counseling techniques ignore the influence of subcultural variables.

Not infrequently, evaluation procedures designed to aid in treatment planning become subtly subverted to serve rehabilitation staff more than the patients or clients. The following exerpt serves to illustrate this process and, at the same time, reflects the problem of overevaluating as a function of the job needs of professionals.

> Most rehabilitation hospitals or units have at least a fledgling psychological service component and some grown quite large, with a dozen or more psychologists on staff. One of the largest is the Psychology Department at Rancho Los Amigos Hospital. The problem is it isn't big enough. The majority of staff time goes into evaluation, leaving little time for treatment. It is not patients who want evaluations, it is other staff; for purposes of planning patients' rehabilitation programs or

coping with day-to-day problems like "refusal to cooperate." The patients get only fragmentary help in a situation which most people—before it happens—are totally convinced they could not handle.

Psychologists from other rehabilitation hospitals report and lament the same experience. When I worked as a psychologist in a rehabilitation hospital it occurred to me that my role was to reduce staff anxiety. Somehow, having test data made us feel we had a better handle on something. If I gave a patient a WAIS and an MMPI and could say with assurance that he was normally smart and wasn't crazy; he was just a little upset over being paralyzed all of a sudden and suspected his wife had moved in with his best friend while he was in the hospital, and he had never done any work except manual labor and didn't see how he could get her and the kids back unless he could support them, and he probably couldn't satisfy her anyway so perhaps he was being selfish to want her back—the anxiety of the staff was relieved. But somehow no one ever said, "Wow! What a heavy trip! I'll do without my evaluations. You should spend your time just talking to people, seeing if you can guide them through this incredible trip, because it seems a lot more important."

I squeezed in as much "just talking," counseling, psychotherapy—whatever you want to call it—as I could. We all did. But we never mutinied and said, "This is ridiculous! We're serving the wrong people. True, it's a heavy trip for them, too, going through this time after time. But the other guys need it worse. Let's reorder our priorities." We just went on assuming that our evaluations were so important they had to get done, and prayed for more staff.

I suspect the marginal status of practitioners of the psychotherapeutic arts has much to do with the explanation. One of the reasons for marginal status is low visibility of effort. One way to enhance status is to get visible. Test protocols and reports containing findings, predictions, and recommendations are visible products. Everyone can see that you're working. How do you prove that you're a necessary member of the team if you just talk to people? Even the chaplain, with centuries of tradition behind him, is seldom regarded as crucial in this role.

A second reason for marginal status is low visibility of success criteria. Physicians have x-rays and blood tests to tell them and the world whether their efforts "worked." Physical therapists, lacking the physicians' hardware, at least have easy-to-describe behaviors to deal with like "puts on own pants—yes or no." Many applied behavioral science fields are beginning to realize that if they are to survive, they will [have to] learn to play the game of "accountability" as well as everyone else. Every effort is being made to remove descriptions of therapy benefits from the abstract (e.g., improved insight) to concrete behavior (e.g., no longer beats wife). Unfortunately, the psychologists' status isn't helped by this as much as it might be.

The reason is one of the bases for the marginal status of practitioners of the psychotherapeutic arts. The benefits of his efforts are not expected at immediate or even intermediate range, but at long range, which further compounds the problem of low visibility of success. If he serves well as therapist, counselor, teacher, guide, or guru, then the individual may be better prepared to deal with exigencies of his altered life, weeks, months, or years after he has left the hospital. That is the hope and intent. But the hospital staff, including the administrators who hold the purse strings, will never witness the "pay-off."

A fourth determiner of status is the extent to which a health profession deals in matters of survival versus "quality of life." When a psychologist correctly predicts, "If you put so-and-so in a full body cast, he'll cut his way out of it and leave the hospital," you can be sure they'll check with him the next few times they're considering using a full body cast. In that case, psychological factors have an impact on physical rehabilitation, the repair of his body—and that's close to a survival issue. When the same psychologist correctly predicts, "His wife really loves him, but he's going to drive her away by continually 'testing' her unless he gets some help," no one gets very alarmed. That only concerns his psyche, a "quality of life" issue. Let's say hospital staff acknowledge the need to deal with psychological problems before releasing the individual. They will not get . . . reimbursement for an extended stay.

It becomes fairly obvious why psychologists in rehabilitation hospitals do evaluation instead of treatment when there is not time for both. They have products which are immediate, visible—both as to effort and outcome—and are believed to impact issues closer to survival than quality of life. "You sure won't be any help to anybody if they close down your department." It's a matter of survival. [Vash, 1975, pp. 154–156]

Thus, evaluation may have expanded beyond its natural limits as an element of service to disabled people. Nonetheless, it often is necessary for official decision making, and it can offer undeniable benefits to those evaluated. In a general way, evaluation data are used to plan effective conduct of the life functions described in Part I: surviving, loving, working, playing, and transcending. More specific uses of evaluation data will be discussed in the following sections.

Screening and Adjudication

Another situation in which staff may be seen as more direct beneficiaries of evaluative information than clients is where data are gathered to aid screening or adjudication decisions. Evaluations help determine whether individuals should be screened in or out of programs or jobs, or judged eligible or ineligible for certain kinds of benefits. In these contexts, evaluators and evaluees often are working at crossed purposes: evaluees want *in*, and evaluators are responsible for screening *out* all but the clearly suited or eligible. As a result, numerous problems, pitfalls, and legal–ethical issues arise. These types of evaluations carry enormous social responsibility for evaluators because the outcomes have critical influence on the lives of evaluees; for example, whether they are hired, permitted to attend college, granted social insurance/welfare allowing them to live outside of institutions, or assigned to public guardians who will control their finances.

These areas have received massive civil rights attention, and the United States Supreme Court has long since ruled that screening instruments containing discriminatory bias must not be used without bias-neutralizing complementary procedures. The section later in this chapter called "How: Evaluation Techniques" will describe selected ways in which such demands are met, plus other methods used for ensuring fairness of decisions based on evaluative data.

Once individuals have been "screened into" designated service systems, the purposes and uses of subsequent evaluations are rather clearly for their direct benefit. It is here that evaluative information is used as a counseling tool and basis for evaluees' personal life-planning decisions.

Tool for Counseling and Stimulation of Self-Evaluation

The evaluation process itself sometimes can have a "therapeutic" effect apart from the uses to which the findings are put. Most notable is the cathartic effect of describing one's history, situation, and problems to an interested interviewer; but responding to psychometric test or questionnaire items can fulfill similar needs. Going a step further, simply learning the findings—before they are put to active use in counseling—is helpful to some people. A client of an alcoholism clinic humorously indicated,

> Somehow, it helped me to know what kind of a nut I am. I got a kind of peaceful feeling that if a picture of me emerged from those zig zaggy lines on the profile sheets, somebody must have a handle on things. For the first time in years I had this surge of feeling, "Hey, everything's gonna be all right." That got me off to a good start in counseling.

Others, of course, have opposite reactions of fearful defensiveness. The difference is probably a function of both the evaluee's personality and the evaluator's manner of presentation.

During any kind of counseling process—from educational advisement through reconstructive psychotherapy—assessment findings may be used to guide the participants in a number of ways. The counselor will keep them in mind when choosing the techniques or style. Both will use them in making decisions about "treatment" (which services to seek or offer) and life in general (what to do about identified problems). The client may continue to use gleaned knowledge of capabilities/limitations and awareness of personal needs/traits for many years after counseling has terminated, when critical life decisions must be made. Moreover, observing the fruitfulness of connecting life decisions to relevant evaluation data can stimulate habits of self-evaluation in introspectively inclined people, and this is often an explicit intent of the evaluator–counselor.

Perhaps most important, evaluative information, both initial assessments and progress evaluations obtained during the course of a treatment process, is used as a springboard to counseling. To illustrate, one demonstration project (Vash & Murray, 1969) was designed specifically to use ongoing assessments of work habits and production in a workshop setting as the "grist for the counseling mill" in weekly group and individual counseling sessions with "hard-core unemployed" disabled men. As a result of experience in this project, the author came to the conclusion that evaluation data not shared with clients—to the limits of their comprehension—constitute serious waste of both the clients' and the professionals' time. Demonstrations such as this are a form of research, the last purpose to be discussed here.

Research

Research efforts in service delivery contexts provide direct benefits to scientists and service providers and indirect benefits to rehabilitation service consumers. Program evaluation, demonstration projects, and other research pursuits—basic and applied—can require extensive assessment of personal variables to discover or document relationships between antecedent conditions and outcome variables. At times, the evaluative data do double duty, serving to guide clinical decision making as well as provide a basis for scientific prediction. At other times, research is the only purpose, and the subject benefits only when findings are translated into program improvements and enhanced techniques of service. In actuality, it is later generations of clients who most likely will be the benficiaries.

Certain ethical issues arise when data are gathered solely for research purposes; that is, the subjects must give consent to provide research data that will not directly benefit them, and they must be informed of the general purposes of the research project. When, in order to protect the soundness of the research design, full disclosure is withheld until after a project is completed, subjects must know and agree to this.

Who: The People Evaluated

It is not only those whose behavior we wish to predict that we evaluate. Sometimes it is deemed necessary to evaluate significant people in their environments, too. The supportiveness of a parent or the emotional stability of a spouse, for example, may be as critical to correctly predicting the behavior summarized as "rehabilitation success" for a given individual as many personal traits. Thus, close family members become likely subjects for evaluation, whether done formally or through casual observation. Close friends, lovers, and sundry "significant others" may similarly become subjects of evaluation.

In addition, rehabilitation personnel may evaluate themselves, or be evaluated by colleagues, regarding the quality of relationships they establish with given patients or clients. To illustrate, when the work climate permits it, a professional who senses s/he has a poor working relationship with a given client may, after evaluating whether the problems are resolvable, ask for the person to be reassigned; or other staff may recommend that a particular professional work with a given individual in the belief that s/he is especially suitable.

Naturally, in the process of rehabilitation, the primary subject is the person with a disability, and s/he may be assessed in a wide variety of roles: patient, client, student, trainee, recipient, worker, and so forth.

What: Objects and Varieties of Evaluation

The facts evaluated can be categorized in several ways. First, we evaluate both independent and dependent variables, that is, resources or deficits that influence rehabilitation outcomes, and the outcomes themselves. In clinical practice, it is generally only the independent variables (resources/deficits) that are measured. Dependent variables (outcomes) usually are assessed only in the context of follow-up research designed to show whether clinically assumed relationships actually hold, or to test the effectiveness of delivered services.

Looking only at the independent variables, certain resources/deficits have been classified previously as personal variables or *inner* resources/ deficits, and the rest are environmental variables or *outer* resources/hindrances. "Varieties of evaluation" refers to specialized sets of independent variables used to predict success in particular life-performance areas, such as in work evaluation, driver evaluation, and evaluation for rehabilitation engineering devices.

Many of the inner resource variables commonly assessed were cited in earlier chapters as requisite to coping, adjusting, surviving, working, and so forth. Intelligence; emotional stability; tolerance for stress and frustration; and ability to handle loss, fear, and anger are assessed rather routinely in rehabilitation settings, sometimes formally, sometimes through casual observation. Personality traits that can help or hinder adjustment also may be assessed in the more psychologically sophisticated programs. Routine evaluation of physical resources/deficits tends to focus on the impaired systems, but "backup systems" (for example, vision for hearing impaired people, hearing for visually impaired people) frequently are included as well. Specialized physical assessment procedures (for example, in work evaluation) reflect still greater emphasis on compensatory strengths in nonimpaired systems.

Fortunately, recent years have seen a positive change in the emphasis placed on assessing strengths as opposed to weaknesses. For several decades, excessive attention was paid to ferreting out deficiencies and liabilities, and too little effort was spent in discovering resources that would be the building blocks of rehabilitation. The bias became known as the "pathology error" and is now on its way toward correction. This altered attitude may have been partly responsible for concomitantly increased attention to personality traits that can help or hinder adjustment, depending on how well they are recognized and responded to; that is, how well they are exploited when they are resources and ameliorated when they are hindrances. Both changes reflect maturation in the PSV disciplines. We no longer are so insecure that we have to mimic the medical model with its focus on pathology; nor must we abjure such unscientific concerns as whether a patient has a sense of humor.

A bias still evident is the concentration of effort on evaluating the mind (emotional, intellectual, personality factors) and the body (physical, sensory factors) and the virtual absence of attention to spiritual resources. In view of a growing belief that experience with disability may have signal importance for spiritual growth, and that spiritual resources may be among the most powerful in integrating disability into one's life, this seems an oversight worthy of correction.

The environment variables most commonly assessed as part of rehabilitation planning are those relating to home and family. Such factors as the family's own coping ability, their capacity for providing emotional and practical support to the disabled person, their occupational tradition or history, and (in the more enlightened settings) their own needs for services all become important data. In addition, the physical facts of the home environment, such as mobility barriers and access to buslines, are essential bits of information.

The following assessment model, originally designed to help allied health staff in a rehabilitation hospital to make appropriate referrals to the hospital's vocational rehabilitation program, will illustrate (1) a comprehensive array of variables that must be evaluated in the process of moving disabled people from the medical to the vocational stage of rehabilitation and (2) some of their important interrelationships.

Drawing from the job demands described in the *Dictionary of Occupational Titles*, it is reasoned that for a worker to have something to offer an employer, s/he must have capabilities in one of the five following "worker resource" areas:

1. Brawn—the ability to use one's body as a "power machine" or a mover of material. This includes such subcomponents as strength, endurance, and agility (coordination plus speed).
2. Brain—the ability to use one's intellect to perform operations on information and ideas. This includes such subcomponents as intelligence, creativity, special aptitudes, and learned knowledge.

3. Hands—the ability to use one's hands to create or manipulate objects. This includes such subcomponents as dexterity, special talents, and learned skills.

4. Personality—the ability to use one's personality to influence the attitudes and behavior of others. This includes such subcomponents as dominance, energy level, and learned interpersonal skills. (It should be stressed that this dimension is limited to that aspect of personality used as a work tool, much as we use our bodies, brains, and hands. Some jobs demand high levels of it—psychotherapist, teacher, trial attorney, receptionist, manager—and some require little or none—statistical clerk, laborer, bench assembler. It does not include aspects of personality that relate to getting or keeping jobs in general, such as poise, adaptability, and grooming habits.)

It is acknowledged that communication skill can be viewed as a subcomponent of the combined brain and personality dimensions. However, because the receptive losses of blind and deaf workers and the transmission deficits of persons with speech disorders affect communication in ways that do not fit with our usual concepts of "brain" and "personality," this has been factored out to form a separate dimension.

5. Communication—the ability to receive and transmit information accurately and efficiently. This breaks down into the subcomponents of visual/auditory reception, and vocal/written transmission. Comprehension and other "data processing" abilities are considered brain resources. Persuasive effect of communications is considered a personality resource. This variable is defined solely in terms of receiving/transmitting abilities.

In addition to the worker resource variables, "emotional stability" must also be considered as a necessary support or background variable in making oneself desirable to an employer. Therefore, this sixth and last variable is added to the list.

6. Emotional stability—the ability to perform a job adequately in the face of stress, and behave appropriately on the job.

These six variables can also form a basis for defining both type and severity of disability. "Type" here refers only to the job-relevant aspect of function that is impaired. For example, individuals can be rated "high," "moderate," "low," or "very low" in each area, compared to the work force population.

A person with a "very low" rating in an area would only be a person having a severe disability. A "low" rating would reflect the presence of a moderate disability. A mild disability would not be expected, by itself, to force a rating below the "moderate" level. Viewed in another way, the functional limitations of a quadriplegic, for example, would always be reflected in "very low" ratings on "brawn" and "hands." Those of mentally retarded persons would reflect "low" or "very low" ratings on "brain" resources. Disabling mental illness would be reflected on the "emotional stability" scale; sensory disabilities on the "communication" scale; and so forth. If a disability reduces a person's reservoir of worker resources to offer an employer, it is reflected in this system. If it does not, it belongs in another part of the predictive equation—perhaps that which treats proximal environment variables affecting the likelihood of a person's working at all, such as social reactions to disability.

This four-point rating scale is only one suggested way of quantifying the data for predictive purposes. An earlier study (Vash & Murray, 1969) confirmed that global ratings made by vocational rehabilitation experts on such simple rating scales do have predictive capability. In that study, two judges rated 100 former clients of an employment project for severely disabled clients on three-point scales (low, moderate, high) in four of the six dimensions—brawn, brain, hands, and emotional stability. Whether or not job placement was achieved was known in every case. The results showed that job placement could be predicted for a client who had one of two rating patterns: one "high" in any of the three worker resource areas plus at least a "moderate" in emotional stability—or—two "moderates" in two of the three worker resource areas and, again, at least a "moderate" in emotional stability. If any other pattern was found, job placement could not be predicted. That is, if a person had only one "moderate" or all "lows" in the worker resource areas, even with a "high" in emotional stability, job placement could not be predicted. Or, even if s/he had "highs" in all three worker resource areas, if s/he also had a "low" in emotional stability, job placement could not be predicted.

It can be seen from the foregoing that whereas "disability" is operationally defined by ratings on one or more of the individual scales, "vocational handicap" (or its obverse, "vocational potential") is defined by the total profile of all the scales. The lack of isomorphism between disability and vocational handicap also becomes readily apparent. For example, quadriplegia would be defined by "very low" ratings on brawn and hands. However, if the individual also had "high" ratings on brain, personality, communication, and emotional stability, his or her vocational potential would be very good (and, conversely, the vocational handicap could be considered mild).

Standardized (standardizeable) measures can be used (constructed) for each of the six dimensions as means of validating subjective, global ratings by experts, or for obtaining more precise predictive indices for clinical use. [Vash, 1973, pp.3–6]

The variety of evaluation that has developed for predicting employability and providing vocational rehabilitation planning data for improving a client's employability is known as "work evaluation." Actually, this is a misnomer; the more accurate designation would be worker evaluation. Work evaluation programs evaluate clients—their potentials to become workers—almost entirely. They seldom assess work—actual jobs, work settings and climates, and other work-life realities that will influence materially the psychological well-being of the client-become-worker. This apparent hairsplitting is worthy of mention because evaluation of the work side of the equation is sorely needed as well, but is seriously and systematically neglected by the field.

Given what it does, work evaluation is awarded high importance in rehabilitation, in terms of program funding and centrality in the vocational rehabilitation plans of disabled people. It encompasses many types of evaluative procedures, from psychometric testing to sampling of actual work performance, and may encompass other varieties of evaluation, such as driver evaluation and evaluation for rehabilitation engineering assistive devices. It has so gained the confidence of the rehabilitation community that work evaluators have emerged as a separate, specialized discipline. This brings us to the next topic for discussion: the people who serve in the evaluator functions.

Who: The Evaluators

Although every rehabilitation discipline includes evaluation among its responsibilities, some are more heavily loaded with diagnostic/prognostic functions than others. Medical doctors, unless they perform surgery or prescribe pharmaceuticals, may serve primarily as diagnosticians after the acute stage has given way to the rehabilitation stage of recovery, delegating the actual treatment to therapists and other allied health professionals. But these personnel have their own evaluative procedures they must complete in order to determine the specific treatment approaches to use. Certain medical specialties, of course, are devoted solely to diagnostic functions; radiology serves as a well-known example.

A similar pattern is evolving in PSV evaluation, although it is less clear cut. Whether psychologists diagnose only, or diagnose and treat, depends sometimes on the setting's policies and sometimes on personal predilections. Social workers and rehabilitation counselors, while lacking a comparably delineated diagnostic role, must—like therapists in medical settings—evaluate both initial status and ongoing progress in order to do their treatment jobs effectively. So far, the work evaluator is the only PSV discipline that has emerged devoted exclusively (or nearly so) to diagnostic/prognostic functions. ("Nearly so" because in some settings they serve on work-adjustment treatment teams.) Rehabilitation counselors delegate a great deal of the evaluation needed to establish a "vocational diagnosis" to work evaluators and psychologists, and some of the consequences of this now will be examined.

Rehabilitation Counselors as Vocational Diagnosticians

Notwithstanding the current interest in habilitation, or independent living rehabilitation, the primary mission of the state–federal rehabilitation program is *vocational*. Consequently, rehabilitation counselors can be viewed reasonably as a specialized variety of vocational counselor. For some reason, however, the profession has not assumed prime responsibility for vocational diagnosis. Major portions of this task are delegated to work evaluators in work-oriented rehabilitation facilities, and psychologists generally are used to administer and "interpret" PSV testing. (The reason for quotation marks around "interpret" will be explained later.) Although the clinical psychological testing undoubtedly should remain in the hands of fully trained psychologists, the vocational testing—abilities, aptitudes, achievement, interests— might be done profitably by rehabilitation counselors themselves. There are several reasons for this.

First, the conceptual base accrued through knowledge of and experience with such testing could strengthen their counseling skills. Second, their greater familiarity with the clients could enhance the accuracy and richness of test information yield. Third, and the reason for surrounding "interpret" with quotation marks, test protocols and profiles can be fully interpreted only with the inputs of the test taker. An expert reviewing score patterns can generate only hypotheses—*tentative* interpretations. Actual, or full, interpretation is a product of interaction between the test taker, the expert, and the record of scores itself. From the score patterns, the expert develops hypotheses that are presented to the test taker. The latter may confirm or disconfirm the hypotheses by providing additional, relevant information—verbally (immediately) or behaviorally (over time).

Thus, a full interpretation cannot be done in the office of a psychologist who has only met the client once. It involves a time-consuming process of determining which findings are valid and meaningful to the test taker; and only the counselor will have the ongoing relationship required to make this possible. To do it effectively, the counselor must be trained, experienced, and fine-tuned; and this could make delegation to another counterproductive. The final reason has to do with the professional status of rehabilitation counselors themselves. As pointed out earlier, possession of software such as test instruments adds to a discipline's professional visibility. It might, then, behoove rehabilitation counselors to consider absorbing the testing function, especially if they wish to move beyond professional certification to state licensure.

Evaluative Biases

A potential problem area shared by all disciplines in their evaluative functions is that of individual practitioner distortions in drawing conclusions from assessment data. The sources are basically two: theoretical bias and unresolved personal problems. To illustrate the first, the Freudian may see sexual concerns, or the Adlerian, power striving, where others would not. To illustrate the second, the practitioner with strong unmet needs in a given area may overstress or avoid that area in evaluating clients. The first source may be the more difficult to deal with, since one person's bias may be another's ultimate truth, and no court exists to prove one of them right. The latter may be correctible, given a practitioner who is open to nondefensive self-examination and, perhaps, a supervisor who is sensitive to the issues and skilled in helping subordinates recognize and correct such problems.

Somewhat akin to evaluative biases is the tendency to prolong the evaluation phase because of professional insecurity about initiating and conducting treatment. Interminable evaluation can be used as a stalling device and is very common among neophyte practicum students and interns. The stall is "covered" by a belief that additional information will make the existing data fall into place, make sense, and provide clear treatment direction. The magical thinking in this usually is obvious to everyone but the uncertain soul caught in the process.

A final bias, also of a behavioral rather than perceptual sort, should be mentioned. Many PSV professionals choose their lives' work partly out of fascination with the intricate interworkings of human nature. Thus, in evaluating, and especially in the interview situation, there is a tendency to gather personal information far afield from what is needed for the treatment program at hand, simply because it is of clinical or scientific (hopefully not prurient) interest. A subtle matter not yet a frequent target of civil rights concern, it may be in the future, as consumer sophistication increases about what information is really needed to plan, say, a vocational rehabilitation program. Civil rights attorneys consider it an invasion of privacy, and psychologists regard it as a counterproductive form of voyeurism that diverts attention from critical issues and wastes client and professional time. Although attended to regularly in psychologists' and social workers' training programs, the problem exists among rehabilitation counselors, too. Thus, this discipline also may need to focus on minimizing it during preservice training.

Nonprofessional Evaluators

It is not only professionals who do important evaluations. The common-sense PSV evaluations of hospital attendants and workshop foremen, who spend far longer hours in direct contact with patients/clients than professionals, can be invaluable. The same is true of the assessments shared by family members and friends. As noted earlier, self-evaluations done by the patients/clients are often the most useful of all sources of diagnostic/prognostic information. Moreover, peer evaluations that emerge from, say, group counseling experiences are beginning to reap the recognition they merit. Discussions of the ways in which these sources of evaluation are used in rehabilitation will be offered later.

Where and When: Evaluation Settings and Timing

Evaluation takes place in virtually every PSV treatment setting: hospitals, rehabilitation centers, work-oriented rehabilitation facilities, consumer-run independent living centers, schools, the state service-delivery arms of the state–federal rehabilitation program, and others too numerous to name. In addition, clinics have come into being that do no treatment per se, but solely offer work-evaluation services, which they sell for a fee to other rehabilitation agencies that perform the treatment functions—most notably, the state rehabilitation agencies.

An overview of the way in which rehabilitation services are organized may be helpful at this juncture. Considering only direct services to specifiable clients (excluding supportive or indirect services that benefit disabled people generally), service-delivery agencies can be assigned to either the public, the private nonprofit, or the private for-profit sector. A large segment of the private nonprofit sector was created by federal grant funding for the expressed purpose of providing evaluation and specialized treatment services deemed infeasible for the state rehabilitation agencies to deliver in their public sector bureaucratic settings. The private for-profit sector is a relatively new phenomenon, existing in states that have enacted "mandatory rehabilitation" laws for industrially injured workers. These laws make available private monies to pay for private services, and PSV rehabilitation professionals have responded by going into private practice—singly or in groups. Here, too, a significant part of the work to be done is evaluation, and it is generally an accompaniment to treatment, not a sole or even primary service.

Some question whether "evaluation *en vacuo*"—not included in a treatment matrix—can provide optimal data. Virtually all rehabilitation clients who raise sufficient questions in their counselors' minds to stimulate referral for evaluation also have treatment needs, whether work adjustment, training, or other. This being the case, use of facilities that can provide both evaluation and treatment, and combine them in ways that enrich each function, would seem preferable to use of facilities that can do only one-point evaluations, with little or no opportunity to observe the rates of behavioral changes that occur as treatment progresses.

Although most of the state rehabilitation agencies have psychologists on their staffs to perform some of the PSV evaluation, most also contract with psychologists and psychiatrists in the private sector to do overflow and highly specialized work. Some may require the referred clients to come to their private offices, while others go to the agency office to interview and test. In short, there is no consistent state-agency model for obtaining psychological evaluations; each agency has the latitude to develop its own system in accord with local need and service availability. Nonetheless, there is considerable dissatisfaction with the various models evolved; difficulties in finding qualified providers, and inability to pay competitively when they are found, are cited as core problems.

The matter of evaluation timing was alluded to with respect to one-point versus ongoing evaluations of worker habits and competencies. Simply, evaluations are conducted before, during, and after treatment services. Initial evaluations give an intake person a basis for screening in or screening out; they then give a case-responsible person some knowledge of a client's status coming into a program—the strengths and weaknesses that shoud be reinforced and corrected, respectively. Ongoing evaluations give evidence of progress and readiness for the next stage of a rehabilitation plan, or needs for additional/changed services not hitherto recognized. These "before" and "during" evaluations generally are conducted by rehabilitation professionals or other providers. Follow-up evaluations may be conducted to determine whether further services are needed, but they usually are done for research purposes—to evaluate program effectiveness or find support for hypothesized relationships between independent variables (for example, client or service characteristics) and outcomes. These "after" evaluations are apt to be done by researchers, who consider themselves scientists rather than professionals or providers.

How: Evaluation Techniques

This is the final and most important issue to consider. It will be examined through an overview of the actual techniques used and some of the problems they present in assessing a disabled population.

PSV evaluation techniques can be classified according to a number of dimensions that may or may not be mutually exclusive. For example, they may be typed by their mode of construction, that is, whether they are standarized or psychometric, versus adventitious situational. They also may be categorized by modes of administration, response, or scoring, that is, whether they are administered to groups or individuals; whether responses are written, oral, or manipulative; or whether scoring is objective or subjective. There are still other ways to classify evaluation procedures, but these distinctions illustrate the breadth of range in use.

The Interview

The interview is generally regarded as the most powerful single tool available to the PSV evaluator. Tests are used as substitutes or supplements when it is necessary to save time or provide objective data amenable to direct comparison with others. In other situations, interviewers' subjective impressions are valued, as reflected in the fabled importance of "the first four minutes" and "listening with the third ear." Moreover, no test can measure the subtle information transmitted through body language, and the instruments required to measure, say, voice stress would destroy rapport. Thus, despite impressive test technology, skillful interviewers attuned to their own affective reactions remain among the best "instruments" available. They are, however, unvalidated, for two major reasons. First, validating professionals' abilities to predict clients' future behavior is costly, mainly in terms of staff time. Second, the process is threatening, so most attempts die aborning from lack of volunteers.

One way to enhance validity is to use two or more interviewers and "triangulate" between their observations and conclusions to arrive at consensual validation. This is also costly. Consequently, it is reserved for such critical situations as hiring decisions or the assessment of potentially dangerous individuals.

Interviewing is particularly important in assessing people with disabilities because many standardized tests/inventories have uncertain reliability and validity when used with a disabled population (to be discussed later). The interview, however, is no less reliable or valid, given an interviewer who is sensitive to disability-related issues without overemphasizing them. Such special competencies parallel interviewers' needs to understand cultural and subcultural values, experiences, and expectations. Despite the known problems, however, disabled people are tested with instruments standardized on general population samples wherein disabled people were probably poorly represented. Next we will explore some of the issues that arise.

Testing

The first problem confronted is the usability of a given instrument, that is, whether a disability precludes its use altogether. At the extreme, a blind person cannot respond to Rorschach cards, nor can a person with paralyzed arms respond to the Purdue Pegboard. In these cases, the exclusion is unequivocal. At the next level, some test makers prohibit use of their tests with certain populations. For example, the GATB (General Aptitude Test Battery) instructions specify that all performance tasks must be done standing, thus excluding wheelchair users even if they could complete the subtests. Here, the exclusion is legal/ethical, and it is sometimes ignored. The most serious problems arise at the next level, where use is nowise prohibited, but a testee's disability raises questions about the reliability and validity of any scores obtained.

Both may be affected by even small changes in test administration, beginning with the presentation of instructions. For this reason, the use of traditional tests with deaf individuals creates problems that sometimes are unrecognized by naive examiners. (Trying to convince psychometrists that makeshift solutions combining miming and scribbling are not sufficient has, on occasion, proved difficult.) If the examiner can sign, the problems are reduced, but the effect of translating is still unknown. The presence of an interpreter introduces yet another unmeasurable difference from standard procedure.

The third-party effect also must be considered when testees must speak, for another to record, answers that usually are written. In personality testing, one may say no more than "true" or "false"; however, when that reflects an emotionally charged confession, there may be less tendency to speak it to another than to record it on paper when working alone. In ability testing, an examiner is more likely to give extra clues to the test taker under these circumstances, leading to an elevated score. On the other hand, anxiety about "performing" for a listener could operate to lower scores. In short, nonstandard forces are tugging on the scores, and their ultimate direction of movement is unknown.

Also in ability testing, a critical problem is timing. Scores on all timed tests may be affected substantially by disabilities that cause either physical slowing or lowered expectations for performing rapidly (Urmer & Balshan, 1960). Most tests of intelligence, aptitude, and achievement are timed, although a few are untimed—or "power"—tests. The problem is sometimes handled by administering a test in both ways; that is, the number of items completed by the time limit is recorded, but the examinee is allowed to continue for an additional number of minutes, until either the test is completed or s/he appears to be making no correct responses. Thus, both "time" and "power" scores are obtained, and the examiner estimates from the difference what an accurate score might be. A highly subjective method at best, it may be more useful than a single score that almost certainly is spuriously depressed.

The attempted use of standardized tests too soon after catastrophic disablement may result in bizarre and meaningless patterns reflecting only the acute state of turmoil the individual is in. The disabled psychologist quoted several times in Part I describes, from personal experience, what can happen later in the adjustment process.

> A few months after I was up in a wheelchair, the high-school psychologist gave me a battery of tests for vocational guidance. The personality tests looked as normal as apple pie because I desperately wanted to impress everyone with how well I was handling things. I "faked good" without even being conscious of it . . . sort of "Oh, that's the healthy response, that's gotta be me;" and I knew better than to "bite" on the faking-detector questions. My IQ, however, unaccountably dropped about twenty points from my ninth-grade scores (which I wasn't supposed to know). Since the psychologist didn't have those tests for comparison, and my score was still good college material stuff, he figured I was in fine shape. However, my personality test scores reflected my intelligence, and my IQ score showed how depressed I was.

Even after a disabled person has stabilized emotionally, certain personality-test findings may have altered significance. An example comes from the Minnesota Multiphasic Personality Inventory (MMPI), where physical symptom responses scored on the Hysteria (Hy) and Hypochondriasis (Hs) scales do not take into account the fact that people with certain disabilities report many critical symptoms for physiologic, not neurotic, reasons. Thus, scores on these two scales may be spuriously elevated. The problem relates to the appropriateness of the normative comparison sample. To get a more accurate appraisal of hysterical or hypochondriacal tendencies in, say, paraplegics, one would need to compare their responses with those of other paraplegics.

The issue of appropriate norms also arises with respect to ability testing, because it has been observed that rehabilitation client populations tend to score lower on aptitude tests than other indicators would predict. From time to time, clinical settings attempt to create "local norms" to compare their disabled clients with other disabled individuals on such tests. However, since aptitude tests are used largely to guide people in the competitive world of work, it is well that most such projects never come to fruition. In this case, it is more useful to know how one scores against actual competitors—most of whom will be nondisabled—than to enjoy more favorable comparisons with peers who also might be at a competitive disadvantage.

The situation is directly analogous to the well-publicized test-validity problems with ethnic minority examinees. Scores are lowered, but low scores do not predict poor performance on criterion tasks as accurately as they do for others. Also in parallel, efforts are being made to ensure that job-screening procedures do not discriminate unfairly against disabled applicants (see Chapter 9). Most efforts are transitional; the ultimate solution will not reside in altering norms. Rather, totally new methods for predicting performance need to be developed. A subsequent section on performance sampling will explore the major current approach to this.

Few, if any, tests are good instruments in and of themselves. Most become good tests only in the hands of gifted examiners who can combine the maximum possible adherence to standard procedure with optimal innovation and skilled interpretation, thus to generate an accurate picture of the test taker's present status and future likelihoods. In some cases, test scores are used without interpretation to make such official decisions as admission to scholastic programs. Where this is done, however, the practice is increasingly being challenged, legally, because of the known validity problems for certain subpopulations. Thus, it is not a good practice to emulate clinically.

The "magic" of good tests resides in the instrument–practitioner interaction. Although the Strong-Campbell Vocational Interest Blank is widely considered one of the best psychological instruments ever developed (research shows it accurately predicts very long-range behavior), it is of little value when used mechanically by practitioners who are only superficially familiar with its construction and potential. The most expert user known to the author, Robert Hadley of the California State University at Los Angeles, is so immersed in the intercorrelations among the subscales that, from a scattering of scores on a profile, he can estimate the rest with an astonishing degree of accuracy. This intimate knowledge of the instrument also allows him to give far richer interpretations than the ordinary user, namely, hypothesizing personality traits or behavioral tendencies that surpass both what generally is deduced from the inventory and what is corroborated regularly by test takers or others who know them.

Harry Grace, of the Pacific University in Hawaii, has a similarly intimate relationship with the Kuder Vocational Preference Record. He uses a "vector analysis" of the extent to which test takers show by their scores that they want to direct, versus be directed by, people, numbers, ideas, and things. He uses the Kuder as a springboard to counseling, and his remarkable ability to do it is based not only on sensitivity to people but extensive understanding of the constituency of the inventory. This is a nontraditional use of a traditional instrument. Other practitioners are using a variety of nontraditional evaluative methods.

Nontraditional Evaluation

Now that it is no longer considered gauche, in intellectual circles, to confess open-mindedness to such paranormal possibilities as extrasensory perception and psychic sensitivity, modalities previously classed with the "occult" and spurned by the psychological mainstream are being explored cautiously. As will be seen in the following chapter, treatment methods that appear to "work" despite unexplained neurophysiological mediation are being taught and used in holistic health/human potential development quarters. The same is true for a scattering of evaluative techniques, with astrological forecasting and psychic readings in the PSV forefront. (Iridology, a system of diagnosing bodily ills from inspection of the iris of the eyes, currently is capturing similar interest in the physical area.)

On the borderline between traditional and nontraditional evaluative techniques are little-used instruments that measure nontraditionally considered traits using traditional tests or inventory methods. Tests of creativity, operationally defined as "divergent thinking ability," have been shown to predict vocational productiveness (Kemp & Vash, 1971), for example. In addition, measures of sensation seeking, including boredom susceptibility (Zuckerman et al., 1978), and motivation to find purpose in life (Crumbaugh, 1977) have suggestive promise for rehabilitation. As research and clinical experience show particular traits to be useful predictors, they may move into the mainstream and become regarded as traditional. Of the three examples cited, only the first has made noticeable headway in that direction. Problems associated with boredom and the will to meaning strike the author as potentially powerful predictor variables and bases for treatment efforts. Each reader probably will think of one or two other traits that seem equally worthy of research and clinical attention.

Performance Sampling

An evaluative approach that has moved recently from the nontraditional area to the traditional is that of performance sampling. Here, the field of rehabilitation has pioneered for more than just the disabled population. Simulated and actual work-sampling techniques were developed as means of solving reliability and validity problems by narrowing the generalization gap when predicting disabled workers' job performance. It was reasoned that the more like the actual work situation the testing was, the less likely it became that predictions would go wrong. Nearly two decades after this was standard operating procedure in vocational rehabilitation, the civil rights movement created changes that required similar generalization-gap narrowing in assessing ethnic-minority job applicants. Thus, the substitution of performance sampling for (poorly predictive) standardized tests—"old hat" in rehabilitation—became the "new thing" in mainstream job-selection screening. It is unquestionably a better way; now efforts need to be directed toward reducing the time required to obtain adequate samples to a cost-effective level.

To add perspective, one type of performance sampling has been practiced by rehabilitation counselors for years: requiring clients seeking artistic training to submit portfolios of their work to agreed-upon experts for talent evaluation. Of more recent origin, videotape feedback offers performance sampling to the clients themselves, for self-appraisal of job interview and other interpersonal skills. This places the evaluative responsibility on the clients themselves, which brings us to the last topic to be discussed in this chapter.

Information and Power

As has been pointed out in many contexts, information is power. Whoever possesses the pertinent information also possesses the power advantage of being equipped to make critical decisions. This is poignantly true with respect to evaluative information. As long as the professionals possess, control, and guard the information yielded by evaluation procedures, they are in more favorable positions than the clients to make decisions about the clients' lives. The solution is simple: give the information to the clients. A way of doing this will be described briefly in the hope that some readers may find it worthy of trying.

The model is borrowed from a practice used by Milton Hahn in his career-counseling work with high-level executives. In a personal communication with the author, he indicated that he prepared a "know thyself" manual for every client, which contained all test protocols and profiles, and summaries of all interpretations and recommendations made to the client during consultation. He commented,

> You have to give clients like these a tangible product of what you've done for them. After all, they've paid you a handsome fee for a job of work [sic] and they expect something to show—literally—for it. They are highly competent people who don't turn their lives over to anyone else, even temporarily. You're just another consultant with the kind of expertise they need at that point to make their own decisions. Those decisions go on after counseling, and the manual can help in making them.

Knowing the different population the author worked with, he added wryly,

> It's a shame we don't treat welfare recipients with the same respect these executives *force* us to show them. Your clients need to be taught how to be as much in charge of their lives—and their own information—as my executives are.

From this remonstrance, a variation was developed for use by rehabilitation facilities that offer staged evaluation, work adjustment, and job-placement programs. Ordinarily, work evaluators report their findings to the work adjustment staff, not the clients; and the work adjustment staff reports to the placement staff at the next transition. The professionals conscientiously transfer information from one to another while the clients wait, passively and powerlessly, for selected bits to be shared with them. It was decided that this situation would be changed by beginning a "know thyself" manual for each client at the outset of the process. Then the clients would be in charge of taking their own information folios to the next type of expert to be seen and would command the information sharing. (Everyone loses things sometimes; file copies would be kept.) Clients would be privy to all evaluative information about themselves; they would be in a position to query the experts about unclear or conflicting findings; they would feel far less the helpless pawns in a game with undeclared rules; and they would be better prepared to serve as their own case managers, a lifelong responsibility that will fall to them after leaving the facility. In short, the advantages of designating clients as the prime repositors of their own evaluative information are considerable. At the end of services, they would have a software product, their "know thyself" manuals, to take with them and use after being trained to do so.

Another power-related issue involves clients' fearing evaluation because the resultant labels may stigmatize the bearer. Labels do have immense power to affect attitudes toward oneself and others; however, their value as shortcuts to understanding can be used, and the distressing aspects avoided, simply by conferring common-sense, neutral terms instead of diagnostic categories that sound clinical and frightening. The public does not resist labeling per se, as the prevalence of "Are you a Virgo? I'm a Leo!" attests. Clinicians can use constructively people's attraction to labeling, toward enhancing self-understanding, if they will apply only terms that accentuate the positive. For example, Skip Heck, a psychologist specializing in problems of loneliness, assigns clients palatable "diagnoses" based partly on Native American typologies, which they use in the process of self-discovery. He points out, in a personal communication, that,

> To be called an "obsessional neurotic" is insulting, but to be called a "visual mouse" can entice you to find out more about what kind of a person you are. Neither term has any meaning to the uninitiated, but the more you know about what is meant by "obsessional neurotic," the less you want to be called one—because only pathology is mentioned. The more you learn about what it is to be a "visual mouse," however, the more you see both the positive and negative features of intense attraction to minute detail, and can intelligently sort what you want to expunge from what you want to keep. When the positive side is highlighted as well as the negative, you don't have to get defensive to keep from feeling like a fool.

The use of evaluative procedures as integral parts of treatment serves as a fitting transition to the following chapter. In it, we will begin to examine treatment techniques, beginning with those aimed at strengthening people's skills and resources for staying healthy—psychologically, socially, and vocationally—despite the "slings and arrows" that may accompany disablement.

11 Strengthening
Psychogogic Approaches

Once a rehabilitation client has been evaluated with respect to psychosocial–vocational functioning, the next step is to select the appropriate training, treatment, or other PSV interventions that will aid the adjustment process and enhance rehabilitation success. This and the following two chapters will be devoted to surveyng some of the issues and techniques considered most important. Although there are countless ways to categorize the welter of techniques currently in use, a simple dichotomy between psychogogic and psychotherapeutic approaches seems most appropriate, especially to reemphasize the point that the psychology of disability is largely the psychology of ordinary people responding normatively to abnormal stimulus situations.

In case the term "psychogogy" is not familiar to all readers, it is a word coined by Abraham Maslow (1965) to denote psychosocial intervention strategies based on an educational, not a medical, model. The suffix "-gogy" denotes teaching, or leading, as in the more familiar "pedagogy." He developed the construct in contradistinction to "psychotherapy," where "-therapy" denotes serving in a curative role. The crux of the distinction can be stated as prevention versus cure. Psychogogic approaches strive to strengthen the individual against the onslaughts of stress, in order to avoid or prevent mental/emotional/behavioral disorder. On the other hand, psychotherapeutic approaches strive to redress or correct disorders that have come about already.

This distinction, like much of Maslow's theoretical work, was influenced by extensive study of Eastern psychology, philosophy, and religious thought. Maslow, like Carl Jung, was responsible for transporting a treasury of ancient Eastern conceptions to spark "new" ways of thinking in the West. The report that in ancient China a physician was paid to keep the "patient" well, and that payment ceased if illness occurred since he obviously hadn't done his job, now is cited frequently by people disenchanted with modern, Western medical care or angry about iatrogenic illnesses induced by curative attempts that backfire. Western health care has developed primarily as a corrective mode, with preventive medicine a tiny subspecialty still practiced en masse (for example, through public health agencies) far more than with individuals who go to see their doctors.

Maslow's infusion of the preventive orientation into Western psychological intervention carried with it two important implications. First, the "patient" has a great deal of responsibility for active follow-through on what the physician teaches, and, conversely, the physician does not so much administer treatment as inform and guide. Second, integral to these Eastern philosophical underpinnings of health care is a holistic conception of human nature that emphasizes the spiritual as much as, if not more than, the bodily and mental components. This contrasts with Western body–mind dualism that either denies spirituality or relegates it to an aspect of mind. Historically, Western psychotherapeutic techniques grew out of the dualistic conception of human nature.

Some general distinctions also can be made between the kinds of clients and practitioners most commonly associated with the two approaches. In the main, clients who receive psychogogic services are psychologically well individuals with severe enough situational problems to need help. Those who receive psychotherapeutic services are experiencing psychological symptoms severe enough to motivate them (or someone else) to seek cure of the symptoms and (it is hoped) their underlying causes. Accordingly, the specialties of practitioners serving the two groups vary somewhat. Counseling and rehabilitation psychologists, rehabilitation counselors, and other counseling specialists provide mainly psychogogic services. Psychiatrists and psychiatric social workers provide mainly psychotherapeutic services. Clinical psychologists and medical social workers may provide either or both, depending on work settings and personal predilections. A summary of these distinctions is presented in Table 2.

It is important to bear in mind that no absolute demarcations exist. As the advantages of holism, attention to spirit, an educative orientation, and patient/client responsibility become recognized as important to cure as well as prevention, psychogogic styles are being adopted by psychotherapists. At the same time, such corrective techniques as behavior modification are taking important places in service to people who are not psychologically ill but who have habitual response patterns that interfere with their lives. Despite the overlap, the distinction may help clarify some of the conceptual polarities involved in PSV service techniques.

This chapter will focus on approaches that are predominantly psychogogic, the techniques most likely to be appropriate for people with bodily disabilites that create difficult situational adjustment demands and problems. We will look at ways in which traditional counseling specialties are, or can be, applied. We also will examine an array of special techniques: those drawing from the transcendent arts; such Eastern techniques as the martial arts, yoga, and meditation; and body-work techniques that seem particularly suitable for a disabled clientele. Finally, we will examine the blending of all of these into rehabilitation-related PSV approaches.

The chapter immediately following will continue to examine psychogogic techniques, but as they are applied by peer, rather than professional, providers. Then, Chapter 13 will discuss psychotherapeutic approaches oriented toward people whose primary disabilities are characterized as mental, emotional, or behavioral, or who have developed serious mental-health problems secondary to bodily disablement.

Traditional, Mainstream Counseling Specialties

The problem with mainstream counseling approaches, for disabled people, is that they often are inaccessible in several ways. First, they exist in settings likely to be architecturally inaccessible. Second, they exist in the mainstream, and if the prospective client has been placed in a "special," segregated track, s/he will not have access to mainstream facilities. Third, when people are or become disabled, professionals tend to refer them to rehabilitation agencies, never thinking of using "regular" resources. Fourth, at the same time, professionals in mainstream settings imagine they cannot work with people with disabilities because they are not rehabilitation experts. As will be seen, these

Table 2

Psychogogy	Psychotherapy
Orientation	
Educational model	Medical model
Prevent	Cure
Teach	Treat
Strengthen	Correct
Inform and guide	Administer to
Strong Eastern influence	Strong Western influence
Holistic	Dualistic
Stress patient responsibility	Stress physician responsibility
Psychologically well clientele	Psychologically unwell clientele
Practitioners	
Counseling and rehabilitation psychologists	Psychiatrists
Rehabilitation counselors	Psychiatric social workers
Other counseling specialists	Clinical psychologists Medical social workers
Clinical psychologists	
Medical social workers	

last two biases combine to create serious gaps in mental health services for disabled people.

Nonetheless, traditional services often may be the most appropriate resources for disabled people, particularly if the counseling need is unrelated or only tangentially related to the disability. Although it seems obvious, this likelihood apparently needs to be stressed: disabled people *do* experience problems in psychosocial and vocational areas that have little to do with their disabilities. Consequently, mainstream counselors only need to be prepared to take a disability in stride and not let it become an artificial focus in their counseling efforts.

Assuming disabled clients can gain access to them, the author sees four basic counseling traditions to be used: (1) educational/vocational counseling; (2) personal or psychological counseling; (3) social casework; and (4) marriage, family, and child counseling. Although some social workers might object to having casework labeled a counseling approach, it is included here for completeness in surveying traditional psychogogic approaches. As noted earlier, some social casework would be grouped with psychotherapeutic techniques under this two-way classification.

Educational/Vocational Counseling

This is the one type of counseling that a large number of people from the general population have experienced. Most people who attend school into the secondary level have at least a passing acquaintance with a school counselor who helps students choose elective courses in line with future goals, such as college versus trade school versus immediate employment. This function usually is called "advisement" rather than "counseling." Because school budgets typically allow for a very small number of counselors to help a very large number of students, the service seldom is recalled with much appreciation. Often, course advisement is all there is time for, and even that is likely to be "mass produced" and mechanical. When genuine counseling and guidance are available, students may get testing, interpretation, and useful consultation on future educational and career choices.

It would be hard to say whether school counseling for disabled students is worse or better than for others. In general, this society has not valued the function enough to provide funding for it. Disabled students probably get a bit more than others, but they need *much* more because of disability-related career barriers. Schools, both segregated and mainstream, usually have liaison arrangements with the local office of their state–federal vocational rehabilitation (VR) program, whereas no comparable counseling resource is available to nondisabled students.

The higher you go in school, the richer the counseling and guidance offerings become. Most colleges and universities have counseling centers for their students, and some offer personal as well as career counseling, especially at four-year schools. However, special counseling programs for students with disabilities are becoming commonplace at community (two-year) colleges as well. Some have more extensive counseling resources for disabled than nondisabled students because stronger funding pressures have been brought to bear. Special offerings for disabled students are sometimes part of, sometimes separate from, the "regular" school counseling center and tread a borderline between the traditional and the innovative. Liaison with the state VR program usually exists. They also may be linked with on-campus consumer organizations devoted to mutual help, advocacy, and related missions (discussed further in Chapter 12).

Personal or Psychological Counseling

College counseling center staff members observe that many students seek educational/vocational counseling when it is actually personal counseling or psychotherapy they need or want. The former simply offers a less threatening entry into the personal-help service system. Such services are likely to be available in either the counseling center or the student health service; thus, college students enjoy better-than-average access to personal counseling. Few practitioners are available in the private sector because few insurance carriers are willing to pay for preventive (construed as nonessential) services. Individuals generally share this reluctance or simply are unable to pay for them. Because of the strong link between disability and poverty, only a few disabled people can afford the hourly rates asked.

Forward-looking employers are beginning to have personal counselors on staff or contract to work with employees whose personal problems seem to interfere with work productivity. Also, a number of churches offer pastoral counseling for members, and community counseling centers and free clinics (usually sponsored by local government and/or a charitable fund) exist in some areas. Most often, personal counseling is available to people involved in some other service system (for example, school, work, or social agency) when the need becomes manifest. Still, even when services are available, people generally are reluctant to admit they need help, seeing such as a sign of "weakness." The need for educational/vocational counseling is considered respectable, but needs for personal help have yet to be fully "legitimized." As will be seen later, transforming/repackaging similar processes and relabeling them "human potential development" has removed this barrier for many people.

Sexual counseling is a particularly important aspect of personal counseling for a disabled clientele, for all of the reasons cited in Chapter 5. It is rare, however, for staff in mainstream counseling centers to have the specialized knowledge required to distinguish disability-related dysfunctions from those with psychogenic origins; thus, they are not well prepared to determine when sexual counseling is all that is needed, or when a more intensive, psychotherapeutic approach should be taken. Ordinarily, it is the author's impression that a psychological practitioner who is good with people in general also is good with people who happen to have disabilities. Part of why they are good is their ability to take a host of human differences in stride, and disability is just one of many they will confront. It is only because of the rather esoteric neurophysiological information base that *may* be involved that sexual counseling presents a few problems. Most physically disabled clients can tell a psychological counselor all s/he needs to know about the disability; but in the emotionally-charged sexual area, s/he may not really know or may "scapegoat" the disability. The counselor may not recognize this unless s/he seeks out "instant training" on the relationships between sexual functioning and (a given client's) specific disease process or injury residuals. If wise enough to know that s/he should do this, and willing to make the effort, a mainstream counselor can do sexual counseling with disabled clients as well as anyone else.

Social Casework

Social workers operating in a psychogogic mode may use a style of service that is little different from the counseling offered by psychologists and other counseling specialists. It seems that the nature of the client's problems and the personality or temperament of the service provider have more to do with what actually takes place in the counseling room—and its effectiveness—than theoretical orientation or training background. Nonetheless, such experience does influence style, and the caseworker may be more prone to deal with the client as part of a larger social system—taking into account socioeconomic and related factors—than the psychologist–counselor. The latter is more apt to use methods evolving from psychological research, such as behavior modification or biofeedback. The social worker also is less likely to be found in employment settings, but more likely to serve in community counseling centers and free clinics.

Virtually the same barriers to utilization exist as were cited earlier regarding personal counseling. These barriers seem to be reduced, however, when a child, rather than an adult, shows evidence of psychological service need—especially when pressure from school authorities is applied. When the disturbance is attributed to family relationships, a fourth variety of counseling may be sought.

Marriage, Family, and Child Counseling

Although the components and typical methods are traditional, marriage-family-child counseling, as a distinct, licensible, disciplinary entity, is fairly new. It appears to have gained impetus in reaction to the elevation of state licensing standards for psychologists from the masters' to the doctoral degree level. This trend has left numerous masters'-level practitioners, who strongly believe themselves qualified to practice unsupervised, with no state-sanctioned means of doing so. In some states, the establishment of licensing procedures for masters'-degree-educated marriage, family, and child (MFC) counselors (or other variants on this title) has created the desired opportunities. Additional impetus grew from concern that the traditional providers—psychiatrists, psychologists, and social workers—lack the specific training, orientation, and experience needed to perform these services well. Unfortunately, it is commonly believed that the licensing requirements for MFC counselors offer even poorer quality assurance than the traditional licenses, at least in some states. On a more positive note, many are known to be excellent practitioners, despite the laxity of the licensing standards.

Perhaps the most significant stimulus to the development of MFC counseling as a distinct discipline is growing societal concern over the threatened dissolution of the American family. Because few pressures can wreck the homeostatic balance and psychological well-being of a family more effectively than disability, these three interrelated areas of counseling are supremely important to disabled people and their loved ones. The White House Conference on Families in 1980 highlighted handicapping conditions as a major stress factor requiring immediate solutions.

As indicated in Chapter 4, the disabled individual has a better chance of getting counseling services than his/her affected family members. S/he is likely to have access to personal counseling through the rehabilitation service system (discussed below), but the spouse, parents, or children are just as likely to be excluded or nearly so. Theoretically, such help might be available through the state VR program, if marriage or family problems were construed as impediments to the vocational rehabilitation of the identified client. Practically, however, agency demands for production of rehabilitation plans and successful closures discourage most rehabilitation counselors from offering time-consuming family services, even when domestic problems are *known* to be sabotaging rehabilitation progress. They are reluctant, too, because they have no more training for it than the other practitioners and far fewer incentives and opportunities to learn by experience.

Awareness of the problem is by no means absent, however. Two counselors in a large state VR agency (Connell & Berkowitz, 1976) proposed and conducted a family-centered program for a severely disabled SSI-recipient population with an extremely low acceptance-for-service rate. They found that by working with the families, instead of solely the disabled individuals, they increased the number of such clients accepted and served by several hundred percent compared with offices not involved in the project. Figures on rehabilitation outcomes are unavailable because the project was not continued past the originally agreed-upon time period for demonstrating changes in acceptance rate.

So far, we have focused on the need for family counseling as an adjunct to rehabilitating a disabled family member. However, as stated in Chapter 4, counseling also is needed for the disabled family members themselves, so they do not become "casualties" of anothers' disability. Kevin (see Chapter 4) described the kinds of interventions he believed would have helped his mother:

> She needed to be *trained* to take care of herself as well as me. She needed *counseling* to eradicate the guilt feelings that led to excessive self-sacrifice. She needed *advocacy*, someone to get across to her that mothers have rights, too; that I wasn't the only one suffering. I didn't have to be protected from the fact that my care was a drag. If she knew that I knew and accepted that, she wouldn't have had to work so hard to pretend it was "no problem" when her ass was dragging, just so I wouldn't feel bad. She also needed a different kind of *counseling for me*, to clarify my supportive responsibility toward her. That would have helped me, too, because my role was all taking and I felt guilty and unworthy. That led me to a very crazy conclusion: "I've used up my dependency quota in the physical area; therefore, I must never expect or accept any emotional support." Naturally, no one can live without it, so every time I sopped up a little emotional support from someone, I felt I was stealing. Suffice it to say, counseling could have avoided unnecessary self-sacrifice on her part and a long-lasting neurotic error on mine. [Emphasis added.]

Clearly, all four traditional counseling varieties have much, potentially, to offer disabled people and their families if the barriers can be broken down. The next section will discuss an approach that has lowered one barrier successfully—that of reluctance to admit the need for help.

Human Potential Development

The human potential development movement was a product of the 1960s—a time when psychologically well individuals began to look inward to cope with unease about a future-shocked world taunted by a war with little meaning to them. Esalen, a resort setting in Big Sur, California, became "Mecca," and dozens of similar "growth centers" emerged throughout the country. No admission of psychological or interpersonal incompetence was necessary; participants had only to acknowledge desire to maximize their inner resources and enhance fulfillment in their lives. They flocked to the centers for training experiences designed to do both. Those who labeled it a passing fad note, with satisfaction, that only a few centers still survive, and their popularity has waned. However, the philosophy, the goals, and the methods have by no means disappeared or even abated. They simply have transformed and continuously reemerge in newer forms—often itinerant rather than center-based—and exert enormous influence on traditional psychological and bodily health-care practices. They are present in such delimited, structured programs as est; and they are integral to the broadly diverse holistic health-care movement.

As indicated in Chapter 8, the disability experience can be a powerful stimulant to developing a coherent philosophy of life that imparts meaning to a source of considerable pain. For this reason, the human potential development (HPD) approach may be uniquely appropriate for people with disabilities; yet it is largely inaccessible to them for reasons of cost and other barriers. Effort is seldom made to house itinerant programs in barrier-free facilities. However, the HPD approach is available to the extent that accessible practitioners, such as rehabilitation counselors, incorporate similar goals and methods into their own counseling approaches; and a growing number appear to be doing so.

HPD is a wholesome approach because it minimizes the "pathology error," and disabled people often are overwhelmed by confrontations with their own pathology—real or exaggerated. The philosophy of accepting oneself "as is" and growing from there is a helpful counterfoil to previous overemphasis on deficits, limitations, and liabilities, coupled with enjoinders to "try to overcome them." Trying to overcome what you are isn't easy for anyone; it is particularly defeating when part of what you are is permanently disabled.

The human potential development movement has been shaped significantly by the importation of philosophy and technique from the Far East. The ancient philosophical, psychological, medical, and religious writings from China and India have had the most notable influence, although Japan and other Asian countries also are represented. Let us look next at some of the specific Eastern approaches that have been adopted in the West, and consider their applicability to a disabled clientele.

Eastern Influences

The martial arts have been familiar in the West for many decades. First jiu jitsu appeared on the Western scene, followed by judo, karate, and now a vast array including tai chi, aikido, and others too numerous to mention. Sometimes they have shown up in customized training for special-interest groups, sometimes in public parlors. The emphasis generally is placed on self-defense, whether for vulnerable clients such as women, senior citizens, or disabled people, or for strong, young, agile males.

Human potential development (HPD) practitioners have been interested in the additional benefits of martial-arts training—those relating to self-discipline, energy utilization, and the enhancement of physical and psychological well-being. The martial arts require development and integration of bodily, mental, and spiritual energies for correct execution. In short, they are holistic. Individuals who never find it necessary to use their arts for self-defense report sometimes minor, sometimes major improvement in the sense of well-being. Terms such as "centered" and "balanced" convey to others who've shared similar experiences what is meant by their claims. Part of it may result from the vigorous exercise plus improved confidence or reduced feelings of vulnerability. An additional part seems to emanate directly from the processes of learning the necessary self-discipline and methods for synchronizing bodily, mental, and spiritual energies.

A few programs, mostly self-defense oriented, exist for teaching martial arts to people with disabilities, particularly wheelchair users or amputees. Although the kung fu master in the television series, "Kung Fu," was blind, there is little martial-arts involvement among blind people. Few mainstream trainers show interest in developing modified approaches to accommodate a wide range of disabilities and degrees of severity; however, such programs could allow disabled participants to enjoy the physical/psychological benefits even though they might never be able to use the art for successful self-defense. A recommendation for future development in this area will be offered in the final chapter.

Yoga has been familiar in the West perhaps even longer than the martial arts, but to a less diverse audience. (One still sees no yoga parlors interspersed among the fast-food stands as is currently true for karate.) Hatha yoga and mantra yoga are the most commonly taught systems. Hatha yoga focuses on body and breath control. Mantra yoga tends to be referred to in the West as "meditation," and the trademarked Transcendental Meditation (TM) has become the most widely practiced variant.

Hatha yoga training is fairly widely available: on televison, in HPD programs, in university extension courses, exercise gyms, and health spas. A major difference from Western exercise approaches is that stretching, rather than contracting, of muscles is emphasized because the goal is fluidity of motion rather than muscle-mass development or increasing muscle strength. Pranayama (breath control) training is less widely available—generally only within HPD programs. This is unfortunate for people with such severe disabilities that most of the bodily postures of hatha yoga are impossible for them to attain. Breath control exercises, even for people with sharply limited vital capacities, would be a feasible form of yogic practice to use to attain the effects of calming, relaxing, and quieting anxieties. These are the primary purposes and benefits of hatha yoga (Swami Rama et al., 1976).

Mantra yoga training is very widely available, at least in the form of TM. It is not only available privately, it sometimes is provided by employers who are convinced it will enhance productivity. It also is available to the clients of some rehabilitation agencies; a few private rehabilitation facilities arrange for such training for their clients, and a few state VR agency counselors have managed to procure such training for theirs. It is important to note that it may be contraindicated for people with spinal-cord injuries (George Hohmann, personal communication) and probably should not be pursued for this population until appropriate research has been done. As is true for hatha yoga, the most palpable psychological benefits relate to calming, relaxation, and reduction of anxieties. Some individuals also report such sequelae as increased creativity, improved insights about themselves and others, and clearer thinking abilities. Mantra yoga is coming to be suggested or even prescribed by physicians treating people with such conditions as hypertension, in efforts to avoid use of medications with unpleasant or unknown future side effects.

Holistic Health Care

The holistic health-care movement evolved out of the human potential development movement, probably as a result of the involvement of health-care professionals in HPD activities. The two movements are now virtually one, with the encompassing goal of fostering total mind–body–spirit health in a self-actualizing person. It is to the totality and inseparability of the mind–body–spirit that the term "holistic" refers. The health of one component cannot be achieved or maintained in the absence of attention to the other two. The Eastern influence is as apparent at this basic philosophical level (the inclusion of spirit along with mind and body) as it is when the actual health-care techniques are examined. Three aspects of the holistic approach are particularly salient to the PSV rehabilitation of disabled people: (1) the emphasis on self-responsibility, (2) the emphasis on nutrition, and (3) the addition of "body work" to the "talk therapy" tradition in counseling and psychotherapy.

After leaving the rehabilitation hospital, many disabled people have been forced to assume more self-responsibility in health care than the average person because so few practitioners in mainstream medical practice know how to deal with disabled patients. For example, a quadriplegic who finds it necessary to use a community hospital needs to explain her/his personal care needs to all levels of staff as thoroughly as to an inexperienced applicant for a job as a personal-care provider. Unfortunately, not all are prepared to do so, and others have found their efforts to inform health providers resented and ignored. Hopefully, the emerging emphasis on self-responsibility will lead to more consistent preparation of disabled people in this respect, and more receptiveness on the parts of health practitioners to being instructed by such patients.

Increased concern over the nutritional quality of food consumed is particularly important among people whose disabilities lower their energy reserves and their caloric needs. A severely paralyzed individual, for example, who needs only 1200 calories per day, can less afford to waste any of them on junk food than a person who needs twice that number to maintain an ideal weight. When energy is depleted by the nature of a disability, or by inordinate effort required to function in spite of it, good nutrition is essential to body–mind–spirit health. A mild case of hypoglycemia might go almost unnoticed by a nondisabled person, yet keep a severely disabled person from making it through the day. The margin of error is too narrow. Few rehabilitation programs give nutrition the emphasis it deserves. Hopefully, the growing social awareness of the relationships between inadequate nutrition and psychological as well as physical symptoms will filter into more rehabilitation programs in the coming decade.

Not so many years ago, psychogogy and psychotherapy were both limited, virtually, to being "talk treatment." Psychiatrists might prescribe drugs or arrange for psychosurgery, but psychologists, counselors, and social workers only talked. The HPD movement brought with it enormously increased interest in exercise and other body work, particularly varieties designed to improve psychological functioning. Intensive efforts to reunite mind and body began and now have exerted considerable influence on mainstream psychological services. The reasons for this are diverse. Because of the noted failure of psychological services to "work" for people who are not verbally oriented, it was finally recognized that the "talk treatment" bias emanated from tendencies of people who enter the involved professions to solve their own problems through rational/verbal explorations, but that other, equally valid ways also exist.

At the same time, specific Eastern techniques incorporating body work (such as the martial arts, yoga, and movement meditations), along with the general, working philosophy of mind–body–spirit holism, were being integrated into Western approaches, first in the nontraditional HPD centers and then into the mainstream. Before long, it was acknowledged that body work was not just an alternative for nonverbally oriented people; it was a needed corrective for people who were too verbally oriented and had neglected their bodies, failing to recognize the impact of bodily habits on their psychological well-being. Naturally, the impact of Western medical sorties to China in the early 1970s, and the ensuing reports that acupuncture "works" although no one could explain how in terms of Western physiological conceptions, was also a great contributor to the wakening realization that at least one path to psychological health is through the body. Countless varieties of body work now have emerged: Eastern and Western, structured and unstructured, aerobic and anaerobic, active and passive, athletic and aesthetic. They are used at the growth centers, in itinerant HPD programs, private consulting offices, and recreation facilities. They move faddishly "in" and "out." The smörgasbord of choices expands daily, so that anyone interested can find just the variety suited to his/her needs or wishes; everyone except people with disabilities, that is.

The same problems exist in the entire range of body-work techniques that were cited with respect to martial-arts and yoga training. Very few efforts have been made yet to study and catalog which techniques, or parts or them, could be used with people with various disabilities. Even fewer efforts have been made to devise adaptations that could allow disabled people to reap at least some of the benefits body work offers. Physically disabled people who attend HPD programs often find themselves sitting on the sidelines during most of the body-work experiences, waiting for the verbal parts to begin again so they can resume participation. A scattering of therapeutic recreation and other rehabilitation programs, as well as consumer-run independent living programs, are beginning to explore these possibilities. It is hoped that published reports will document their experience and findings and will serve to spread such efforts. Dance and movement "therapies," as well as martial-arts training, seem to be the most frequently tried. Dance therapy also can be grouped with another set of nontraditional approaches that are gaining momentum in the psychological services field—those based on the transcendent arts.

The Influence of the Transcendent Arts

The fields of recreation and psychology are turning virtually every artistic discipline known to humankind into "therapies," most notably, music and the visual, performing, and writing arts. Sometimes they are therapies in the corrective sense used here; at other times they might be classed better as psychogogy. Central purposes in all such approaches are relaxation and renewal; facilitation of self-expression; enhancement of self-understanding; and the improvement of mental focusing, self-esteem, and feelings of psychological well-being. The discovery of substantial creative talent and drive is generally a peripheral concern.

As reflected in the familiar quotation from William Congreve's *The Mourning Bride,* "Music hath charm to soothe a savage breast, To soften rocks, or bend a knotted oak," music therapy is used often with people who need to have intense or pervasive fears quelled but find other relaxation methods threatening. Thus, it is used most widely in psychotherapeutic settings, but it has psychogogic applicability as well. Music therapy usually implies listening, or music appreciation, rather than singing or playing instruments. Accordingly, the latter activities are grouped here with the performing arts.

Traditionally, the visual arts have formed an important basis of occupational therapy activities in both psychiatric and medical rehabilitation settings, with crafts and painting the most commonly employed. When budgeting allows, sculpture and various graphics techniques also may be used. It seems to this author that sculpture offers greater potential for psychogogic work with blind individuals than has been exploited. Also, life-history murals—a technique created at SAGE, a highly progressive senior citizens' program in Berkeley, California (Luce, 1979)—might be used profitably with people who are coping with life changes imposed by disability, as well as aging.

Among the performing arts approaches, psychodrama now has a long-established history in psychotherapeutic settings. The minidrama techniques associated with Gestalt therapy and transactional analysis, for example, are included here, generically, as psychodrama. They are used fairly widely with psychogogy clients, disabled and nondisabled. An unusual form of psychodrama has emerged recently in which clients become the "directors" and professionals do the "acting." Increasingly, professionals and students are being exposed to role-playing opportunities in which they learn something of what it is like to be disabled. Spending a day or a week blindfolded or in a wheelchair are the most common simulations. Through these techniques, nondisabled providers gain better understanding of the frustrations encountered and the trust that must be developed by people whose disabilities generate and demand them. The disabled participants in such programs gain greater confidence in the empathy of those who serve them, plus a sense of mastery, of having something important to teach or share.

The potential of dance and movement therapies for people with disabilities is being noted by many providers. The newsletter of a consumer-run independent living program (Darrell McDaniel Independent Living Center, 1980) describes a "Dance Mystique" program conducted at the annual convention of a state association of disabled people:

> The evening begins in darkness as the Dance Mystique group enters with light swords invented by DJ Brad Pierce. They instruct everyone on the floor not to dance until they are touched by the light swords in the still darkened room, and they are to dance without partners. As the number increases, the lights start coming up, and by the end of the piece, everyone is dancing in the light.
>
> The group explains that the use of the lights is symbolic: When the light swords touch them, people are freed to come together without fear or inhibition and express the light of their own being, in an environment where the inner dancer is released. And it is the inner dancer who is the one who truly dances. You don't need to be able-bodied or know the latest steps when, as "Dance Mystique" says, "the heart is open." They go on: "The inner dancer once freed can express the light within all souls, and that is the dance mystique."
>
> Those who were at the dance the last night of the CAPH convention did not spare their enthusiasm. Said Willy Jackson: "You did an excellent job of making people love and share together. It was the perfect way of getting people to respond to each other." "I've never really seen us this loose before . . . " said Ed Rambo. [pp. 4–7]

Singing, especially group singing, and playing musical instruments, especially small stringed instruments and recorders, are used occasionally in psychogogic or psychotherapeutic work but have not been developed systematically. This may be more a function of their auditory intrusiveness than lack of psychological service potential. Singing is used sometimes as a means of improving breath control, but it is regarded more often as a physical or inhalation therapy than as a psychological technique. Mime has been explored as a means of encouraging self-expression among people with mental or speech disabilities, but no systematic programs are known to have been reported. Each of these areas seems worthy of additional investigation, especially singing, because of the apparent relationship between breath control and control of anxieties. Lowered vital capacity and poor breath control are found among people with numerous physical disabilities.

The writing arts have long been used in psychological services, both in the passive (reading) and active (writing) modes. Currently, bibliotherapy is being elevated to a high level of importance in pain-management programs, where well-stocked libraries of self-help books on stress management, meditation techniques, spiritual development, and related subjects are often part of the service offerings for clients/patients learning to manage their own pain. Autobiography writing, for the dual purposes of diagnosis and treatment, has enjoyed long usage; but it now is undergoing a renascence wherein greater emphasis is placed on its treatment potential and relevance for psychogogy clients. Poetry writing is a relative newcomer but already has been the object of considerable theoretical development and technical systematization.

All of these techniques based on the transcendent arts should be considered for disabled clienteles because of their potential for supplying new mechanisms for emotional discharge and new sources of reward and pleasure after familiar mechanisms and sources have been lost. These are just two of many special issues PSV practitioners must consider in serving clients with disabilities.

Special Issues in Counseling Disabled People

Three clusters of special issues will be discussed here: common problems, common skill-training needs, and the applicability of selected group counseling approaches.

Common Problems

Very early in the recovery process, emotional support is needed to cope with the shock, fear, and anger experienced over what has taken place. People born with disabilities, or acquiring them while still very young, need similar support when they begin to realize that they are disadvantaged, compared with others, by their disablements. The central theme of the support needed in either case is assurance of unimpaired self-worth and hope for a gratifying future. If these assurances are offered by individuals who sincerely believe that disablement in no way reduces a person's human worth or obviates chances for a fulfilling life, it may matter very little how they are delivered. When permanence of disability is known to be likely before the affected individual is ready to acknowledge that, the holding out of false hopes regarding prognosis can be avoided, somewhat, when the assuring messages suggest, "Sure, it's conceivable that you could recover; but whatever the outcome in that regard, your human worth is unchanged and opportunities for fulfillment will be many."

Many disabled people who have attained outstanding success in life say this was the consistent message they got from their loved ones, often nonexplicitly. It was felt, and it was transmitted in one way or another. This has important implications for hospital and other rehabilitation personnel. However disability is viewed, it is likely to be communicated to the individual; thus, more important than learning techniques for providing emotional support is gaining personal perspective so that a sense of tragedy, the belief that irreparable damage to human worth has occurred, or feelings of dread will not be conveyed because they do not exist.

Somewhat later in the adjustment process, more specific aspects of loss must be dealt with. Three highly significant areas confronted by people with the full range of disabilities are: (1) the loss of emotional discharge mechanisms, (2) the loss of reward or pleasure sources, and (3) the loss of physical and economic independence. These frequently lead to what might be termed "secondary losses" in self-esteem and the sense of meaning, or purpose, in life. They also may lead to such secondary disabling conditions as alcoholism or boredom-induced amotivation syndrome. For example, the loss of emotional discharge mechanisms appears to be a frequent contributing factor in excessive drinking among people with disabilities, a problem now eliciting great concern from both peer and professional providers. An individual who has relied on vigorous activity to discharge emotional/physical tensions may resort to dulling their impact with alcohol when such physical "exhaust" methods become impossible.

The supports needed to counteract such maladaptive behavior patterns are practical help and consultation in finding more effective, less debilitating ways of coping, laced liberally with the kind of emotional support described previously. First, information is needed in the form of exposure to other ways of discharging tension, other sources of reward and pleasure, and available opportunities for gaining/regaining economic independence. Second, consultation is needed on how to use the new information, coupled with "supervised practice"—opportunities for action and self-expression followed by accurate feedback on the effectiveness of such efforts in developing constructive insights and responses to altered circumstances. Third, cognitive/attitudinal restructuring is needed to (a) help the person separate real losses from imputed but unnecessary ones; (b) avoid equating physical dependency with total dependency; and (c) understand that temporary confusion does not harbinger life-long disruption of purposes, meaning, values, and goals.

An achievement-oriented society such as ours stresses goals of accomplishment, and goals of acquisition are associated with materialism. Such biases can be defeating to people with disabilities that limit their potential for success along these dimensions. It is particularly important, therefore, for them to know that other kinds of goals—at least as worthy—also exist and are reachable. Life goals can be grouped roughly into three general categories: goals of *doing*, goals of *getting*, and goals of *being*.

Goals of *doing* relate to activities, achievements, and accomplishments. The person says, "This is what I want to *do* in life—to achieve or accomplish." S/he might conceive it in terms of an epitaph: "I want it to say s/he did such and such well." The specific goals might be as common as wanting to do a good job of child rearing or as unusual as wanting to devise a testable theory of the origin of the universe.

Goals of *getting* relate to acquiring, gathering, and accumulating. The targets of striving may be material or nonmaterial. Material goals range from garnering the barest survival basics of adequate food and shelter to enjoying opulence that requires vast accumulations of wealth. Examples of nonmaterial goals are reputation, prestige, status, power, and fame. They are externals to acquire in that their existence lies in the perceptions of others. The material and nonmaterial aspects of "getting" goals are interdependent; attainment in one aids attainment in the other.

Goals of *being* relate to developing attributes of character, which reside within. Here, the individual says, "I want to *be* a certain kind of person, one who is (honest, tough, spontaneous, firm, loving, fiery, fair, critical, sensible, reverent, wise, courageous, or countless other valued qualities)." The characteristics sought for may be unrelated to reputation; the individual strives for an inner surety that the prized attributes are (being) attained.

Most people set goals in each of the three areas—sometimes without realizing it—but concentrate on one or two. To illustrate, individuals who move quickly to the tops of corporate ladders focus heavily on goals of doing and getting. Creative artists who pursue painting or writing despite poverty and ignominy may disdain the executives' goals of getting while sharing with them a deep commitment to goals of doing. Spiritual aspirants and leaders may concentrate mainly on goals of being.

It is important to help people realize that disabilities need not interfere with attaining goals of being. A totally paralyzed person with impaired vision, hearing, and speech could succeed as well in this realm as anyone else. As pointed out in Chapter 8, the disability experience can block this type of goal seeking, but it can catalyze and foster it equally well. In order to facilitate the latter, skill training in the goal-setting process may be required.

Personal and Interpersonal Skill Training

At some point in the course of adjustment, either the disabled person or a rehabilitation consultant may realize that formalized training in specific personal/interpersonal skill areas is needed. Disability creates unusually heavy demands for assertiveness, decision-making and goal-setting abilities, and life- and family-management skills. Training programs have been developed in each of these areas for the general population, and for disabled people in particular. Assertiveness training is perhaps the best known, but all of the mentioned varieties are offered widely by rehabilitation facilities and individual practitioners.

Although little is available yet, more is being said about the need for programs to enhance physical attractiveness, ranging from basic grooming tips, at the simplest level, to cosmetic surgery, at the far extreme. Variations on the "charm school" theme are a frequent middle ground. This seems to be a hard area to address without tempers flaring. The "pros" indicate improved attractiveness and poise will better a disabled person's chances for success and it is thus irresponsible to ignore the matter. The "cons" want to avoid emphasizing shallow concerns better left unstressed in society at large, as well as any implication that disability makes one less attractive. Conversely, they point out that disabled people could be hurt by being tempted to compete in an attractiveness market where they are predetermined to come out second best. The "pros" counter that if a person gets a job within a month after attending "attractiveness school," following two years of previous turn-downs, that speaks for itself. By the very fact of providing service, counselors tacitly acknowledge an opinion that clients could profit from behavior change. The controversy over confronting clients with the possibility that changes in grooming behavior or social presentation also might yield rewards seems deeply ingrained in our own insecurities about whether *we* make the grade as beautiful people. Any issue powerful enough to generate so much discomfort and resistance must be important to deal with in counseling!

People whose disabilities interfere with communication and, therefore, interpersonal relationships have uniquely important skills to learn. First, they must learn to transmit and receive messages as accurately and rapidly as possible. For this, speech therapy or training, sign language and lip reading training, and sensory/communication aids usage represent three major approaches for people with speech, hearing, and vision disabilities. Beyond such basic assistance, subtler aspects of interpersonal communication must be attended to. For example, nonhearing speakers must learn to use others' facial responses in monitoring their voice modulation. Blind individuals must learn to discern, from auditory cues, all those nuances of interpersonal and group dynamics that others deduce from body language. People with extremely slow or labored speech must learn to capture their listeners' attention and patience and also put them at ease. Actually, speech therapy or training could be construed as an additional psychogogic variety in view of the central use of psychological principles and counseling methods entailed. The feelings, especially anxieties, of speech therapy clients are as important in their speech training as the physiological difficulties presented. For this reason, relaxation training techniques are being adopted by speech practitioners as quickly as those more typically considered "counselors."

Group versus Individual Approaches

Regardless of the type of counseling or skill training involved, the question arises: can it be done more effectively with individuals or in groups? Group techniques are popular because of their apparent cost effectiveness, but it is important to determine whether sacrifices in quality will be made or whether a group approach will produce equal or enhanced effectiveness.

In the author's opinion, group approaches are frequently the modality of choice for psychogogic work, for several interrelated reasons. First, by comparison, one of the primary reasons for choosing to work privately with individuals in psycho*therapy* is that their ability to trust other human beings is often so impaired that it is more feasible to begin rebuilding it with one other person (who is professionally skilled in nurturing trust) than with a group of several people (some of whom may have attacking tendencies). In psycho*gogy*, severely damaged trust is not at issue. Second, both a mechanism and goal of psychogogy with disabled people is augmenting their understanding that they are not alone; others are experiencing similar facts and feelings, others have useful insights they can share, and others can profit from *their* insights— they are helpful persons as well as persons needing help.

One of the few published group approaches developed specifically for use with disabled clients is Structured Experiential Therapy in Rehabilitation (SETR) (Lasky et al., 1977). Although labeled a "therapy" by its creators, it is more akin to what is classified here as psychogogy, because of the target clientele and the nature of the problems addressed. Its central theme is the reduction of interpersonal stress between disabled and nondisabled people, especially that arising from disability-related stigmatization.

The structured group format highlights goal orientation, accountability, mutual help, and the development of coping skills. Sessions consistently include about half disabled and half nondisabled members, all of whom are striving toward more effective problem solving, better use of their resources, psychological growth, and satisfactory living. Two coleaders work with eight to ten members and attempt to establish strong group cohesiveness and mutual concern. The job of the members is to identify, explore, evaluate, and act on specific problems. Written contracts are used to facilitate the process, as are such other practical approaches as establishing contact with resource people, organizations, events, and articles. Members are exposed to role models, and the value of incidental learning from each other is stressed. The process is seen as comprised of three fairly distinct phases. The first is individualistically oriented and includes goal identification, exploration, and evaluation, with some didactic interventions, such as recording behavioral base rates. The second phase is group oriented, utilizing the group cohesion and felt mutual responsibility to help the members attain their goals. This phase also includes feedback from the group to help members assess their levels of goal attainment. The final phase stresses generalization of what has been learned to other (or future) problem areas, consolidation of learning, and recapitulation of learning in follow-up sessions after the group has formally ended. "Booster" sessions can be planned if the members wish.

Similar philosophy is evidenced in an unpublished group approach used at Rancho Los Amigos Hospital in the early 1970s. Several clients of the vocational rehabilitation program there expressed interest in a singles group, to deal with their fears about dating and forming intimate relationships. The program designed to respond to these requests had two somewhat unusual features. First, it used a taped course on heterosexual relationship issues as a springboard to group discussion. Second, it recruited nondisabled participants from a nearby community college in an effort to deter disabled group members from imagining that their singles' problems were irrevocably tied to their disabilities. The use of the taped course appeared to serve well as a means of breaking down barriers to open sharing, especially when course material triggered disagreement. The inclusion of nondisabled participants was broadening for both disabled and nondisabled members. The desired effect of illustrating that nondisabled participants shared virtually all of the same fears, problems, and preoccupations, with minor variations, was clearly accomplished. In addition, hospital staff and clients alike were gratified by the number of new student referrals that followed feedback from early participants. One disabled client expressed the feelings of many by saying, "This is amazing. I really didn't think they'd want to come and get counseling with *us*." A nondisabled client similarly reflected his peers' views in commenting, "Don't get me wrong, I don't want a disability; but I'm not sure you guys really appreciate how much you've learned from yours. You all seem so together, so mellow, compared to everyone else I know. I'd sure like to find some other way to get to where you are!" Such observations offer validation to the Lasky et al. (1977) premise that matters of stigma must be addressed, and in groups including both disabled and nondisabled participants.

Individual counseling's greatest value may be its potential for spontaneity. When someone needs help immediately, an ad lib counseling session can be invaluable, and convening a group would be farcical or impossible. Counselors, like therapists and medical practitioners, are in the habit of scheduling standard periods of time for working with clients. It has been done that way for so long that everyone imagines it *should* be done that way; alteration may even be seen as reflecting faulty professionalism. The pattern was set, however, to conform to the comfort, convenience, and income maximization needs of private practitioners. After the fact, it was rationalized as somehow better for clients or patients. This given should be reassessed. The concept of dealing with issues while they're "hot" has considerable common-sense appeal. Moreover, demand-responsive service systems, such as crisis intervention hotlines, have proved to be effective in the treatment of drug abuse and suicidal compulsions. In these situations, the inadequacy of a delayed response becomes immediately obvious. In less dramatic situations, the need for immediate reckoning may be just as great, although the consequences, when no help is available, are less public. Thus, programs that make counselors available as needed, who can respond with alacrity when a client's issue is hot, may be as vital to effectively helping people adjust to disability as in preventing drug recidivism or suicide.

The PSV Melting Pot

Any combination of the psychogogic approaches and techniques discussed so far may be brought together in the highly eclectic field of PSV rehabilitation. Rehabilitation psychologists and counselors must help disabled people deal with the full array of ordinary human problems, as well as the special issues related to disabilities.

Influences of the Rehabilitation Milieu

Regardless of the specific type of rehabilitation setting being considered, the psychological impact of the milieu is of foremost importance. This is not a statement about milieu *therapy* for people in rehabilitation hospitals (see, for example, Kutner, 1977); it is a statement about the quality of the ordinary social environments in which disabled people find themselves when needing services.

The importance of emotional support has been cited many times already and is appropriately reiterated here. Capacity for emotional supportiveness is not only important for professional staff, it should be a screening variable for every person hired to work in a rehabilitation setting. Clients spend considerable periods of time with secretarial, attendant, and housekeeping personnel, too.

One aspect deserving of special mention—because it is so often underemphasized—is the need for massive support when disabilities impair cognitive functioning. For example, patients with traumatic head injuries, strokes, or multiple sclerosis frequently mention that their physical (motor or sensory) losses are less frightening to them than the realization that their mental (intellectual or emotional) abilities are "out of control" to some degree.

The infusion of certain language habits into the rehabilitation milieu is almost as basic as creating an emotionally supportive environment; and they are the same language habits that should be stressed in public education designed to reduce disability stereotyping. The following five provisos can set the stage for more positive ways of thinking about and reacting to people with disabilities. The earlier a person is exposed to such "cleaned up" language, the less undoing of destructive attitudes will be required later on.

1.   Avoid the shorthand terms "the handicapped" and "the disabled." These phrases are prized for their brevity, but they carry the hidden cost of summarizing the individual(s) described as nothing more than one of their many characteristics, one that conjures a negative image in the minds of most. They also may be republicans, democrats, lawyers, homemakers, Catholics, Buddhists, beautiful, homely, or play any number of other roles and possess any number of other traits. All that is lost and forgotten when they are "collapsed" into the sole category of "the handicapped/disabled."

2.   Avoid the imprecision of describing a person as "handicapped" when what is meant is "disabled." As pointed out in the introduction to this book, it makes sense to refer to "a disabled person" when that is a consistent, permanent condition for him/her; however, it does not make sense to speak of "a handicapped person" because virtually no one is handicapped, by a disability, in every activity. References to handicaps always should make clear in what pursuits the individual is handicapped.

3.   As often as possible, avoid use of the verb "to be" and its conjugations in discussing people with disabilities or handicapping conditions. For example, "Sally *has* arthritis" is preferable to "Sally *is* an arthritic," when the subtleties of language-induced stereotyping are examined. The latter construction, like "the handicapped," summarizes Sally as nothing more than her arthritis; the former implies that she is more, that Sally, among other things, has arthritis. The "name-calling" quality of using the verb "to be" becomes very evident in speaking of people with disabilities that arouse social disapproval. For example, some people who have maladaptive drinking patterns resist being labeled "alcoholic" because they fear being reduced to nothing more than this in the conceptions of others. Their preference for admitting to "*having* a drinking problem" is derided in some quarters as denial of the problem, but it may equally well be a sensible avoidance of socially destructive stereotyping.

4.   Whenever possible, put the person before the disability in sentence construction. "Person with a disability" is preferable to "disabled person." The first thing to stress is the personhood of the subject (or object) of the sentence. After that basic mental image has been set, the modifying adjectival clause "with a disability" is less likely to dominate the conveyed concept of the person.

5. Abjure passive constructions such as "person *in* or *confined to* a wheelchair" in favor of such active constructions as "person who *uses* a wheelchair." The former conveys an image of passive sitting and victimization. The latter suggests a person who is actively using a wheelchair as a tool for living life. The difference is that between the "helpless invalid" of fifty years ago and the "consumer activist" of today.

The rehabilitation milieu also should provide support for patients/clients to develop their inner resources. For this reason, the pathology bias must be overcome so that staff will be alert to discerning existing or potential resources. Very important in this is to avoid misdiagnosing resources as pathology! A commonly acknowledged area in which this can happen involves aggressiveness and uncooperativeness, which are signs in some people of their determination to stay in charge of their own destinies, even while institutionalized. It may be troublesome to the staff while it's happening, but the same traits may harbinger better adjustment later on.

Another resource often misconstrued as pathology in institutional or agency settings is manipulativeness. When it is noted that a patient/client attempts to manipulate others, staff are resentful and quickly focus their efforts on blocking the individual from successfully manipulating *them*. This is a reaction, not a response, and it is self- (ego-) serving rather than client serving. Alternatives are possible. First, severely disabled people who are unable to manipulate the physical world have no other way to operate on it except through other people. It may be neither reasonable nor kind to try to block their only avenue toward mastery. Second, if manipulativeness is noticed, then part of the problem is that the manipulator's not doing it right. A good manipulator doesn't get labeled; part of the skill is escaping detection.

If manipulating other people is the only path toward mastery, and if a skill level that avoids offending others is possible, perhaps part of PSV rehabilitation is teaching clumsy manipulators to be more adept. Manipulating does not necessarily imply exploiting or harming those manipulated. Manipulation of others' feelings, perceptions, and behavior is central to an immense array of respectable occupations: psychology, teaching, trial law, counseling, the ministry, management, fund raising, sales, and the entire entertainment industry. If manipulation training for disabled people stressed the importance of being fair to the targets of manipulation and of offering them rewards for what they do (as much as occurs in the just-mentioned occupations), perhaps it would become an acceptable alternative to extinguishing one of the most useful survival traits a severely disabled person might have. The study in which school children with behavior problems were trained to condition their teachers—using behavior modification techniques—to treat them with more affection and respect, proved to make life much pleasanter for the teachers as well as the students. Rehabilitation personnel might find themselves reaping similar rewards.

Special Issues in Vocational Rehabilitation

A problem with state VR program effectiveness is that it attempts to focus too narrowly on the vocational aspect of rehabilitation without sufficient attention to the psychosocial needs of its clients. As one rehabilitation psychologist pointed out, "They don't do PSV rehab; they just do V rehab and hope the PS will take care of itself! It would be more likely to work the other way." The 1978 amendments to the Rehabilitation Act of 1973, which added provisions for independent living rehabilitation, acknowledge and respond to the S (social needs), but the P (psychological needs) continue to be underemphasized in this program. The needs for personal, sexual, marriage, or family counseling may be recognized, yet rehabilitation counselors feel constrained by vocational rehabilitation production demands from devoting the requisite time or case-service funds to them.

One reason for this is the peculiarly diverse role of the rehabilitation counselor. As documented by Kemp (1981), the typical job is more accurately that of "case manager" than "counselor" and entails numerous functions that may be antagonistic—both in terms of activity demands and worker temperament—to the counseling function: coordinating, expediting, procurement, reporting–accounting, and "sales" or job placement.

Complicating the basic problems of interfering demands and too little time and money to expend on psychological services is the very fact that VR agency counselors *have* case-service funds—to expend on behalf of clients or to withhold—and this strains counselor–client relationships in ways not confronted by others who do personal counseling. Counselors seldom are prepared for the impact of this in their preservice graduate training. They are in unique power positions. They can choose to be "good guys" and spend large amounts of case-service funds for private training, personal vehicles, monthly maintenance allowances, or whatever is needed/desired by their clients; or they can choose to be "bad guys," conserving agency funds and requiring clients to find other ways to meet these economic needs. Because of their fiscal discretion, they can choose to be "good guys" with some clients and "bad guys" with others. Then, because of the ethical constraints against discussing one client's situation with another, they may be unable to explain their professional rationales for differential treatment. Thus, the potential for their fiscal role eclipsing their counseling function in the eyes of the clients, and for being seen as autocratic, parental authorities rather than helping persons, is introduced and must be dealt with directly before a rapport conducive to personal counseling can develop.

The agency role also creates a philosophical dilemma for many counselors. They may wonder, "Whose agent am I? Do I work for the taxpayers/state, or do I work for the client? Am I here to reduce the welfare rolls and increase the number of disabled people paying taxes, or am I here to help disabled people achieve equity, dignity, and improved quality of life?" Some are able to choose or otherwise reach a comfortable resolution; others report that the schism interferes with serving effectively and consistently in either capacity and consider it a major cause of burnout.

Two recent client-service trends offer to provide some relief for these interrelated problems. First, experience with independent living rehabilitation is leading to heightened awareness, within vocational rehabilitation, of the need to attend to psychological as well as social/survival needs of clients. This is reflected in (a) increasing independent living programming within the state VR agencies and private-sector facilities and (b) the burgeoning consumer-run independent living centers.

Second, job clubs—an approach to job finding developed by behavioral psychologist Nathan Azrin in the early 1970s—are being used increasingly in vocational rehabilitation, to the psychosocial as well as vocational benefit of both clients and counselors. Job clubs combine job-search training with mutual help, much of which is comprised of motivational/emotional/moral support, as well as job-lead sharing and other practical assistance. A series of side benefits emanate from this approach. Counselors who fear and avoid doing job placement can work in teams, with other counselors and job-club members, thereby receiving the support *they* need to confront this difficult part of their jobs. Their active involvement in helping with job search then alters the clients' perceptions of them; they come to be seen as more genuinely helpful. This, in turn, has a positive effect on the likelihood that clients will seek their counsel when they need to and are ready to deal with personal problems. When clients initiate such services, they are unlikely to be withheld.

The Self-Help Philosophy

Job clubs and consumer-run independent living programs are but two highly significant manifestations of the self-help philosophy that is spreading rapidly throughout the industrialized world. Others mentioned earlier are the holistic health movement, pain-management clinics, and, of course, Alcoholics Anonymous—the prototype organization for mutual helping among people who share similar problems. Toffler (1980) traces the pattern by which the same social forces—notably, skyrocketing advances in electronics technology, with a resultant explosion of data-processing and telecommunications capabilities—are giving impetus to both the "self-help" and "do-it-yourself" movements. He arrives at a prediction that future society will reunite production with consumption at the individual level; that is, each of us will tend to produce more for our own consumption and less for the market, or for consumption by others.

Within the broadly-conceived health-and-human-service field, we are seeing already that the watchwords are, "Know thyself" and "Heal (serve) thyself": we all are becoming our own "physicians." Mutual-help approaches can be seen as barter-economy variations on the self-help theme, and the following chapter will examine the self- and mutual-help phenomena that now loom large in rehabilitation. Specifically, peer-provided psychogogic services and the psychological impact of other peer-provided service approaches will be reviewed.

12 Coaching

Peer Counseling and Related Services

Like several other human-service innovations mentioned earlier in this volume, a prototype for organizations operated "*by* the disabled, *for* the disabled" germinated in the fertile social soil of Berkeley, California. The Center for Independent Living (CIL) came into being when a number of severely disabled graduates of the University of California at Berkeley (UCB) discovered that college degrees had not made them independent. Unable to find jobs even as college graduates, they had to find ways to survive in the community if they were to avoid custodial institutions or returning to their parental homes. Thus, in the early 1970s, CIL was essentially a community extension of the Physically Disabled Students Program on the UCB campus. Partly because there are so many more disabled people struggling to survive out in the community than on college campuses, it was destined to outgrow the size and fame of its parent organization within five years.

The Zeitgeist was right. The same phenomenon was beginning to appear elsewhere at about the same time. Massachusetts, Texas, Ohio, and, gradually, more and more other states developed independent living programs (ILPs) operated by and for the disabled. In California, they multiplied quickly after CIL's prime mover was appointed by the governor to head the State Department of Rehabilitation. The new director encouraged the development of similar centers throughout the state by funding grants and giving technical assistance. Other states began equivalent campaigns. In 1978, the Rehabilitation Act was amended to provide for independent living as well as vocational rehabilitation, and a new era in rehabilitation was under way.

A highly significant aspect of the new era is the provision of some rehabilitation services by people who have experienced disability themselves. The embracement of this concept by rehabilitation professionals represents a greater shift in values and attitudes than some veteran providers care to remember. Well into the 1960s, disabled applicants to many academic programs for professional training in rehabilitation disciplines were not welcomed by screening committees unless they demonstrated unusual ability to avoid "identification" with clients' or patients' problems. Nondisabled professionals feared disabled providers would be unable to separate their own problems (and resulting emotions) from those of their clients, reducing their objectivity and helpfulness. The (largely unrecognized) assumption underlying this prejudice was that a person who is disabled must be so pervasively damaged by it, psychologically, that recovery of objectivity and emotional control, when the subject is touched, is virtually impossible. This attitude was tempered first by the increasing realization, within the entire psychosocial/ behavioral helping field, that "identification" is neither so rare nor so deadly as previously imagined. Second, it was quelled by the rising voice of an increasingly political disabled constituency. The "customers" began to insist that they could do the job better in some respects, and they demanded the right to try. The ILPs provided a mechanism for them to do so.

Peer Services

To the extent that ILP staff members have disabilities, often their rehabilitative offerings are construed as peer services, regardless of their professional backgrounds. Here, peer status is defined clearly in terms of disability. In other contexts, the term "peer" connotes the absence of professional training; it is used in contradistinction to "professional" (provider). Thus, peer status sometimes relates to professionalism. It may be helpful to keep this dual nature of peership in mind when considering peer-provided services. In this chapter, the terms "peer provider," "peer service," and similar variants will connote both personal experience with disability and the absence of professional training requirements for providing services. This definition allows for disabled professionals to do peer counseling when to relate as a peer rather than as a professional seems more appropriate. It also allows for peer-helping relationships among family members of disabled people, as well as the disabled individuals themselves.

This distinction can be made rather clearly, but the existence of a middle category—paraprofessional providers—blurs the lines. Since some training is needed for most peer providers, at what point do they become paraprofessionals? This may be resolved best by noting whether certification has been obtained. For the purposes of this chapter, the distinction between professionals—whose main qualification is full, formal training in a rehabilitation discipline—and peer providers—whose main qualification is disability experience—will suffice. A major difference resides in the prominent use of coaching techniques by peer providers. Certain rehabilitative tasks appear to be better done by life-experienced helpers than formally trained professionals; and the coaching relationship seems particularly suitable for many of these tasks.

The Coaching Concept

Psychogogy relies on teaching methods, and coaching is one of them. Typically, coaches are or have been players in a given game and their teaching power resides in their deeply ingrained understanding of both the game's demands and the players' needs. This holds true whether the "game" is athletic competition, artistic performance, or virtually any other activity. It is important to distinguish coaching from tutoring. A tutor may not have learned through experience; in fact, the subject matter is often didactic rather than experiential. Also, tutoring is a one-to-one process. While coaching may be, it is not limited in this respect. Group (most likely a team) coaching may be combined with adjunctive individual coaching.

Coaches employ a vast array of teaching methods. They instruct; that is, they provide factual information. They advise; that is, they offer judgments and make recommendations based on the facts. They counsel; that is, they attempt to motivate and provide emotional support. They do role modeling; that is, they demonstrate how given activities should be performed.

Coaches also provide ongoing feedback during and after the learner's performance. They don't deliver lectures and leave the performer to incorporate suggestions and correct errors without further guidance. They stay with the learner, instructing, advising, encouraging, demonstrating, and supporting as the performance unfolds. This aspect of coaching makes it time consuming and therefore expensive. As a result, it has been used mainly in the sports world, which society is willing to subsidize, and the performing arts, which highly motivated individuals will scrimp and save to finance. It has not been considered feasible for PSV rehabilitation providers.

The advent of ILPs staffed with volunteers or modestly paid workers has made the cost of coaching feasible in PSV rehabilitation. As a result, its unique power in preparing disabled people for independent living has come to light. People who themselves have adjusted emotionally and practically to disability can coach others—using both their abilities to "identify" and their parallel experiential bases. They coach sometimes as effectively and sometimes more effectively than professionals whose knowledge is "second hand."

Varieties of Peer Service

Peer counseling is explicitly psychogogic in nature. Before examining it more extensively, however, it would be well to explore the psychogogic effects of other peer services, many of which carry "counseling" in their titles. Financial, attendant, and housing counseling, although referred to as "counseling," are actually more akin to ombudsman services. That is, they combine coaching (instruction, advisement, role modeling) with advocacy (agency intervention). Psychological growth is enhanced in part through the process of incidental learning; clients observe that disabled people can learn to solve their practical problems and then teach others how to do it. This message alone can contribute to a client's growing self-confidence.

It also must be recognized that the facts of resolving financial, attendant, and housing problems have enormous impact on psychological well-being; even having an aware person to talk with about them can be helpful. None of these benefits were readily available to disabled people in the community before ILPs and their peer-provided services came into being. In the hospital, there were social workers to help with such matters; but once home again, unguided trial and error coupled with unchanneled worry soon eroded any acquired sense of well-being. Now, peer providers are attending to psychological health, both in these indirect ways and directly through the medium of peer counseling.

Peer Counseling

Selection of Peer Counselors

Although the professionals of an earlier era may have misjudged both the degree to which "identification" interferes with good counseling and the degree to which disabled counselors might project their own problems onto clients, they were attuned to a real, potential pitfall; that is, having experienced disability is not, in itself, sufficient qualification for functioning competently as a peer counselor. Just as the best football, drama, and other coaches typically have been good performers, the best peer counselors ("living-with-disability coaches") perform well in their own lives with respect to emotional and practical adjustment to disability. No one wants as a coach the player who couldn't make the team; and no one needs a person who is bitter, ineffectual, and unfulfilled as a counselor.

Selection of peer counselor candidates, by programs that use them, is made even more difficult than ordinary employee selection by two factors. First, unlike the situation in hiring professionals, there is no long and arduous preparatory process that can be relied on to either correct problematical habits or eliminate individuals clearly unsuited for the work. Often, decisions must be made on immediately available data plus, at most, a very brief period of preservice training. Since the peer counselor will be drawing mainly from effective life experiences and good personal adjustment, methods for quickly and correctly assessing such notoriously hard-to-assess matters must be developed.

Second, sometimes people offering to work on a voluntary basis have to be rejected. It is doubly hard to turn away free services when the "employer" knows the applicant is searching for a way to be and feel useful; no one wants to be responsible for aborting such efforts. Nonetheless, if the requisite personal qualities are absent, other ways to encourage such an applicant must be found if harm to that individual and those s/he would attempt to help is to be avoided.

Settings

Like the ILPs themselves, peer counseling as a service entity took root on college campuses. When disabled students joined forces for mutual aid and political amplification, informal counseling among peers was a natural result of their coming together. Today, campus programs for disabled students and community-based ILPs are the major settings in which formalized peer counseling services can be found. Undoubtedly, the reason is that both tend to be operated by and for the disabled. The genre seems to be here to stay and has, in fact, generated several subvarieties.

At the same time, an increasing number of traditional, professionally-operated rehabilitation settings—hospitals, centers, and agencies—are adding peer counseling to their own selections of service alternatives. While this reflects a view that peer counseling has something unique to offer, its addition has been met with mixed reviews from both sides. For example, some disabled activists charge "tokenism" and insist disabled people with the talent for peer counseling should be encouraged instead to pursue full, professional training so they can reap the economic benefits of mainstream work. This does happen for some; for example, peer counseling experience gained as an advanced rehabilitant working with more recently admitted clients/patients has been a stepping stone toward professional training for a number of people. Another problem is that peer counselors in traditional settings tend to work under the supervision of largely nondisabled PSV professionals who reportedly treat them as "patients" rather than as "colleagues." This same complaint, however, is voiced by fully trained professionals who have disabilities, about nondisabled coworkers in rehabilitation settings.

In the state VR agencies, peer counselors are most apt to be used in ombudsman roles, dealing with complaints about service rather than operating in the mainstream of service delivery. This is particularly difficult duty, requiring consummate diplomatic skill overlaid on a serenely objective nature, if problems are to be resolved rather than escalated. When underqualified individuals have been hired, polarization has arisen between disabled and nondisabled staff simply because of their respective roles.uu13A few voluntary rehabilitation agencies and work-oriented rehabilitation facilities are making limited use of peer counselors, but greater use could be made. Nontraditional employees can be integrated better into these more flexible organizations than into the rigid confines demanded by hospital or large bureaucracy structures.

Training

Although the term "peer counselor" connotes "untrained," this reflects a matter of degree. Initially, training was resisted in the belief that "having been there" provided more salient preparation than the professionals had and that professionals urging or offering training were acting out of self-interest. However, on finding that totally untrained peer counselors too often were unequipped to either help others or protect themselves in the demanding, emotionally charged relationships that sometimes developed, this resistance weakened. Now, most programs using peer counselors either have combined screening/training methodologies or are making concerted efforts to develop them. A few use professionally-trained disabled counselors in the role of peer counselors, to maximize the quality of counseling; however, these people still retain the title "peer counselor" because of its greater consumer acceptance.

As previously noted, candidates are screened primarily on the basis of personal qualities, that is, their apparent potential for *learning* rather than their possession of skills. This is partly a function of the newness of the role—no sizable pools of experienced candidates yet exist—and partly a function of a design to give many disabled people opportunities to fill the role because of its power to aid their own growth. The truth of the maxim, "One learns best by teaching," is accepted here.

Available training ranges from structured, rather sophisticated programs that train groups of candidates and last for several weeks, to single orientation sessions conducted by volunteer professionals from such disciplines as social work, rehabilitation counseling, or psychology. An example of the former comes from Howard Community College in Columbia, Maryland (Corn, 1978). Their training prerequisites include (1) having experienced a physical limitation due to surgery, injury, or illness; (2) having adjusted to this limitation to the point of living a productive, rewarding life; (3) wanting to help others achieve an optimal personal and social adjustment following a similar handicapping loss; and (4) being willing to make a definite commitment of time and effort to the peer counseling program after training. The training goals are to enable each learner to (1) establish a warm, genuine, empathic relationship that enables another to develop more readily new understanding and self-acceptance following a sudden loss; (2) provide practical guidance and information about available community resources for help in coping with a physical disability; and (3) further their own personal growth through self-understanding, improved interpersonal skills, and the rewards of reaching out to help others. The specific learning objectives are to:

1. Share personal experience
2. Listen effectively
3. Express feelings

4. Respond to feelings
5. Accept others' experience
6. Encourage independent living
7. Be aware of sexuality and family issues
8. Provide resource information
9. Work with professional helpers
10. Understand peer counseling responsibilities and limitations.

Both peer counseling and the various professional counseling varieties are referred to regularly as "the art of forming helping friendships." The friendship entails the elements of relating with warmth, genuineness, and empathy, and also of having a usable reservoir of knowledge about community resources. While it is true that they share this characteristic, the Howard training program highlights a significant difference in that it excludes coverage of principles and techniques relating to basic psychological intervention strategies (for example, behavior modification and nondirective counseling). It is possible that, in time, peer counselors will wish to upgrade their discipline to the paraprofessional level. At that point, such material might be added profitably to their training.

Peer Counseling as the Service of Choice

Although peer counseling often is relied on when professional staffers are in short supply or too expensive, there also are times when it is clearly the service of choice. A prime factor has been alluded to already: consumer acceptance. Many consumers, who do not acknowledge the need for professional psychological services (perhaps because the psychogogy–psychotherapy distinction has never been made clear to the general public), are very willing to admit that peer counseling might be useful. Coaching by a peer is bereft of the threat associated with accepting a psychologist's help, so at least some help is accepted.

It follows that peer counseling might be the service of choice for people who need to be prepared to accept more intensive psychological services. A peer counselor who has profited from professional help and can relate about this comfortably may have far greater credibility and influence than a professional. Also, disabled people who have had little opportunity to be with, and develop positive identification with, other disabled people can profit especially from helping friendships with disabled peers. For many such individuals, shared facts about coping possibilities come as revelations and have the power to alter motivation levels, belief systems, and behavior. Generally, peer counseling is the service of choice when a good-quality, helping friendship is all that is needed. There is no point in bringing out the "heavy artillery" of high-level professionals unless their sophisticated knowledge of psychological principles and their finely tuned skills are actually required.

Peer counselors carry a unique set of credentials: credibility as an ordinary person who has been able to "make it," special insights that come only through experience, a capacity for forming a special rapport that stems from shared experience, and a potential for role modeling that emanates from the first three. Each of these credentials deserves further examination.

Credibility as an *ordinary* person who is succeeding in life is extremely important to at least the middle two-thirds of any normally distributed population. For this reason, efforts to hold out the success of disabled professionals as inspirational examples often backfire, as illustrated in Part I. Only people in the top ten percent of the population, intellectually, could hope to emulate them, and when such other requisites as drive and interpersonal support are taken into account, the percentage dwindles further. This suggests that the very best peer counselors might be part-timers who tread another occupational path during the rest of their working hours. This would expand the range and depth of feasible options to which counselees would be exposed.

The issues of special insights and the capacity for special rapport also must be viewed with a degree of caution. Counselor and counselee are two different people, and a valid charge still can be made that "You don't understand; you're not *me*." Peer counselors who invest a great deal of their feelings of confidence and competence in their capacities for special insights and rapport building may be particularly vulnerable when such charges come, and they inevitably do. Lowering peers' expectations for automatic rapport based on similar demography is an important part of the preservice orientation. It is equally important for peer counselors to learn when to share their own experiences and when not to. Those who are still reckoning actively with their own adjustments may be especially prone to "taking over," sharing too much too soon, in ways that inhibit rather than facilitate counselees' progress. It was overgeneralization of this realistic concern that led earlier professionals to discredit the concept of peer counseling.

Similar caveats attach to the matter of role modeling. Role models are chosen, not imposed. For example, able-bodied, white males have had a vast array of potential role models to select among throughout history, but their own inner needs will determine whom they pick. Recent efforts to present potential role models to nonwhite, nonmale, or nonable-bodied individuals sometimes overlook this fact, assuming that the proffered role model *is* a role model rather than only potentially one. Thus, peer counselors may or may not prove to be lifestyle role models for given clients. However, at a more mundane and practical level, modeling—or demonstrating—effective techniques for, say, contacting agencies can be emulated whether or not clients wish to pattern their lifestyles broadly after the counselors'. It is this level of role modeling that can be striven for consciously.

Peer Counseling Approaches

Peer counseling is construed generally as a one-to-one interaction with psychogogic intent, and it often takes place in offices not unlike those used by professionals. However, it is no more limited to this than is professional counseling. Six major variations will be discussed.

Adventitious Peer Counseling

This occurs when psychogogic purposes are added to the practical goals of advisement on such matters as managing finances, procuring attendants, obtaining suitable housing, and meeting recreational needs. The natural dovetailing of personal-growth counseling into the context of such practical planning has advantages in terms of reaching people who might not ask explicitly for this kind of help, as well as in clarifying the importance of personal growth to success in day-to-day coping. Peer counseling can happen adventitiously in a less formal sense, too. People who learn how to form helping friendships can use their skills in ordinary contacts with disabled friends and acquaintances as well—and be better friends than before. Hopefully, this may have a cumulative effect akin to that which TM practitioners claim for their discipline; that is, as the number of practitioners increases, anxiety-induced social aberrations will decrease exponentially. It is reasonable to imagine that each disabled person skilled in helpfulness will transmit her/his ways of being to several others; thus, the effect would magnify. This is another reason for maximizing the number of individuals admitted to the field.

Of all the peer-service specialties focused on specific coping skills, attendant counseling creates the heaviest demands for psychogogic inputs. To be done effectively, the employer–employee relationship must be examined thoroughly. This is because attendant turnover problems are often the result of disabled employers' failures to (1) empathize with attendants' needs and frustrations, (2) create rewarding job situations to counterbalance the low pay levels, (3) maximize flexibility in procedures without becoming subject to exploitation, (4) communicate effectively about job demands and performance satisfactoriness, or (5) confront potential relationship problems in timely, effective ways. Attendant counselors who display solid understanding and helpfulness initially may be called on to mediate if relationship problems arise after an attendant has been hired. The needed skills and conceptual framework have much in common with marriage counseling and conflict resolution among workers in organizational settings. Sometimes, professional intervention will be required, and it is important for the attendant counselor to discern when this is true.

Rap Groups

It is the intensity and complexity of interaction between (or among) individuals being counseled that determine whether professional skills are needed, not simply the fact of working with more than one person at a time. The success of "rap groups," for limited purposes, attests to this.

Peer counselors frequently conduct rap groups as a central activity, with individual counseling sessions evolving from needs discerned in the groups. The term conveys "nothing heavy-duty going on here." Opportunities to ventilate, exchange ideas and experiences, obtain moral support, and other relatively nonthreatening interchange are cited in publicizing such groups. Support and relief may come from sharing "war stories" with people who can understand immediately the subtle ironies that often must be explained to nondisabled associates; shared belly laughs feel good. Because of this psychodynamic "lightness," the rap group sometimes is disparaged as a psychogogic tool. However, while it may have little direct impact on serious psychological problems, Norman Cousins (1979) has made a convincing case for the value of feeling good and happy in improving both bodily and mental health. It is easy to overlook the obvious. The psychological essence of Cousins' highly acclaimed book is a single message: laughter is the best medicine. Many sophisticates have responded to this as if it were a revelation, although *The Reader's Digest,* one of the country's most popular (but unsophisticated) periodicals, has carried a feature by this title for years. Thus, the rap group's greatest strength may lie in its ability to improve feelings of well-being temporarily, because this improved state of consciousness makes further, deeper changes more feasible.

Consciousness Raising

An important feature of some rap groups is consciousness raising (CR). In addition, groups explicitly designed for this purpose may be conducted along the lines of CR groups for women. Here, emphasis is placed on helping participants enhance their self-concepts or feelings of self-esteem through clarified recognition of their rights as members of a given class of people. Individual frailties are separated conceptually from responses to externally-imposed constraints, in the hope that participants then can perceive expanded vistas and greater degrees of freedom with which they can operate.

Obviously, this relates to what was called "the other half of the psychology of disability—the *politics* of disability" in the introduction to this book. Accordingly, consciousness raising as a psychogogic modality is not confined to CR groups: it occurs as an integral part of advocacy by the disabled, for the disabled as well.

Disabled people of both sexes who become involved in advocacy efforts have equivalent opportunities for the kind of CR that accompanies learning to fight for sociopolitical rights. However, CR groups as a peer counseling function still are oriented most commonly toward the needs of disabled women. Since the CR phenomenon grew out of the women's movement, this is not surprising; but the approach seems so appropriate for disabled people generally, it probably should be made more available to the men.

An independent living center once sent out its monthly newsletter with the motto, "Crippled is beautiful" emblazoned on the cover. The number of negative responses from recipients showed how much more CR needs to be done. Good consciousness raising can help people become desensitized, in the sense of being less vulnerable to hurt, to uncontrollable words and actions on the parts of others. Once this is accomplished, vistas can be expanded "safely" because fewer fears remain of vulnerabilities that might take one by surprise and prompt withdrawal from other challenges.

Hotlines

Occasionally, in nearly everyone's life, the challenges of living threaten to overwhelm coping abilities. When this happens, still another peer counseling service, the hotline, may be used to help disabled people—especially those who are isolated/immobilized—to handle such crises.The use of the telephone for crisis intervention grew from programs designed for people in such serious trouble—psychologically and physically—that the telephone might be as far as they could reach out for help. The term "hotline" grew out of the urgency of these situations.

Alcoholics Anonymous has long offered "twelfth step" work: when tempted to drink, call another member and talk it out instead. Later, suicide prevention and drug rehabilitation programs developed techniques for telephone diagnostic screening, as well as refined methods for remote treatment intervention. Now, hotlines have been instituted in a wide range of programs for an increased range of purposes, from truly "hot" issues such as defusing urges to batter children, to such "cooler" needs as the dispelling of loneliness. A few ILPs now have hotlines operated by peer counselors, and more are working to establish them. When the counselors are willing to do so, residence numbers may be provided to give potential callers extended hours of telephone coverage.

Peer counseling by telephone is uniquely appropriate for homebound disabled people, simply because of the difficulties in arranging transportation. The potential of telephone counseling is not limited to that provided by peers, however. The author began using this method in the early 1960s when working as an outpatient psychologist with homebound, former patients of a rehabilitation hospital. No implication is intended that telephone counseling is superior or even equal to in-person contact; however, it is vastly superior to its realistic alternative of *nothing* for people unable to get to a service location. If Toffler (1980) is right, telephone counseling may be the wave of the future. Transporting people's bodies from place to place is becoming almost unmanageable because of energy shortages and uneven population distribution. At the same time, the electronic age is making the movement of information so much easier with each passing day that the need for transporting bodies—to central work locations, for example—is diminishing rapidly. This could be good news to people unable to gain access to public transit systems or afford private means.

Just as necessity has motivated many physically disabled people to develop unusual intellectual skills (for example, memorizing telephone numbers because looking them up is difficult), the necessity of using telephone counseling if in-person contact is infeasible may motivate users to develop the skills for making the most of it. At the same time, counselors undoubtedly can learn ways of exploiting the features of telephone communication while circumventing its constraints.

Peer-Provided Body Work

This area of peer service is just beginning in a few ILPs. Several have disabled staff members who have had martial-arts training and offer informal training, in karate or other disciplines, to program participants. Also, several centers have instituted movement and dance therapy programs. For example, in one, a staff member whose dance career was interrupted by mental illness provided a variety of dance and movement experiences for people with either physical or mental disabilities. Another program began with professionally-provided dance experiences aimed at opening up relationships among participants; it now has a cadre of experienced staff and clients who are passing the approach on to others.

A more fully developed approach comes not from an ILP but from a conceptually similar program for senior citizens. Luce (1979) describes the body-work program that has evolved at SAGE (Senior Actualizations and Growth Experiences) in Berkeley, California. In addition to martial arts and dance/movement offerings, a highly valued program of massage—administered by self, staff, or other participants—has been established. Although SAGE is described here as "conceptually similar" to ILPs, it should be pointed out that it, in a sense, reverses the usual priorities of ILPs; that is, practical survival and coping skills seem to place second in importance compared with personal growth and inner development.

The goals are similar in all of the just-mentioned programs: (1) to learn that the body, even if it is disabled or aged, is a source of pleasure, beauty, and grace and (2) to use body work as a means for improving one's psychological well-being and ability to connect with others. The SAGE program has found that nude body work is particularly powerful as a means of helping participants unlearn the misconception that old bodies are no longer beautiful or a pleasure to touch. The same goal is clearly relevant to people who believe disabilities and/or deformities have rendered their bodies unbeautiful.

This illustration also brings out a desirable new direction for peer services of a psychogogic nature: the potential inherent in a coalition between seniors and disabled people of all ages. Many of the needs and issues are the same, and more are at least comparable. A few programs are beginning to tap this symbiotic potential, such as foster-grandparent programs for disabled (or nondisabled) children who lack loving families and for older people who need to give love, and programs wherein mentally retarded students make regular visits to convalescent hospitals to entertain and socialize with elderly, disabled people. In another example, a small rehabilitation hospital found it necessary to discharge two young paraplegic men to a nursing home populated solely by elderly patients, because independent living situations in the community could not be arranged for them. Viewed as potentially catastrophic for them at first, it was later regarded as divinely inspired. One of the young men changed within a month from morose and apathetic to a self-ordained recreation director for the elderly. The other, following this lead, helped to conduct the activities. The morale of the elderly patients was affected similarly. In about three months, both had made their own independent living arrangements in the community and moved on. The nursing home now is asking for more such young men to be sent to them, and the hospital is considering doing so.

Peer-Provided Three-Quarter-Way Houses

The final peer-service approach to be discussed here is currently at an even more rudimentary stage of development than the coalition of aging and disabled people. It is peer-operated group living arrangements for people needing continuous emotional support to avoid rehospitalization in neuropsychiatric settings. The traditional half-way house is professionally staffed and managed; however, a nontraditional approach was developed by four extremely intelligent individuals who met while they were patients at the same neuropsychiatric hospital. Each had been discharged to the community on two or more occasions but had succumbed to the stress of trying to survive alone and so required readmission. Two of the four had tried traditional half-way houses and left them because they found it intolerable to have their lives "managed" by professionals.

With assistance from hospital staff, they arranged to rent jointly a large, older house and moved into it at approximately the same time. All four worked in community jobs; none of their employers knew of their psychiatric histories. All had learned the rudiments of mutual helping during their hospitalizations, and they developed their skills remarkably while living together. For example, one woman, emaciated as a result of anorexia nervosa, loved to cook but refused to eat. Her housemates established a rule whereby for her to earn the privilege of cooking for the group, she was required to gain one pound per week. Any week in which she failed to meet the criterion meant no kitchen privileges until the pound was gained.

They have become known to the author because they are seeking funding to replicate the model for other groups. They enunciate their philosophy clearly: although professional expertise is respected and *consultation* is welcomed, having their homes and lives *managed* by professionals is abjured. Unfortunately, because they fear "going public" would jeopardize their jobs, their efforts to encourage replication have not been very successful. They are convinced, however, that without the emotional support, informal behavior modification programs, and other help they offer each other, none of them could have remained out of the hospital for what now has been quite a long period of time. It clearly has worked well for them, and it appears to have potential for other small groups with similar needs.

This chapter has focused on the kinds of psychological services that can be used by people who are healthy or stable enough that professionally-trained providers are not (or not always) required. By contrast, the following chapter will examine issues and practices relevant to people with such severe psychological problems that professional intervention of a curative or psychotherapeutic nature is required.

13 Correcting
Psychotherapeutic Approaches

This chapter will provide an overview of psychotherapeutic services, primarily for rehabilitation professionals who are not fully familiar with their scope and purposes; and it will show how they fit into a general PSV rehabilitation context. Because a massive research and clinical literature exists in the field, a comprehensive synthesis would require more pages than have been allotted for this entire volume. The scope of the chapter will be clarified further, but, first, several definitional distinctions should be made.

The psychogogy–psychotherapy distinction was made earlier (see Chapter 11) in terms of whether the intent is preventive—to strengthen the person so psychological breakdown will not occur—or curative—to correct psychological disorders that have developed already. Whereas the term "psychogogy" might be applied to any methods employed in prevention, psychotherapy is but one of three paths that might be chosen for treating existing disorders. The other two are psychosurgery and the use of drugs or nutrients. Psychotherapy, like psychogogy, generally is mediated by a learning process, in contradistinction to surgery, medication, and nourishment, which operate directly on bodily tissues in the attempt to bring about psychological change. This does not mean that all psychotherapy is verbal. As recently as the 1960s, psychotherapy was referred to as "talk therapy" by its practitioners; however, since that time, many new techniques have been adopted, including an array of nonverbal body-work techniques. In these, exercise, massage, and other bodily procedures are used as media for *teaching* such behaviors as relaxation; there is no attempt to correct the problem through direct bodily intervention. Biofeedback training (used increasingly in the cure of phobic reactions and maladaptive habit formation) and other behavior-modification procedures lie on the borderline; they are not construed as talk therapy but they do use varying degrees of spoken and inner verbalization.

For simplicity, "psychotherapy" will include here any curative approach to psychobehavioral disorder that excludes surgery, drugs, and nutrients. No effort will be made to examine the latter approaches, leaving their discussion to authors with the appropriate medical or physiological training. The focus here will be on psychological approaches of either a verbal or nonverbal nature.

Whether or not an intervention qualifies as either psychogogy or psychotherapy depends on the nature and severity of the client's problem. When problems are severe, establishing acceptable nomenclature is made doubly difficult because the area is still weak with respect to empirical grounding and people react emotionally to any terms used. In fact, it is the author's prediction that the new, third edition of the *Diagnostic and Statistical Manual (DSM:III;* American Psychiatric Association, 1980) will fail ultimately in one of its aims: to generate nonthreatening terminology. It is likely that, with time and experience, the common-language terms it substitutes for today's clinical-sounding terms simply will become the clinical-sounding terms of tomorrow. It has been pointed out, not totally in jest, that other common-language terms may have to be invented so that rehabilitation professionals not sanctioned by state licensing to establish psychodiagnoses will be able to describe their clients' problems without breaking the law. The *DSM:III* is a very new "dictionary," and it will take some time to make uniform the nomenclature used to designate even the general phenomena addressed in this chapter, whether now called psychological disorder, mental illness, behavioral dysfunction, or another combination of such words.

Proponents and critics of all alternatives can be found. The disagreement extends to the issue of *what* is "ill," "disordered," or "dysfunctional." Is it the individual's body, mind, spirit, or a combination of these, or is it the family or even the larger society? Some say all must be "diseased," "deranged," or "aberrational" for symptoms to appear. The term "psychosomatics" is fading from use as more practitioners become convinced that all disease is produced through the interaction of soma and psyche. Psychogenic substrates are suspected in virtually all organic disease; physiological substrates are suspected in virtually all psychological disorders, particularly those labeled "psychoses."

Recognizing that such definitional controversies exist, this chapter will select arbitrarily the term "psychological disorder" as the most general rubric encompassing psychoses, neuroses, behavior disorders, and other classifications conceived to indicate that something has gone wrong mentally, emotionally, behaviorally, or psychologically. (Whatever the root causes, the symptoms tend to be perceived by others in these terms.) "Mental illness" here will imply psychosis. "Emotional disability" will be used to distinguish the preceding varieties from mental disabilities affecting primarily intellectual functioning, such as mental retardation and learning disabilities.

Given these definitions, for purposes of discussion in this rehabilitation context, the populations served can be distinguished along two dimensions: (1) whether a psychological disorder constitutes the primary disability or arises as a secondary disability in conjunction with physical or intellectual impairment and (2) whether the disorder is in the acute stage or has passed that and the individual is undergoing rehabilitation. These distinctions can be summarized graphically as follows:

	Psychological disorder is *PRIMARY* disability	Psychological disorder is *SECONDARY* disability
Acute Stage	Cell 1	Cell 2
Rehabilitation Stage	Cell 3	Cell 4

A detailed examination of the intervention issues associated with Cell 1 is clearly beyond the scope of this rehabilitation-oriented volume. Here, discussion will be limited to matters of relevance to subsequent rehabilitation efforts. The remainder of the chapter will review the basic parameters of psychotherapeutic services, specific approaches used in selected settings, and common problems encountered, with primary emphasis on Cells 2, 3, and 4. In addition, certain implications for rehabilitation counselors will be discussed.

Parameters of Psychotherapeutic Services

Although the nature of the problem and the state of the art might seem the logical determinants, the general goals of psychotherapy are likely to be decided by such practical exigencies as time, funding, and provider availability. Arising from this, a major goal distinction is made between symptom removal and/or emotional support on the one hand, and correction of underlying causes on the other. The more limited the resources, the more likely it is that symptom removal or emotional support will become the treatment goal. There is no point in contemplating reconstructive therapy, which is generally reckoned in years, if the funding allows for a maximum of ten sessions per client. (It should be noted that some thinkers view symptom removal as all that is possible or desirable; the concept of underlying, psychodynamic causes is considered a meaningless issue. For these professionals, symptom removal is always the goal of choice rather than a practical necessity.) Beyond this level of general goal setting, cost and availability factors often alter choices on such other basic parameters as the types of providers, the specific objectives and treatment modalities, and the timing and settings of treatment. We will review salient issues relating to each of these factors before discussing a selection of specific treatment experiences.

Types of Providers

Although licensing requirements for practicing psychotherapy vary widely among the states, the primary providers are considered to be clinical psychologists, psychiatrists, and psychiatric social workers. The labels applied to their practices may be "behavior modification," "psychoanalysis," "social casework," or other designations, but if the intent is to correct problems in psychological functioning, it is regarded here as psychotherapy. Especially in institutional practices, psychologists and psychiatrists are apt to delegate actual treatment to others working under their supervision, and social workers are frequently those to whom psychiatrists delegate. Others to whom treatment is delegated are so varied and numerous as to defy documentation; they span a range of PSV professionals, paraprofessionals, peers, family members, hospital attendants, and job supervisors. The less training and experience the person has had, the more structured and delimited the assignment.

Thus, psychotherapy providers comprise two distinct groups: the "official" therapists and the highly important ancillary personnel. Although the division of labor often is dictated by cost and availability factors, use of ancillaries is by no means always "second best." One increasingly hears comments, within the field, to the effect that the doctoral-level experts may be best qualified to establish diagnoses and prescribe the forms of treatment, but they are not necessarily the best qualified to conduct therapy. One might speculate that traits of temperament required for successful completion of doctoral-level studies (for example, theory mindedness, scholarliness, and achievement and power needs) actually could interfere in the helping process. In any event, routine use of psychologists and psychiatrists to conduct psychotherapy may be as counterproductive as using orthopedists to do physical therapy instead of delegating it to specifically trained, less costly, more temperamentally suited physical therapists.

Specific Objectives and Treatment Modalities

Psychotherapy objectives are only beginning to be articulated clearly by treating professionals. The age of accountability has been late in impacting this area, partly because it is difficult and partly because it is considered dangerous to compartmentalize human beings into discrete, measurable units of psychosocial functioning. Efforts to force psychotherapists to separate conceptually and explicitly state the component parts of their global efforts to "improve psychological functioning" or "enhance insight and behavioral control" have thus met resistance. The counterforces toward it are stronger, however, and psychotherapists are joining educators and rehabilitation counselors in attempting to meet control agencies' demands for this basic level of accountability. Since such claimed outcomes as improved insight or enhanced feelings of psychological well-being are not subject to validation by public consensus, associated changes in observable behavior are becoming the subjects of the documentation.

The targeted behavior changes are as multiform as problem behavior itself, and the treatment modalities used to create change can be categorized along numerous dimensions. Examples are verbal–nonverbal, individual–group, traditional–nontraditional, and countless finer breakdowns within such general categories. Characteristically, the dimensions are much as described in Chapter 11; thus, it is mainly the intent and therefore the specific techniques that differ. However, two points relating to the individual–group dimension warrant mention here because of their potential impact on rehabilitation.

First, when serious psychological problems develop, severely impaired ability to trust the good will of others is often at issue. When group treatment totally supplants individual psychotherapy because of cost and provider availability factors, a foundation stone of recovery may be neglected because fledgling trust often needs to be nurtured initially in the safety of a one-on-one treatment environment. Second, in institutional treatment, "groups" sometimes resemble throngs—entire wards or filled auditoriums—not the dozen or less people usually envisioned in a group therapy session. The efficacy of such groups for institutional control may far exceed their usefulness in inducing functional improvement. This is not to suggest that large groups are without treatment utility, however. Throng groups are used very effectively in postinstitutional "networking" meetings of all the potentially helpful associates of an identified patient who can be assembled in that person's home. At the other extreme, a group might include only a couple of participants and a therapist, as happens when patients with similar problems are brought together spontaneously for a specific purpose. Thus, it is important to bear in mind that "group approaches" may encompass a momentous range of sizes and purposes.

Treatment Timing and Settings

Ideally, the best time for intervention is before the fact, in time for effective preventive measures. In fact, however, the problem usually becomes so severe as to be apparent to others before treatment is sought and initiated. Beyond this, funding and personnel shortages, coupled with procedural delays—inherent, it seems, in service-delivery organizations—further impede effective timing. It may be hyperbole, but one agency director has declared that "waiting lists can kill"; many others believe they are damaging to motivation for treatment by allowing the moment of peak readiness to pass. When these directors cannot serve individuals immediately, they prefer to arrange a referral if that is possible, or just to give them an honest "No" over lulling them into believing that help is imminent when it may be many months away. Naturally, others disagree, saying the reassurance of being on a waiting list can be "therapeutic" by reducing anxiety and stimulating increased self-exploration.

The treatment modalities and specific techniques used vary, according to whether the disorder is in an acute or a later stage and whether it is getting worse or better. These, in turn, influence the types of settings selected for treating the individuals. Thus, timing and setting issues are inextricably interrelated.

Psychotherapeutic Services

Rehabilitation and Primary Psychological Disability

A clinical psychologist who owns and operates two small, private, psychiatric hospitals states an essential issue thus:

> If I know an applicant for admission has previously been hospitalized for as long as two weeks in a state mental facility, I am very cautious about admitting the person. Especially if electroshock treatments have been used, I find that the damaging consequences of the entire experience are so pervasive that we have little chance of really helping them. The use of electroshock is the worst problem, but more is involved. The impersonal, regimented milieu, coupled with a greater sense of responsibility for protecting the people outside than for treating the people inside, [do] irreparable harm.

He volunteers that he may overstate the case, somewhat, to make his point, but the problem is clear: what happens during acute-stage intervention can make or break success in subsequent rehabilitation efforts with people whose primary disability is psychological.

Discussions with numerous PSV rehabilitation professionals who have had extensive experience in this area yielded little in the way of service approaches believed to be effective and a great deal of frustration over the problems encountered. Most of these professionals are known to be positive and optimistic in their general outlooks on life, but a sense of futility permeates their descriptions of rehabilitative work with people who have chronic psychological disabilities. Jacqueline Sanchez—nurse, rehabilitation counselor, administrator, and holistic healing expert—has worked with emotionally disabled people in all of the major types of settings (state mental hospital, state VR agency, private psychiatric hospital, half-way house, and work-oriented rehabilitation facility). Her words (personal communication) summarize the essence of what virtually all professionals expressed:

One of the first problems encountered is having to "label" the person psychiatrically to establish eligibility for benefits or insurance, knowing it will later create problems for them in job discrimination. Often, the hope of receiving benefits is the only reason the person is participating. If clients said they wouldn't work, they got cut off—so they said they wanted to work. But no diagnostic tool can tell you if a person *can* work, much less whether they want to. At the hospital, judgments were made that a person could work if they watched TV, but animals watch TV so that is no indicator. At the half-way house, I knew that if I cut off patients' benefits they'd *have* to go to work; but if it turned out they couldn't, they'd be returned to the hospital. I was tempted constantly, but never tried it.

Most patients didn't actually manipulate the system because their intellects were so dulled by either meds or the disease, but they had no self-motivation that comes from having a self-image in the community. Motivation was the whole issue—and that was dulled by drugs or disease. Maybe there's a hormone that motivates us—like endorphin kills pain—and is destroyed by the disease process.

As to treatment, maybe biochemistry is the answer; I know I didn't find psychotherapy appropriate for chronic schizophrenics—neither group nor individual. Groups were conducted, but they were efforts to motivate for work, not provide psychotherapy. The whole treatment effort is aimed toward getting the person off the welfare rolls—motivate them to work—not helpling their psychological functioning. For normals with acute situational problems, group support helps—especially group acceptance of "bad" parts of a person. But this doesn't work for chronic schizophrenics—they neither give it nor get it. There are no breakouts from mental institutions like there are from prisons because there is no group support, no social community. When you get riots in mental hospitals, you have people who don't belong there. The hero in *One Flew Over the Cuckoo's Nest* wasn't crazy. I tried running groups at the first two places I worked, but by the time I got to the third, I had grown up. It's easier to motivate staff than patients.

Frankly, I think rehabilitation counselors would be devastated if they ever faced the total futility of working with mental patients within the system that exists now. Let me explain what I mean. I found the people in Micronesia are motivated by a different value system. They're not labeled "crazy" but they're not motivated by the work ethic. Unfortunately, publicly supported programs *are*. So they don't work for Micronesians, and they don't work for people here who happen to reject the work ethic. The Micronesians needed medical and restorative services but they didn't need to be put to work—which was seen as a penalty—but the VR system out there required it. I think the analogy is clear.

Something is needed here, but it may not be work and I question whether it is psychotherapy for people who are chronically disabled by mental illness. For acute, situational reactions, that is a different story. Ironically, VR tries to work mainly with the former because the latter aren't eligible since their disabilities are temporary. I don't know whether chronically ill clients really belong in VR, but VR becomes a "dumping ground" for welfare and mental health agencies to demonstrate that they've done *their* jobs! They've made referrals, and only VR can do what's needed next. VR has become the good shepherd of the government agencies in trying to save the lost souls no one else can do anything for. And so many mentally ill clients are scored as successes on the 30th day of a job, are back in the hospital again on the 35th day, and a VR client again on the 40th day—to be "successfully rehabilitated" time after time after time.

The methods used don't work. Electroshock is used as punishment, whether or not it's admitted or even conscious. Traditional psychotherapy doesn't work. I don't really think body work or the esoteric therapies could work either, given the amount of drugs the people are on. For awhile, I put everyone in a workshop just to give them someplace to go and see if they'd follow through on anything. When they didn't, whether they wouldn't or couldn't was always a question.

There are a few success stories, but most of them are found among acute situational reactions. These don't seem to be on the same continuum with chronic psychoses—they seem to be different varieties. Acutes bounce back. Chronics have nothing to bounce back from. The ones who succeed seem to have needed more *time* than the service system allows for. Sometimes a counselor will hear that a former client is about to get situated in a sheltered setting with the interpersonal support needed that might "work" and [the counselor will] quickly re-open the case to claim credit—but the system doesn't tolerate having them on a caseload for years with no training going on.

It is important to bear in mind that these observations reflect the viewpoints of PSV professionals whose primary concern is vocational rehabilitation—a complex and demanding goal. A recent volume (Talbot, 1980) chronicles an array of treatment programs that have achieved varying degrees of success in improving the general psychological functioning and independent living potential of chronically mentally ill people. However, widespread agreement exists that vocational rehabilitation success is undermined frequently by premature referral from mental-health agencies, where staff perceptions of success may be biased in an overly optimistic direction. When drugs or disease processes interfere with clients' abilities to function in evaluation, training, or work, individuals who appear improved when they exit the mental-health system may prove unsuccessful in a vocational rehabilitation context.

A relatively new phenomenon—employee assistance programs (EAPs) in private industry and government—offers limited psychological services to employees experiencing psychological problems that interfere with work productivity or on-the-job behavior. The major emphasis in these programs is substance abuse—mainly alcoholism—but employees undergoing acute psychological distress also may refer themselves or be referred by supervision. At the present time, the concept of EAPs is ahead of the practice. Many are staffed by recovered-alcoholic former managers who are comfortable working with alcoholics as peers but lack psychotherapeutic skills. A few EAPs secure contract psychotherapists, however, who can help such employees deal with acute reactions without having to leave their jobs.

Rehabilitation and Secondary Psychological Disability

In rehabilitation circles, it is not uncommon to hear such comments as, "His physical disability is less of a problem to him than his emotional reaction to it," or, "Her attitude is more handicapping than her blindness." These remarks illustrate the typical level at which psychological problems are seen to complicate rehabilitation, or personal adjustment and growth, following bodily disablement. More severely incapacitating instances occur, too. For some individuals, the stress of bodily disablement and its accompanying disruption of personal and familial homeostasis are sufficient to nullify coping efforts, at least temporarily. It generally is assumed that other stress of comparable magnitude would have similar effect; that is, it is not the disablement per se that leads to emotional breakdown, it is a degree of stress that exceeds the person's coping resources. In a sense, the secondary disability becomes primary. In many instances, an emotional disability of impaired stress tolerance may have preceded the physical disability, but it becomes apparent only after physical disablement.

Herbert Rigoni, who directed the psychological services program at Rancho Los Amigos Hospital for many years, expressed the view that, at one extreme, psychosis can be a reasonable coping strategy that should not be tampered with by rehabilitation professionals (personal communication). To illustrate this, he cited a woman so severely disabled by amyotrophic lateral sclerosis that she was unable to move, was barely able to speak, and spent all her time in a tank respirator. With death only days or weeks away, she falteringly recounted hallucinatory images of young people engaged in sexual activity in her hospital room. It is his opinion that this constituted meaningful, end-of-life psychological work for her, and that staff desires to "cure" her psychosis were misdirected and reflected their own discomfort with the sexual material.

When severe psychological disorders threaten to nullify physical rehabilitation efforts that otherwise might be fruitful, intervention is necessary; however, many factors militate against intervention happening, at least effectively. If the symptoms of psychological breakdown occur while the individual is undergoing intensive rehabilitation for the primary disability, it is unlikely that the facility will be staffed adequately to deal with disorders of a psychological nature. Concomitantly, transfer to a psychiatric hospital may be impossible because of that facility's inability to meet the needs associated with the person's primary disability. In practice, it often seems that the signs of psychological breakdown are only beginning to be recognized by rehabilitation staff when discharge to the community is imminent. At this point, extended stays, to take advantage of whatever psychological support services are available, are likely to be denied by third-party payers. The option of serving the person as an outpatient also is plagued by problems. A pyramiding effect exists, wherein all people who have ever been inpatients are potentially eligible for outpatient status; but virtually no hospitals are staffed to handle such caseloads in the psychological service area. Community mental health resources are typically inaccessible to people with bodily disabilities—socially, physically, or economically (American Psychological Association, 1980)—so there may be, *au fond*, no place to go.

The problems are compounded further by the reluctance of those needing service to admit to their needs. They collude, as it were, with agencies' failures to supply such services by rarely confronting the lack. This is partly due to fear of acknowledging two disabilities and partly a reluctance to forfeit secondary gain. Many psychological disorders, it must be recalled, are defense-oriented adaptive attempts that must "work" to some extent to be retained in the behavioral repertoire.

Despite the problems and the frankly low probability of getting psychotherapeutic help in a timely manner when one is otherwise disabled, exemplary services do exist. Most are oriented toward people in the rehabilitation stage of their primary disabilities. Some selected examples follow.

Rehabilitation Hospital Programs. Rigoni indicates (personal communication) that the most outstanding successes he has observed in treating serious psychological disorders in tandem with physical rehabilitation have involved patients with paranoid symptoms that could be addressed best by open confrontation during routine contacts. Regardless of the nature of the disturbance, however, he stresses the singular importance of interdisciplinary cooperation among all direct service providers in dealing with psychological problems during intensive rehabilitation: all must be involved in planning the approach, and all must be attuned to each phase of progress in order to provide assistive continuity.

Behavior-modification programs conducted in rehabilitation hospital settings have shown considerable promise. A uniquely successful one provided assertiveness training for behaviorally disturbed children. Explosively aggressive behavior in several youngsters was corrected effectively by teaching them appropriate techniques of self-assertion with care-givers, including skill training in articulating their requests precisely and understandably. As their frustration levels dropped, their aggressive behaviors became subdued. Although the ward staff was resistive initially ("Teach *those* kids to be *more* assertive?"), they came to appreciate the difference between assertiveness and aggressiveness, and were highly gratified by the results.

A different type of program used videotaped instant feedback in correcting ororverbalization in a group of brain-injured participants of a hospital-based vocational rehabilitation project. Several group members learned to monitor and curtail excessive talking well enough to succeed in job interviews after treatment, whereas countless previous efforts had failed. In general, a variety of behavior-modification techniques have proved successful in treating the psychological sequelae of brain injury. Token-economy programs for reducing distractibility, shaping appropriate work behavior, and improving productivity are notable examples.

Insured Rehabilitation. When rehabilitation costs are covered by worker's compensation or other insurance, the likelihood of getting help in dealing with psychological sequelae may be somewhat better than in other cases. When an attorney is involved, s/he generally will fight to ensure that the psychological as well as physical consequences of an illness or injury are recognized as compensable. This brings private-practice psychotherapists within financial reach. By contrast, when publicly supported services are the only ones accessible, often all that can be expected are symptom-ameliorating medications and perhaps minimal contact with ancillary personnel offering supportive counseling aimed only at maintaining present status. This reflects the positive side of what an advocate can do. The negative side is that people involved in litigation often are observed to develop psychological symptomatology that might not have come about in the absence of (1) potential monetary rewards for being as disabled as possible and (2) active encouragement by a respected legal professional to maximize symptoms. Some believe this reflects a guilt mechanism, with power to create actual sickness in the wake of illness that is feigned; others consider it a straightforward result of suggestion.

Substance-Abuse Services. A psychological disorder frequently found among people with bodily disabilities is alcoholism. Alcohol becomes a means for dulling what an individual sees as unpleasant realities, easing tensions that arise from the loss of more active "exhaust" mechanisms, fighting boredom, and escaping confrontation with other aspects of disability that have not been accepted. Although service availability falls far short of the need, the problems are beginning to draw planning attention in many communities, and numerous disability-related organizations are urging alcoholism-treatment resources to accept and work with otherwise disabled clients. Robert and Patricia Hadley, of California State University at Los Angeles, specialize in the study and treatment of alcohol problems associated with physical disability. They indicate (personal communication) that identification of individuals needing help is one of the most serious problems they confront. Patricia Hadley summarized the situation by saying,

> Statistics show that nearly ten percent of the workforce has alcohol problems—so we can assume that about one out of ten general-caseload rehabilitation clients does—yet their counselors are totally unaware of it unless alcoholism's the primary diagnosis. Counselors have no training in what to look for, so they make no effort to get these clients to services.

It is fairly common practice for work-oriented rehabilitation facilities to require clients with known drug and alcohol problems to obtain treatment for those conditions in order to be eligible for the facility's vocational services or job opportunities. Many expedite the referrals and keep abreast of progress, which creates a mutually reinforcing partnership between the vocational rehabilitation and psychotherapeutic efforts.

Mental-Health Services for Deaf People. Geno Vescovi, a deaf psychologist who specializes in psychotherapeutic services for deaf individuals, indicates that the issue of mental-health services for the deaf receives more explicit concern than is true of other specific disability groups because of the high frequency of illiteracy and resulting dependency found (personal communication). He stresses that there is no unusual or characteristic psychodynamic content to be dealt with in psychotherapy; rather, the unique aspects of treatment for a deaf clientele relate to communication. Very simply, if none is taking place, then there will be no therapy. He considers the situation little different from that in which the therapist speaks only English and the client speaks only Spanish or another foreign language. He stresses that the therapist must be able to communicate at the client's level of comprehension if diagnosis is to be valid and therapy effective. This may or may not call for using any formalized system of manual communication, since clients have different, sometimes fragmented, ways of expressing themselves. Moreover, they have widely divergent abilities to comprehend others—just as is true in the non-deaf population. Thus, therapists must be able to assess all individuals and follow their leads.

Vescovi further believes that to combat the two root causes of psychological problems among deaf individuals (illiteracy and dependency), a very close relationship between therapist and client is required. In addition, the therapist must be a teacher as well as a therapist. Therapy is needed to help clients increase their independence, but teaching also is needed to help them increase their literacy. He does not concur with the opinion of some that, ideally, deaf therapists should work with deaf clients. He believes anyone able to communicate well with the client can serve effectively. Gregory Kimberlin, a deaf psychologist who directs a mental-health program for the deaf at a community hospital, expresses agreement with this premise but suggests that communication of the subtle nuances of affective material may be most accurate when the therapist's primary language matches that of the client (Kimberlin, personal communication). Obviously, in a deaf clientele, this would exclude most therapists other than those who are deaf or who grew up with deaf parents.

Vescovi does not suggest the use of third-party interpreters as a reasonable alternative. This relates to the signal importance of the one-on-one relationship with deaf clients, due to the severe relationship deprivation deafness can cause. He spells out a stepwise process in which the therapist's ability to communicate at the client's level leads to greater client comfort in the relationship, leading in turn to a better rapport. He believes that, when all factors are in place, the relationship itself may be the major contributor to effective therapy.

Kimberlin, however, sees some justification for interpreters. He prefers to avoid using the term "illiteracy," pointing out that the problem is actually a limited grasp of English, and the person may be highly proficient in American Sign Language. He cites several key factors that influence the course of psychotherapeutic treatment with deaf and hearing-impaired persons: (1) the etiology and degree of loss, (2) the age of onset, (3) the mode of communication used and level of primary language development, (4) educational background, and (5) family dynamics. The last includes both psychodynamics and communication dynamics. Kimberlin stresses the importance of the therapist's understanding of the psychosocial implications of deafness. Given this, he supports the use of interpreters as a means of allowing treatment to take place until a therapist is capable of using signs.

Both psychologists indicate that the oft-mentioned conception of "deaf paranoia" (the notion that because deaf people cannot hear what others are saying they frequently come to believe themselves to be the topic of conversation) is a myth. Their observations are that the incidence of paranoid thinking is no higher among deaf people than in the nondeaf population.

The Role of Psychotherapy in Vocational Rehabilitation

Just as medical intervention, or physical restoration, is sometimes a critically needed element in a client's vocational rehabilitation plan, so, too, is psychological intervention or restoration. Accordingly, the laws and regulations governing the state VR programs allow for case-service funds to be expended on psychotherapeutic treatment for clients whose employability is predicted to be enhanced by it. Although the various states and territories differ in the extent to which they purchase psychotherapy for their clients, it seems fair to say that there is a general disinclination to commit a significant portion of case-service funds to this purpose.

The reasons given by agency administrators and counselors are essentially the same: it is a costly form of service and the responsibility for it should be borne by mental-health rather than vocational rehabilitation agencies. The fact that in the main it is *not* is treated as an unfortunate reality that is also up to the mental-health agencies to correct. It is pointed out further that most states are constrained to pay for psychotherapy at levels commensurate with their state's Medicaid allowances, and that excellent practitioners seldom can be procured for the sanctioned rates. Thus, the expected benefits of psychotherapy, if provided, are also called into question. Although many state agencies have psychologists and psychiatric consultants on their staffs, their expertise and/or job responsibilities often are limited to diagnostic functions.

As a consequence of these cost-related barriers, very little psychotherapy is provided, at least in comparison with the need expressed by direct service providers, state administrators, and federal officials. A high degree of consensus exists, at all of these levels, that untold numbers of rehabilitation plans are sabotaged yearly by the lack of appropriate attention to the psychological service needs of clients (Vash, 1977b). Some evidence for this widely held opinion exists. An unpublished review of cases closed in "Status 28" (client not rehabilitated into gainful employment), conducted jointly by the author and a state VR supervisor in 1973, showed that counselor errors in the psychological area occurred in sixteen out of the thirty-three cases reviewed. (The other error categories studied were vocational, relationship, and medical, with findings of twenty, nine, and three instances of error, respectively.) The nature of the errors in the psychological area included (1) failing to recognize the need for psychological services, (2) recognizing the need but failing to respond to it, (3) attempting to meet the need through own counseling efforts when greater expertise was required, and (4) referring the person for psychotherapy but failing to confer with the therapist at least once during or following treatment. The sixteen instances of error were distributed rather evenly over these four categories.

When many workers make similar errors, more than individual competencies must be examined. The system within which work is done tends to make the commission of errors more or less likely. System deterrents to correct handling of psychological service needs among vocational rehabilitation clients probably include low agency priorities for (1) using limited case-service funds for psychotherapy, (2) developing rosters of competent, affordable therapists in given communities, and (3) providing both pre- and in-service training for counselors in the psychological area. At the same time, high agency priorities for moving directly toward job placement with minimal attention to related issues (especially when construed as belonging in another agency's domain) may contribute equally to the kinds of oversights observed.

Ironically, agency pressures to produce a large volume of job placements encourage counselors to accept clients with what appear to be mild psychological disabilities, in the hope that they will be easier to place than clients with visible, severe, physical disabilities. However, if the needed psychotherapeutic services are not supplied, these clients may prove to be more difficult to place, not easier. Plan after plan may be discarded in favor of altered approaches that also will prove ultimately to be destined to failure. Related to this, psychologists who examine applicants for vocational rehabilitation services express the opinion that many "mentally disabled" clients who are successfully rehabilitated by state agencies—without benefit of psychotherapeutic intervention—are not, in fact, psychologically disabled. Rather, they have been tutored to exaggerate mood-state complaints that are within the normal range, and the examiners succumb to pressures from referring counselors to apply diagnostic labels rendering them eligible for services.

On the other hand, just as psychotherapy has a role in vocational rehabilitation, vocational rehabilitation often is seen by mental-health professionals as having a crucial role in psychotherapy. Unquestionably, this is true; however, as pointed out earlier by Sanchez (personal communication), labor shortages in mental-health agencies cause clients to be referred while their emotional conditions are not yet sufficiently stabilized, or drug dosages are so high that their abilities to function in evaluation, training, and work are impaired seriously. If the vocational rehabilitation and mental-health professionals worked jointly with their mutual clients, early entry into the vocational rehabilitation system might, indeed, have the intended therapeutic effect. It is seldom done, though, since a prime value of the referral, for the mental-health professional, is to open up a caseload vacancy for a person on a waiting list. Thus, the rehabilitation counselors must try to resolve, alone and in a service environment that is only tenuously appropriate, problems to which their training was never addressed.

Implications for Rehabilitation Counselors

The issues cited in the foregoing pages have far-reaching implications, some of which have been described, for rehabilitation counselors working with clients who have psychological disabilities. This section, the last of this chapter, will highlight four additional implications considered highly significant in avoiding frustration on the parts of counselors and in maximizing chances for success on the parts of clients.

Accepting Recidivism

When the primary disability is psychological, and especially when it is a chronic condition, a mind-set that accepts the reality of probable recidivism may be the most wholesome attitude for a counselor to take. The administrator responsible for services to mentally ill clients in a state VR agency observed a marked reduction in signs of burnout among her counselors after she began reassuring them actively that they had not failed when their clients became ill again, lost their jobs, and returned for further services. She stressed the success entailed for both clients and counselors when chronically mentally ill clients were able to stay on jobs, working responsibly, for as long as six months or a year. She further stressed that the counselors were not mental-health experts, and, given the state of the mental-health arts, they were doing the best they could. She indicated that, when the counselors stopped feeling like guilty failures, they welcomed returning clients and again did the best they could; whereas, before, they had rejected and attempted to avoid them. It is important to note that all of the PSV professionals who were queried on exemplary practices but expressed feelings of futility instead, worked in agencies that held a different working philosophy. Their agencies viewed chronically mentally ill clients no differently from stabilized physically disabled ones when they returned for more services: they were agency failures.

Avoiding Pushiness

Several of the professionals queried cited counselor overdirectiveness as a frequent saboteur of rehabilitation success with passive people, regardless of whether the passivity is tied to chronic mental illness, "disenfranchised" social status (common among ethnic minority clients), or other origins. Excessive directiveness in counseling is thought to reinforce a passive orientation of following orders while remaining uninvolved. Because of agency pressures, a "hurry up," directive stance often is assumed by counselors who may find later that an appearance of compliance masks an absence of useful learning. Thus, with clients who appear to be passive/compliant, it is important to avoid directiveness. Instead, use approaches that require their active involvement in decision making and follow-through.

Recognizing Danger Signals

The importance of noting that a client has a passive/compliant personality exemplifies a more general need to be aware of "red flags" that can warn alert counselors of danger ahead in the rehabilitation process. A casework evaluation team, armed with "magnifying retrospectoscopes," always can see evidence, right in the case files, of danger signals that the counselors who built the files somehow didn't see at the time. Recorded hints that a physically disabled client also had serious emotional problems and clues that more expert psychological help was needed stand out in clear relief once the outcome is known. It also is possible to *foresee* such negative outcome potentials if sufficient attention is paid to psychological data at the time counseling is taking place. Often, the demands of large caseloads tempt counselors to ignore the red flags that are there for them to see and respond to if they only will.

Setting Realistic Limits

After the problem or need has been noted, it is important for the counselor to appraise realistically his/her limits as a psychotherapist. After-the-fact case evaluations also reveal instances in which counselors attempt psychotherapeutic duty that exceeds their skill and knowledge levels. A frequent type of error might be encapsulated as "treating a psychotic or prepsychotic as if s/he were neurotic." What this means, in practice, is that "uncovering techniques" designed to bare unconscious material assumed to be neurotically repressed are used when, in fact, the individual already is being flooded with material from the unconscious and is being overwhelmed by it—a psychotic process. Similarly, techniques entailing high degrees of therapist self-revelation, especially feelings of positive regard for the client, may be used with clients who are terrified by interpersonal intimacy. Both errors are common among counselors trained in settings influenced by theoretical models designed for use with middle-class, privately paying, normal or mildly neurotic clienteles.

Obviously, these same issues also have significant implications for counselor educators and program administrators. In the next and final chapter of this book, a wide range of policy implications will be addressed in the context of looking forward—to the research, prevention strategies, training, service programs, and other changes needed to ameliorate the experiential problems described in the foregoing chapters and to make the best use of available intervention resources.

14 Looking Ahead

Considerations for the Future

The previous chapters of this volume have attempted to describe today's realities—sometimes contrasted with those of the past—surrounding the psychological experience of disability, plus the intervention techniques used to resolve some of the problems. This chapter will look to the future and discuss events, trends, and changes that seem necessary or desirable for reducing unproductive psychological suffering and improving the quality of life for people with disabilities.

Five basic areas will be considered. The first is research. In order to achieve needed changes, the knowledge base must be extended into areas not currently understood well. The second is professional training. Once the knowledge is available, it must be used in training the experts who provide services to people with disabilities. The third is public education. Not only the professionals, but the public as well—especially those experiencing disability directly—must have access to both old and new information that can help them deal effectively with the problems they confront. The fourth is environmental change. Once armed with the needed knowledge and skills, all concerned can bring about more effectively changes that are needed in the physical, sociopolitical, and other aspects of the world without. The fifth is "the work within." The external world simply cannot be improved enough to solve *all* of the problems associated with disability; thus, each affected individual has inner work to do to resolve the dissonance, disappointment, and pain that issue from losses of functionality.

The author does not pretend to offer an exhaustive view of what the future should bring; rather, selected issues—which appear to have had less attention elsewhere in the literature than they deserve—will be discussed, in the hope of elevating future concern for their importance.

242

Research

Four different research varieties need to be considered: basic, applied-demonstration, applied-development, and market analysis. Since these and similar terms are used with varying shades of meaning, their usages here will be clarified.

Basic Research

This implies controlled *hypothesis testing* for the purpose of establishing lawful relationships among independent and dependent variables. Moreover, although ultimate utility of discovered knowledge is assumed, specific applications of it are not included in the research design, and immediacy of applicability is not deemed essential to the worthiness of the research pursuit.

A great deal of the basic research conducted into the psychological aspects of disability has focused on identifying personality correlates to specific types of disablement. This approach is viewed by some as an important avenue toward prevention and by others as a vacuous waste of time. To the extent that findings of such studies actually can be used, someday, to aid prevention of disability and/or secondary emotional complications following disablement, their importance is undeniable.

Three lines of investigation seem particularly promising in this regard. The first is the study of stress-induced disabling conditions, undertaken to improve understanding of the relationships among environmental stressors, individuals' perceptions of and responses to stress, and the development of stress-related illnesses with disabling residuals.

The second is the study of the relationships between attitudes and disablement. Kemp (1976) cites four examples of ways in which attitudinal predispositions can increase the likelihood of disablement: (a) high risk-taking attitudes and impulsiveness can lead to traumatic injuries; (b) reluctance to express feelings or poor communication abilities can lead to muscle tension resulting in disabling pain conditions; (c) an attitudinal predisposition toward "conspicuous consumption" appears to have led to increased injury rates among children of blue-collar workers who purchase overpowered toys in their quests to secure prestigious material goods; and (d) the attitudinal constellation of time urgency, competitiveness, ambition, and energetic activeness seems to be a precursor to cardiovascular disease.

The third line of investigation is the study of learning-mediated disability development. Kemp (1976) illustrates how the development of disease with disabling residuals can be mediated by the learning process, as when hypochondriacal behavior, seizure activity, or pain are reinforced inadvertently.

Buck & Hohmann (in press) report on a fairly extensive clinical literature detailing imagined pitfalls and problems ahead for disabled people who are or choose to become parents—and the virtual absence of research documentation for the opinions expressed. Clearly, this is an area that has come to light as needing extensive study in order to learn what the real relationships are and are not. Readers undoubtedly can cite many additional areas in which they are aware of discrepancies between the clinical folklore and the facts they have experienced, discrepancies that also call for carefully controlled investigation.

Applied-Demonstration Research

While there is significant need for basic research in the future, of the four research varieties mentioned, the need for applied-demonstration projects may be the greatest. Demonstrations do not test hypotheses, they attempt to *demonstrate the validity of assumptions*. That is, rather than start with an open-minded question as to whether an hypothesis can be ruled out, or which of alternative hypotheses might receive more confirming evidence, demonstrations begin with assumptions that certain intervention approaches will result in greater benefit to subjects (for example, clients, patients, students, recipients) than alternative approaches or the absence of intervention. More simply stated, demonstrations assume certain techniques will *work* and that the projects will provide convincing evidence of this to others.

Two cautions are in order regarding future demonstration projects. The first has to do with replicability in the absence of special project funding. In the past, many demonstrations have involved enriched funding levels that few, if any, service agencies could hope to continue—however effective a demonstration proves to be—after grant funding ends. An example from the author's own experience will suffice (Vash & Murray, 1969). A project that successfully moved into employment forty-five percent of a large group of hard-core unemployed ghetto residents with severe disabilities proved, in retrospect, only that it can be done *if* the clients can be paid a $45-per-week stipend for participating, be given the opportunity to earn up to minimum wage for part- or full-time employment in a training workshop, and be permitted to retain their full Aid to the Totally Disabled benefits despite these other sources of income. Project staff concluded that many of the clients became "addicted" to having ample money to spend and were willing to do whatever they had to do, including finding and keeping jobs, in order to satisfy their "habits." When the grant funding and special provisions ended, the success of the remaining program elements was not comparable. This situation can be summarized succinctly: it doesn't help to know what works if you can't afford to do it. True, the information concerning the relationship between income experience and job placement success is important information that still could be put to use, but both funding and funded agencies must attend to replicability under ordinary conditions when the goal of a demonstration is to develop workable service methodologies.

The second point of caution relates to making it easier for publicly-supported VR agencies to use portions of their base program budgets to conduct small-scale tests of new psychological service techniques—or, indeed, any other new techniques or procedures—before attempting to implement them agency-wide. Currently, government regulations prohibiting agencies from offering unique services to special groups that aren't available to all constituents are used by control agencies to deter service agencies from doing such needed testing in microcosm. The inordinate length of time required to secure grant funds exempted from such strictures has the effect of quashing staff motivation and sterilizing projects that begin long after the timing was right in terms of an agency's optimal operation. This policy problem needs attention and correction if the business-as-usual syndrome is to be avoided and the state of the service arts is to advance.

Program evaluation is a common form of demonstration research. Although, on the surface, it might seem to reflect an open-minded question ("Is it working?") rather than an assertion ("I believe it will work and I'll show you."), the fact is, agencies don't establish programs not expected to work. Thus, in practice, "demonstration projects" can be seen as services receiving especially thorough program evaluation, and "program evaluation" can be seen as ongoing demonstration research.

Unfortunately, too much program evaluation consists of little more than statistical reporting of services rendered and outcomes achieved, without efforts to assess relationships. This is a wasteful practice because the ongoing client-service activities within agencies of all types and sizes offer rich opportunities for studying cause (services rendered) and effect (client outcomes) relationships—what works and what doesn't—but these "laboratories" typically remain unused. A major reason is that service providers seldom are requested and rarely are trained to do manageable, day-by-day documentation of client behaviors that could be studied later when research questions arose. Regular recording of key observations on behavior change is a simple, nonthreatening example of potentially useful data for subsequent study. Going a step further (somewhat threatening but still simple), records on service providers' feelings toward clients and their jobs, studied against elsewhere-documented organizational events, could yield potentially invaluable information about interactions among agency policies, worker morale, and the rehabilitation progress of clients. Myriads of other examples could be given to show how easily recorded observations—which have side benefits of helping service providers maintain high levels of awareness regarding client relationships and professional decision making—could enhance the growth of the PSV professions. Still, however limited the recording task might be, service providers generally feel so beleaguered by paperwork demands that the prospect of additional recording is greeted with jeers whenever it is proposed. At the same time, if the useless redundancy in most agency records were eliminated, providers could save more than enough time to do documenting that might lead to significant state-of-the-art advancement through ongoing clinical research.

Applied-Development Research and Market Analysis

To some extent, the research areas labeled "applied-development" and "market analysis" must be discussed together. Development here relates to technological applications, such as rehabilitation engineering and the construction and refinement of evaluation instruments/systems and service models. The author's favorable view toward utilizing modern technology on behalf of people with disabilities has been made clear in earlier chapters. No end is foreseen yet to the quality-of-life-enhancing possibilities offered. Nonetheless, while many useful products have resulted from the generous federal funding for rehabilitation engineering that recent years have seen, some of these funds, and untold private funds, have been wasted because projects were not based on sound market research—which in this case means assessing the needs of potential disabled product users. Too often, engineering experts start with intriguing (to them) bits of new technology and try to imagine rehabilitation-related uses that might be made. Working in this backward fashion generally fails, and exquisite solutions to nonproblems have been the expensive result. If the needed market research is done, such projects will start with known priorities of actual product consumers, not vain imaginings of what the theoretical "average disabled person" would like. Development of service models also requires market research. If the known needs and wants of PSV service consumers had been used to guide the development of rehabilitation services many years ago, we probably now would see job clubs in every community and the need for sheltered workshops much reduced. We also might be less preoccupied with avoiding "duplications of services," since involved consumers tend to see nonduplication as monopolistic and regressive, and we might be more concerned about the service gaps. The general populace wants a choice between, say, car manufacturers or physicians. The disabled person needing services usually will have only one resource to turn to, and no alternatives if service is unsatisfactory. The best the consumers can hope for is that the providers in the sole service agency will be well trained and genuinely desirous of helping them.

Professional Training of PSV Experts

Training is construed here in a very broad sense, encompassing the many avenues by which information—old or new—comes to be utilized in service agencies. Similarly, PSV experts include not only peer and professional service providers, but also agency administrators and public policy makers, who influence the nature and quality of service programs. Changes in agency policies, programs, procedures, services, and techniques all come about through the efforts of people who have absorbed information—through formal training or informal educational channels—that they believe merits utilization. Thus, organizational improvements, like direct service advancements, occur as a result of informational inputs to PSV experts. The remainder of this section will be devoted to a sampling of selected issues that might be included profitably in formal training or self-prescribed continuing education with a view toward eventual incorporation into agency operations.

Breaking the Ice at State VR Agencies

Having visited VR agency offices in numerous states, the author always has been struck by the quiet, the scarcity of clients seen on the premises, and the lack of interaction among clients in waiting rooms or between clients and staff persons other than the assigned counselors. The ambience seems so unlike what is found in most rehabilitation centers visited, where hordes of interacting staff and clients make considerable noise. Perhaps the author's strongest wish for the future is to see VR agency offices look less like decorous rows of frequently empty cubicles and more like the bustling rehabilitation centers where clients help each other as well as receive help from staff. For this to happen, staff will need to alter their perceptions of client needs and their expectations about how helpful agencies function.

The advent of job clubs in VR agencies has begun, in a few locations, to break the ice. It seems that when half a dozen counselors and half a dozen clients roll up their sleeves and work together, in a room filled with desks and telephones, to get job leads and interview dates for all of the clients, the camaraderie and interactive styles developed spill over into the waiting room and the rest of the office. It looks like a place where human beings give and get help; it comes to life.

This wholesome trend could be extended. The VR office could be a place for clients to come when they want to be part of a rap group or hear a speaker on independent living or seek counseling to counteract despair. Once the process of loosening up begins in the bureaucracy, perhaps weekend or evening hours—for postemployment counseling—could become common occurrences instead of rare exceptions. Top management might even allow middle managers who are so inclined to institute such changes, without being distressed by the fact that other of their offices are operated differently. The demand for uniformity among all offices of multilocation agencies may be the deadliest blow of all to innovation, fresh ideas, creative experimentation, and, therefore, state-of-the-art advancement in the PSV services.

Overuse of Client Evaluation

This comparison between VR offices and rehabilitation centers is not meant to imply that the latter have, generally, more effectively solved the problems of delivering quality PSV services on time to their clients. The hospitals and other facilities have their share of shortcomings to correct, too. The most notable one, to the author, is the apparent imbalance between the amount of time and effort directed toward client evaluation, as compared with that invested in psychosocial treatment services for clients. The perceived genesis of this imbalance was described in detail in Chapter 10 and need not be reiterated. Suffice it to say here that a serious effort to correct the situation seems a worthy goal for the future.

People with Disabilities

Both types of agencies appear to ignore, or at least underestimate, the need for counseling of family members as well as the disabled individuals who are their identified clients. This issue also was discussed earlier, in Chapter 4. What remains to be pointed out with respect to future correction is that, in many cases, serious bureaucratic disincentives exist to dissuade counselors from working with families, even when the needs are patently manifest and recognized. Pressure for high quantities of "employed" case closures, without counterbalancing pressure or credit given for high quality of either casework or outcomes, inhibits workers' willingness to expend the additional time required to work with families. Failure to do so may lead to clients' losing their employment after agency credit for attaining it has been taken, but no penalties exist for this either, for agencies or individual workers. Even when such explicit production demands do not exist, the pressures of large case-loads in almost every type of setting serve similarly to inhibit work with families. Clearly, sufficient information is available now to support the necessity for making policy changes that will reduce these disincentives and facilitate increased attention to the service needs of the entire family experiencing disability.

Early Intervention in Industrial Injuries

Family counseling is a mechanism for preventing secondary emotional disabilities among clients and their loved ones. Another is early intervention, as described by Akabas et al. (1980) in cases of industrial injuries. These authors point out that VR agencies flexible enough to accept injured workers for services *before* they have stabilized can avert, for the government, lengthy, costly periods of benefit payments and can prevent, for the client, the emotional complications accompanying loss and uncertainty after employment ties have been severed. Along similar lines, an iconoclastic but interesting and successful effort to avoid reinforcing injured workers' beliefs that they were "totally and permanently disabled" was developed by a creative workshop counselor doing eligibility evaluations on disability insurance applicants. After a year of inviting all such clients to return for vocational rehabilitation services when they felt strong enough to consider returning to work, and having none do so, he began to add twenty minutes of "Dutch Uncle counseling" to the exit interviews. His way of describing the content was this:

> I essentially told them to be psychopathic if they had to, but not to get neurotic about it. In other words, if they needed to take whatever money they could get from the system so they could have a little breather from work and responsibility, I said, "Fine, go ahead; but don't get to feeling so guilty about 'ripping off' that, in order to justify it, you convince yourself that you really *are* permanently and totally disabled. If you feel you need some paid time off badly enough to go through this miserable process, then you probably do. But that doesn't mean you'll never feel like getting back to it again . . . and when you do, come and see me." And guess what? They started coming back . . . three months later, six, a year . . . seven or eight of them within a year.

Perhaps Dutch Uncle counseling should be added to the PSV professionals' training curricula.

A New Approach to Medical Aspects Training

A serious concern relating to the formal training of PSV professionals is that of preservice coursework and inservice training on the medical aspects of disability. Although PSV professionals clearly need to be familiar with principles, issues, and, perhaps, the most commonly confronted facts, there seems to have been, in certain quarters, an overemphasis in this area. Continuing-education programs find "medical aspects" courses among their most popular offerings, and they tend to repeat what is most appreciated. Because of the unavoidable "shotgun" nature of the content coverage, however, the benefits to students appear to be greater in terms of their personal interests and prestige—since knowing about medical matters carries social status—than their on-the-job decision making. Charges of PSV professionals playing "junior physician" sometimes are heard.

Without a doubt, one basic course in the medical aspects of rehabilitation is needed to alert students to the potential psychosocial and vocational implications of their clients' health and disability status. Such a course should prepare the students to know what questions to ask, but it need not give them prepackaged answers, as this may tempt PSV practitioners to *inform* clients about their medical conditions rather than *teach* them the techniques they need in order to obtain medical information for themselves. The latter seems a more appropriate and valuable function for a PSV professional. If a counselor needs to know the information, the client needs to know it even more. The author envisions the following scenario reflecting a wholesome state of affairs: the counselor asks the client to seek and supply the needed information, demonstrating from the onset the client's role of responsibility in the rehabilitation process. If the client is questionably capable of doing so accurately, the counselor can "cover" by obtaining the information independently, providing a check as to the client's ability. In this way, on a case-by-case basis, the counselor adds to his/her store of transferrable information and, at the same time, makes each client responsible for his/her own. When a client fails to extract the needed information from a taciturn physician, the counselor can demonstrate effective interviewing techniques by telephone or, if time permits, in a joint visit to the physician's office. This approach exploits the PSV professional's primary area of competency as an expert in interpersonal relations and is preferable to relying on a secondary knowledge area. It also helps to give the client a skill s/he can make use of for a lifetime, and it uses the "teaching case" method of learning for the counselor—which is infinitely more effective than the classroom lecture method.

Professionalism

To date, the concept of "professionalism" has been a mixed blessing; at times it has encouraged practitioners to follow high standards of performance and ethics, and at other times it has been used to justify refusal to perform needed work that seems, somehow, beneath one's station. In addition, while registration, certification, and licensure are the official hallmarks of professionalism, their intended aim is to protect the public from harm. In practice, however, it too often seems that it's the professionals' turf that is really being protected. It is to be hoped that these negative outgrowths of a worthy concept will be reduced among future generations of practitioners.

The first problem, the "we don't do windows" syndrome, can be corrected only within the field, through alterations of practitioners' attitudes. If lesser-paid clerks, hospital attendants, employment officers, or others can do a task competently and are available to do it, then it is only sensible for more highly paid professionals to preserve their time for plying their special skills. However, it is often the case that if the PSV professional doesn't do it, no one will. When this is true, the author believes the helping professionals' credo should be, "You do whatever needs to be done to help the client." Illustrations from the author's experience of true helping professionals include a speech pathologist who took turns with family members doing continuous cuddling of a semicomatose brain-injured girl because hospital attendant staff were too busy caring for other patients, and a vocational counselor who caught up on his report writing while babysitting for a job-hunting client. The brain-injured girl's degree of recovery astounded hospital staff because it so far surpassed expectation, given the extent of damage. The job-hunting client, a paraplegic ghetto resident with no prior work history outside of a training workshop, got a job as a lead man in the electronics industry. The high degree of caring evidenced by professionals who would do "whatever was needed" was surely a factor in both success stories.

The second problem may need to be resolved through improved consumer education so that the public will not be unduly restricted in its range of sound choices by professional turf guarding. The mechanism by which this must happen is improved education of legislators and other government policy setters so that licensing will function more purely to safeguard the public from harm. In practice, this will necessitate closer attention to (1) a broader range of alternative academic and experiential patterns that may be equally qualifying and (2) more rigorous standards of licensible competency levels in a number of fields.

Public Education

Additional future thrusts with respect to public education will be needed. Many devolve upon helping the general populace to understand that the advent of disability does not harbinger a cataclysmic change in the affected individual's humanity. This is necessary for the purpose of reducing obstacles placed in the way of disabled people by a general public that views them as somehow less than human, exempt from usual considerations, or discrete from the mainstream. It is also necessary as psychological preparation for the high number of nondisabled members of the general public who will, within their lifetimes, also become disabled.

The mass media have begun to report on events associated with disabled people's efforts to attain their civil and human rights; they also have devised feature stories about the experiences of disabled people. What is missing still is the ordinary portrayal of people, who just happen to have disabilities, going about the business of ordinary living in very nearly ordinary ways. Only this will interrupt the stereotypic images of disabled people as chronically caught up in disability concerns, either tragically or heroically, and seldom having the time or ability to live life pretty much like everyone else. To illustrate, disabled people are seen rarely in bit parts or crowd scenes in fictional film and television presentations; moreover, when a disabled individual is depicted in a key role, the disability is virtually always a foreground matter, rather than the background concern it is in real life. Judging from the TV commercials watched by the average citizen for more than an hour every day, disabled people don't brush their teeth, fry chicken, wear perfume, eat pudding, or wax floors. The combined messages from TV programming and advertising suggest they are too busy being abjectly miserable or heart-wrenchingly courageous. This is not helping to break down stereotypes that result in highly destructive us–them distinctions. A few disabled people, like a few nondisabled people, may be courageous, but the matter of dealing with their disabilities and handicaps more likely reflects a very ordinary instinct for survival.

Needed in the future are more images of disabled people as "plain folks," without overdramatized attention to a single aspect of their lives, disability, which creates dissociating reactions in viewers or readers whether the differentness is portrayed as pathetic or heroic.

It is important for those of us in rehabilitation to acknowledge that we have contributed to this state of affairs. Two phenomena have probably done as much to set people with disabilities apart, in the minds of the public, as anything that can be attributed to faulty attitudes among mass-media decision makers. These are (1) fund raising for charitably supported rehabilitation efforts and (2) the infamous "Hire the Handicapped" slogan. The first will not be dealt with easily. When fund raisers have attemped to respond to disabled activists' demands that they be portrayed more realistically and positively in fund-raising campaigns, contributions have plummeted. The director of one affected agency reports receiving "hate" mail after a telethon that was widely acclaimed by the disabled community as a superb model. One writer asked, "Why should I send my money so *they* can play basketball and tennis when *I* can't afford to play tennis?" Clearly, if the funding base of a large number of organizations that are providing valuable services is to survive, the pathos cannot be extracted from the fund-raising campaigns. Activists are still trying to decide whether they would prefer to let these organizations go or continue to suffer the social damage done by their admittedly necessary methods of securing funds, hoping instead to counteract it through other messages to the public. The matter may resolve itself. As disabled people become an increasingly powerful political force, and their demands for equity cost more and more public dollars, the sympathy base of charitable fund raising for them may be progressively eroded.

The second matter, the plea to businesspeople's social consciences to "Hire the Handicapped—It's Good Business," could be dealt with more swiftly. This outmoded rhetoric could simply be put away and replaced with the more pertinent message of today—"Don't Discriminate against Workers with Disabilities—It's Illegal." That makes sense. It does not make sense, nor is it good business, for an employer to hire someone who is handicapped, implicitly, at performing the job in question. It is quite reasonable, however, to hire someone who is qualified despite a disability that is demonstrably nonhandicapping—either from the outset or after reasonable accommodation. The message, in the future, should stress "workers" rather than "the handicapped" and should not carry within it such blatantly contradicting terms. A few efforts in local areas to invent something better have done worse, in the author's opinion. Cute catch phrases, such as those playing on the "able" within the word "disabled," have the effect of infantilizing the individuals designated. In the future, it probably would be very wholesome to say directly what the issue is: nondiscriminatory employment of workers with disabilities.

Environmental Change

The elimination of discriminatory hiring practices constitutes a good example of the many environmental changes to be hoped for in the future. The "environment" is construed here as encompassing everything outside of the individual: the physical world, the sociopolitical milieu, service and product resources, and other salient elements. Given so vast a range to consider, only a few, additional, high-priority hopes for the future can be mentioned here. Among the highest is greater mainstreaming of the political influence of disabled people. While representation on rehabilitation-related advisory committees, oversight commissions, and policy boards is fairly good, it is still rare to find disabled individuals on such general-interest bodies as health-planning boards, transportation and energy commissions, and committees on the status of women. Until disabled people are involved in this way, their inputs will be absent from the mainstream of citizen concerns, and disabled individuals will see disability as their only realm of expertise and responsibility. This is not a sound basis for developing one's total personality or citizenship.

Even fewer disabled individuals can be found in elective offices. The rare activist who shows interest in running for office is likely to be seen as too parochial in perspective and limited in scope of interests to represent *all* of the people in a given locality. Whether or not this is true, few gather sufficient support to launch campaigns. For the future, a recent, positive event was the establishment of the League of Disabled Voters based in Washington, D.C. This organization promises to provide a forum in which people with disabilities can combine their efforts and amplify their influence over a greatly extended range of political decisions, not solely those relating specifically to disability. In addition, its existence can be expected to aid in the development of disabled candidates to run for public office.

At the time of this writing, numerous observers are expressing the opinion that the Education for All Handicapped Act and implementation of regulations for Section 504 of the Rehabilitation Act may have attempted to do too much too fast. Backlash has become fairly strong, in the forms of defiant noncompliance and concerted efforts by economically affected groups to weaken the demands on them to make their offerings to the public accessible to people with disabilities. Social integration is no less important for disabled people than for people belonging to ethnic minorities, but it is considerably more costly when building modifications, unique instructional procedures, or "reasonable accommodations" must be made. Some assert strongly that demands for building accessibility should be limited to new construction, and that the equal education of the most severely disabled individuals is too costly to be justified. Also, there is little consensus on the kinds and extent of accommodations that can be considered "reasonable." The future may shed light on whether a more cautious gradualism might have yielded faster progress in the long run, or whether today's doubters should try harder to adapt to pressured change.

The Work Within

Adapting to inevitable, relentless changes may be the essence of the inner work that people affected by disabilities are called on to do. Part of this adaptation has been encapsulated by Ken Keyes (1975) as recognizing that, while you don't always get what you *want* in life, you always get what you *need*. Keyes, a nationally-known spiritual leader and teacher, illustrates the principle personally when he professes the belief that the experience of permanent quadriplegia was one that he needed in order to foster his own spiritual development, although at the beginning it was by no means a wanted or welcomed turn of events (Keyes, personal communication). Once one observes the serenity and happiness that he appears to both possess and radiate to those around him, doubts as to whether this might be a case of "sweet lemon rationalization" melt away. Keyes' perspective, like that of Maslow and Mittelman (1951) and generations of Far Eastern mystics before them, is that the ultimate human needs relate to the spirit, not to bodies or their materialistic acquisitions. This is no longer an isolated or eccentric point of view. An increasing number of other individuals who have been touched by the disability experience are beginning to demonstrate and share comparable attitudes.

Carolyn Strite, a rehabilitation counselor–administrator who developed multiple sclerosis early in her career, prepared an open letter to send to the many inquirers who sought helpful advice from her following the publication of a newspaper story citing her as a person who had learned to live by almost dying. In it, she says,

> In a way, I may have "virtually licked" multiple sclerosis, yet medically and diagnostically, I have M.S.
> The questions have all been centered on "What have you done to get rid of it?"

or "What can you prescribe for others to feel better and less depressed?" Unfortunately (or fortunately, depending upon how you view life's challenges) I have no secret cure or wonderfully helpful steps to health to pass on. What I can do is simply tell you about my experience, my growing awareness, my continual efforts to become more balanced and centered in living. My life, personality, disease, and coping behavior are as truly unique, individual, and personal as each person's. Hopefully, there is some room for sharing and generalization of what we each learn from our life experiences!

My M.S. exacerbations and symptom elevations are something I live with daily. I am currently mostly symptom free from an observer's perception. However, I think I have become more and more acutely attuned to my body's subtle messages to me to take notice of the fact that there is "something out of balance" at times when I feel symptoms. I can only say that it is a little like an alarm clock going off to warn me that I am not attending to all that is important. If I shrug the warning aside, the alarm gets louder or the symptom becomes more apparent and stressful. The message is in learning to listen to my body language and, often, even dream language.

Just as brief background, I have had growing M.S. difficulties since 1963 during my first and only pregnancy. From that time until 1971, I had numbness of extremities, total body numbness, loss of vision, loss of sensation and function in both legs, disequilibrium, staggering gait, loss of bowel and bladder control, and slurred speech. I mention this to tell you of my body's messages. I went through the first few years scared, angry, depressed, resentful, in denial, until I became acutely depressed and actively suicidal. I very carefully studied and planned how I could "go to sleep and not have to awaken to the constant fear and more personal losses."

When my symptoms were at their worst, and I was diagnosed, my life literally collapsed about me. My husband left; my son was placed with another family; I lost my home (could not make the payments); my job retention was in question; my body did not seem to be my own anymore. My previous outlets for anxiety, frustration, and anger had been tennis, running, and bicycling. Those were out of the question at that time. Yet, when I attempted to write one last note to my exceptionally caring boss to explain why I had chosen this way out of my pain, I could not do it.

Instead I found myself reliving and reviewing my whole life, and I was amazed to discover that *I* cared about me. I realized that my boss had faith that I would come to grips with the trauma; he repeatedly refused to discuss my resignation, asking that I "talk about it (with him) next week," then the next week, then the next. During the hours of that "suicide weekend," I found out that who I am is inside me. I made a pledge to my inner self that I would find a means of continuing to express what I had to give, regardless of my changes. These extreme changes gradually became exciting challenges to me, full of endless struggles AND tremendous rewards and satisfaction.

As I continually learn to question and test my daily abilities and limitations, I find that my reality, my wellness, my happiness is of my own making. I can literally make myself sick, depressed, nonfunctional, by my attitude and outlook. Conversely, the same thing works in the positive direction. What works for me is to remember, rediscover, remind myself, that it is QUALITY of life, not QUANTITY of life's gifts that truly count. When I have pushed myself beyond my limits for that moment, I may have to restructure everything for awhile, and I am forced to find a creative way to handle simple tasks. Sit down for a whole day or weekend, write letters or reports instead of walking, driving, or working; simply find another way to stay actively involved in the world with people. That has made a huge impact on my progress and growth, physically, mentally, and spiritually. I get worse in all aspects when I close myself off, hole up, give up, quit trying to find new ways to BALANCE my life activities, energies, gifts. This is a difficult undertaking to express without sounding simplistic and overly general. If I make it sound obvious and easy, it is not. It takes constant attention, continual refinement or "listening inward/upward," and a growing trust in intuitive/all-knowing/en-lightened/brave SELF.

Through working with M.S. (mine and others'), I have been led to many marvelous "teachers," wonderfully helpful books, helpful and growth producing holistic health seminars, lectures, classes. My work in rehabilitation is a daily validation that I learn as much, if not more, from my clients as they from me. And that each person must discover his own path to understanding and acceptance of illness, limitation, and loss. I can share what helps me, what I have learned from others that has made a difference, and we can search together and learn from each other. But there is no one solution or cure for anything, not even life—the most terminal of all conditions. I guess that to me the most essential element lies within us, the will to keep searching and discovering and growing. Sometimes that bright spark gets clouded over or ignored, but eventually it can be re-uncovered. Some-times it takes asking or going for help. Sometimes I find that I have had to surrender all that I want to make happen or keep the same in order to find something better than I could have imagined. [Strite, 1980]*

Not only those who experience disability directly reach such levels of affirmation of *all* their life experiences; the loved ones of disabled individuals may find their forms of loss serve comparably. A remarkable illustration was shared with the author, following an address touching on these subjects, by a member of the audience. A young woman related that after her brother, Mark, was discovered to have serious intellectual limitations, her entire family underwent a lifestyle transformation. Her father was a nuclear physi-cist in the defense industry; her mother worked as a homemaker. They had not been a particularly happy family. Her father was at once absorbed and bothered by the nature of his work; her mother felt neglected and unfulfilled. The upward spiral of consciousness development stimulated by her brother's diagnosis eventuated in a totally new way of life. Her mother became a special-education teacher and her father left his job, saying he no longer could contribute to war endeavors that create disability. He took a position as custodian at the school where her mother teaches and her brother attends class. She says,

*Reproduced by permission of the author.

Mark is the most loving child any family ever had. Because of him, we see beauty everywhere. And we don't do what we don't believe in just because it has "status." My folks work together at the school; it just doesn't matter that one is a teacher and the other is the janitor. We are happy at home in a way that, before Mark, none of us ever imagined was possible. Some people think my Dad is weird for giving up a big job to work as a janitor. *We* think it was pretty weird for him to devote his life to blowing things up.

In cases such as these, one could speak of "transcending transcendence." To "transcend" denotes rising above an experience—which, in a sense, implies that perhaps elements of it are best left behind. The individuals just described have taken a further step. They have retained and *transformed* their catastrophic experiences into positive features in their lives. By sharing as much as they can of the processes and outcomes with others, they offer, not roadmaps, but topographical maps of a new psychological territory that could be inhabited by anyone who would venture to go there. It appears to be a clean environment for both disabled people and the rehabilitation professionals who serve them. Perhaps the future will see more of us migrating there.

References

Akabas, Sheila, et al., 1980. Preventive Rehabilitation: Untapped Horizon for VR Agencies. *American Rehabilitation,* 5:2.

American Psychiatric Association, 1980. *Diagnostic and Statistical Manual.* Third edition. Washington, DC:Author.

American Psychological Association, 1980. Mental Health Services for Handicapped Fall between Agencies. *APA Monitor,* 2:4.

Bach, George, & Deutsch, Ronald, 1970. *Pairing.* New York, NY: Peter H. Wyden.

Beisser, Arnold, 1979. Denial and Affirmation in Illness and Health. *American Journal of Psychiatry,* 136:8.

Buck, Frances, & Hohmann, George, in press. Parental Disability and Children's Adjustment. In Pan et al., eds., *Annual Review of Rehabilitation.* Volume 3. New York, NY: Springer.

Connell, Caroline, & Berkowitz, Howard, 1976. Rehabilitation for the Disabled Family in Stress. Research proposal prepared for the California State Department of Rehabilitation at Los Angeles, CA.

Corn, Roger, 1978. Aiding Adjustment to Physical Limitation: Training Manual. Prepared for Howard Community College at Columbia, MD.

Cousins, Norman, 1979. *Anatomy of an Illness.* New York, NY: Norton.

Crumbaugh, James, 1977. The Seeking of Noetic Goals Test (SONG): A Complementary Scale to the Purpose in Life Test (PIL). *Journal of Clinical Psychology,* 55:3.

Darrell McDaniel Independent Living Center, 1980. Dance Mystique at 1980 CAPH Convention. *Hub,* 4:6.

Frankl, Viktor, 1970. *The Will to Meaning: Foundations and Applications of Logotherapy.* New York, NY: Plume Books.

Fromm, Erich, 1956. *The Art of Loving.* New York, NY: Harper & Row.

Goffman, Erving, 1961. *Asylums.* Hawthorne, NY: Aldine.

Hall, Calvin, & Lindzey, Gardner, 1957. *Theories of Personality.* New York, NY: John Wiley.

Harris, Thomas, 1967. *I'm OK, You're OK.* New York, NY: Harper & Row.

Hayman, Barbara, 1975. Man in Search of Meaning. Term paper prepared for United States International University at San Diego, CA.

Henderson, David, 1979. Therapeutic Recreation Center. *American Rehabilitation*, 5:1.

Institute for Information Studies, 1980. *A Guide to Financial Resources for Disabled Individuals*. Falls Church, VA:Author.

Institute for Information Studies, 1980. *Rehabilitation Engineering Sourcebook*. Falls Church, VA: Author.

Jung, Carl, 1929. The Problems of Modern Psychotherapy. In Read et al., eds., *The Collected Works of C. G. Jung*. Volume 16, 1966. Princeton, NJ: Princeton University Press.

Kemp, Bryan, 1973. Client Perceptions of Production Staff Attitudes in a Rehabilitation Workshop. Research report prepared for Rancho Los Amigos Hospital at Downey, CA.

Kemp, Bryan, 1976. Psychological Aspects of Disease, Disability, and Rehabilitation. Syllabus prepared for Harbor Community College at Los Angeles, CA.

Kemp, Bryan, 1981. The Case Management Model in Rehabilitation. In Pan et al., eds. *Annual Review of Rehabilitation*. Volume 2. New York, NY: Springer.

Kemp, Bryan, & Vash, Carolyn, 1971. Productivity after Injury in a Sample of Spinal Cord Injured Persons: A Pilot Study. *Journal of Chronic Diseases*, 24:2.

Kerr, Nancy, 1977. Understanding the Process of Adjustment to Disability. In Stubbins, ed., *Psychosocial Aspects of Disability*. Baltimore, MD: University Park.

Keyes, Ken, Jr., 1975. *Handbook to Higher Consciousness*. Berkeley, CA: Living Love.

Kutner, Bernard, 1977. Milieu Therapy. In Marinelli and Dell Orto, eds., *The Psychological and Social Impact of Physical Disability*. New York, NY: Springer.

Lasky, Robert et al., 1977. Structured Existential Therapy: A Group Approach to Rehabilitation. In Marinelli and Dell Orto, eds., *The Psychological and Social Impact of Physical Disability*. New York, NY: Springer.

Lewin, Kurt, 1935. *A Dynamic Theory of Personality*. New York, NY: McGraw Hill.

Luce, Gay, 1979. *Your Second Life*. New York, NY: Delacorte/Seymour Lawrence.

Maslow, Abraham, 1965. *Eupsychian Management*. Homewood, IL: Richard Irwin.

Maslow, Abraham, & Mittleman, Bela, 1951. *Principles of Abnormal Psychology: The Dynamics of Psychic Illness*. Revised edition. New York, NY: Harper.

Masserman, Jules, 1955. *The Practice of Dynamic Psychiatry*. Philadelphia, PA: W. B. Saunders.

Nelson, John, 1975. *The Wheelchair Vagabond: A Guide and Goad for the Handicapped Traveler*. Santa Monica, CA: Project Press.

Nelson, Nathan, 1971. *Workshops for the Handicapped in the United States: An Historical and Developmental Perspective*. Springfield, IL: Charles C Thomas.

Nesbitt, John, 1979. Recreation and Careers in Recreation for Disabled People. *American Rehabilitation*, 5:1.

Richter, Curt, 1958. On the Phenomenon of Sudden Death in Animals and Man. In Reed et al., eds., *Psychopathology: A Source Book*. Cambridge, MA: Harvard University Press.

Roberts, Edward, 1977. Mealtimes in an Institution: A Disabled Person's Experiences. In Perske et al., eds., *Mealtimes for Severely and Profoundly Handicapped Persons: New Concepts and Attitudes*. Baltimore, MD: University Park.

Shaul, Susan, et al., 1978. *Toward Intimacy*. New York, NY: Human Sciences.

Shushan, Robert, 1974. Assessment and Reduction of Deficits in the Physical Appearance of Mentally Retarded People. Doctoral dissertation prepared for University of California at Los Angeles, CA.

Strite, Carolyn, 1980. Dear Friend. Unpublished letter, Los Angeles County–University of Southern California Medical Center, 1935 Hospital Place, 2B–10, Los Angeles, CA 90033.

Swami Rama, et al., 1976. *Yoga and Psychotherapy: The Evolution of Consciousness.* Glenview, IL: Himalayan Institute.

Talbot, John, 1980. *The Chronically Mentally Ill.* New York, NY: Human Sciences.

Toffler, Alvin, 1980. *The Third Wave.* New York, NY: William Morrow.

United States Department of Labor, 1965. *The Dictionary of Occupational Titles.* Third edition. Washington, D.C.: U.S. Government Printing Office.

Urmer, Albert, & Balshan, Iris, 1960. Aspiration Level and Handicap. Research report prepared for Rancho Los Amigos Hospital at Downey, CA.

Vash, Carolyn, 1973. A Predictive Model for Vocational Rehabilitation. Position paper prepared for California State Department of Rehabilitation at Sacramento, CA.

Vash, Carolyn, 1975. The Psychology of Disability. *Rehabilitation Psychology,* 22:3.

Vash, Carolyn, 1976. Psychological Growth and Acknowledgement of Disability. In *Proceedings of Training Seminar: Psychological Aspects of Disability.* Wright Institute at San Francisco, CA.

Vash, Carolyn, 1977a. The Rights of People with Disabilities. Paper presented to the Annual Convention of the Occupational Therapy Association of California at Costa Mesa, CA.

Vash, Carolyn, 1977b. Re-focusing Psychological Services in Vocational Rehabilitation. Paper presented to the Annual Convention of the American Psychological Association at San Francisco, CA

Vash, Carolyn, 1978. Disability as Transcendental Experience. In Eisenberg and Falconer, eds., *Treatment of the Spinal Cord Injured.* Springfield, IL: Charles C Thomas.

Vash, Carolyn, 1980. Sheltered Industrial Employment. In Pan et al., eds., *Annual Review of Rehabilitation.* Volume 1. New York, NY: Springer.

Vash, Carolyn, & Murray, Bruce, 1969. Employment Demonstration Project: Final Report. Research report prepared for the Office of Manpower Policy Evaluation and Research, United States Department of Labor, Washington, D.C. Downey, CA: Rancho Los Amigos Hospital.

Zuckerman, Marvin, et al., 1978. Sensation Seeking in England and America: Cross Cultural Age and Sex Comparison. *Journal of Consulting and Clinical Psychology,* 46:1.

Appendix

Suggestions for Further Reading

The books that follow are recommended as resources for further information in the areas covered by this volume. General readings, those covering all or many of the topics covered here, are listed first. Specialized readings, those addressing specific aspects of the disability experience or psychosocial–vocational intervention approaches, are listed in the order in which the topic appears in this volume.

General Readings

The Psychological and Social Impact of Disability, edited by Marinelli and Dell Orto. Published by Springer Publishing Company, New York, 1977.

> A collection of readings gathered primarily from the journal literature of the 1960s and 1970s. The contributors are respected leaders in the rehabilitation field.

Social and Psychological Aspects of Disability, edited by Stubbins. Published by University Park Press, Baltimore, 1977.

> Very similar to the volume described above, this one includes a large selection of articles from the 1950s as well as more current works.

Physical Disability and Human Behavior, by James McDaniel. Published by Pergamon Press, Elmsford, New York, 1969.

> Presents concise descriptions of psychological/behavioral theories helpful to understanding human responses to the disablement and rehabilitation processes. Relevant research findings are also discussed.

Physical Disability—A Psychological Approach, by Beatrice Wright. Published by Harper & Row, New York, 1960.

> Describes a wide range of disability-related experiences in terms of social psychology theory, notably the conceptualizations of Kurt Lewin's field theory. Uses highly readable language and numerous illustrative examples.

Medical and Psychological Aspects of Disability, edited by Cobb. Published by Charles C Thomas, Springfield, Illinois, 1973.

> Provides a basic overview of medical and psychological factors associated with heart disease, hemiplegia, stroke, cerebral palsy, amputations, respiratory diseases, kidney disease, gastrointestinal disorders, epilepsy, and hearing impairment.

Annual Review of Rehabilitation, Vol. 1, edited by Pan et al. Published by Springer Publishing Company, New York, 1980.

> A yearly review that provides a regular, periodic mechanism for summarizing the state of the art in the wide range of rehabilitation issues and disciplinary concerns. Coverage of psychosocial–vocational rehabilitation is particularly thorough.

Specialized Readings

Handicapping America: Barriers to Disabled People, by Frank Bowe. Published by Harper & Row, New York, 1978.

> Describes the nature, genesis, and effects of the societal barriers confronting people with disabilities. It is written from the wide-ranging perspective of a Director of the American Coalition of Citizens with Disabilities.

Rehabilitating America: Toward Independence for Disabled and Elderly People, by Frank Bowe. Published by Harper & Row, New York, 1980.

> Viewed as a sequel to the volume described above, Bowe describes a plan for societal rehabilitation to head off what he considers a potentially uncontrollable upward spiral in costs related to elderly and disabled people.

The Role of the Family in the Rehabilitation of the Physically Disabled, edited by Power and Dell Orto. Published by University Park Press, Baltimore, 1980.

> A collection of readings that covers a wide range of issues related to family involvement in the rehabilitation process. Includes numerous suggestions of specific ways in which families can help their disabled loved ones.

People Making, by Virginia Satir. Published by Science and Behavior Books, Palo Alto, California, 1972.

> Provides a system for families to deal with the family process, finding that all of the ingredients in a family that count are changeable at any point in time. Presented with clarity and free of jargon. Not specifically written for families dealing with disability, but highly relevant.

Who Cares? A Handbook on Sex Education and Counseling Services for Disabled People, by the Sex and Disability Project. Prepared by George Washington University, Washington, D.C., 1979.

A handbook that is the result of a year-long research project aimed toward compiling available information on needs and services in the area of sexuality. Covers issues of attitudes, training needs, providers, and settings, and offers recommendations for the future.

The Sensuous Wheeler, by Barry Rabin. Published by Multi Media Resource Center, San Francisco, 1980.

Focuses on issues relating to spinal-cord-injured individuals who use wheelchairs, but includes an excellent and extensive bibliography in the general area of sexuality and disability.

Foundations of the Vocational Rehabilitation Process, by Rubin and Roessler. Published by University Park Press, Baltimore, 1978.

Surveys the rehabilitation literature and then integrates the findings into the rehabilitation counseling model developed by the Arkansas Rehabilitation Research and Training Center. The chapter on evaluation is considered especially valuable.

Who's Hiring Who, by Richard Lathrop. Published by Ten Speed Press, Berkeley, California, 1977.

A primer on how to get a good job that is addressed to the general population of job seekers. It is a thorough, upbeat, self-help manual that can also help counselors interested in developing unconventional approaches.

The Psychological Aspects of Physical Illness and Disability, by Franklin Shontz. Published by Macmillan Publishing Company, New York, 1973.

Ways in which rehabilitation facilities and hospitals both help and hinder people dealing with illness and disability are described. A very clever, imaginary case study is used to illustrate potential problems arising from poor interdisciplinary communication and understanding.

Born to Win: Transactional Analysis with Gestalt Experiments, by Muriel James. Published by Addison-Wesley Publishing Company, Reading, Massachusetts, 1971.

Provides a system for increasing a person's awareness of the power to direct his/her own life, to make decisions, develop ethical systems, and understand what it means to "win." Aimed at both professionals and lay persons, it is well regarded in private-sector rehabilitation.

Index